YOUNG PEOPLE
IN OUT-OF-HOME CARE

YOUNG PEOPLE IN OUT-OF-HOME CARE

Findings from the Ontario Looking After Children Project

Robert J. Flynn, Meagan Miller, Tessa Bell,
Barbara Greenberg, and Cynthia Vincent

University of Ottawa Press

2023

University of Ottawa **Press**
Les **Presses** de l'Université d'Ottawa

The University of Ottawa Press (UOP) is proud to be the oldest of the francophone university presses in Canada and the oldest bilingual university publisher in North America. Since 1936, UOP has been enriching intellectual and cultural discourse by producing peer-reviewed and award-winning books in the humanities and social sciences, in French and in English.

www.press.uOttawa.ca

Library and Archives Canada Cataloguing in Publication

Title: Young people in out-of-home care : findings from the Ontario Looking After Children Project / Robert J. Flynn, Meagan Miller, Tessa Bell, Barbara Greenberg, and Cynthia Vincent.
Names: Flynn, Robert J. (Robert John), 1942- author. | Miller, Meagan (Research associate), author. | Bell, Tessa, author. | Greenberg, Barbara (Research assistant), author. | Vincent, Cynthia (Research associate), author.
Series: Health and society (University of Ottawa Press)
Description: Series statement: Health and society | Includes bibliographical references and indexes.
Identifiers: Canadiana (print) 20230203108 | Canadiana (ebook) 2023020452X | ISBN 9780776638010 (softcover) | ISBN 9780776638027 (hardcover) | ISBN 9780776638041 (EPUB) | ISBN 9780776638034 (PDF)
Subjects: LCSH: Foster home care—Ontario—Evaluation. | LCSH: Foster children—Ontario—Social conditions—Evaluation. | LCSH: Foster children—Services for—Ontario—Evaluation. | LCSH: Child welfare—Ontario—Evaluation.
Classification: LCC HV887.C3 F59 2023 | DDC 362.73/309713—dc23

Legal Deposit: Second Quarter 2023
Library and Archives Canada

Production Team
Copy editing   Tanina Drvar
Proofreading   Robbie McCaw
Typesetting   Édiscript enr.
Cover design   Lefrançois, agence marketing B2B

Cover Image
Yan-Éric Côté, *Ce qui est en moi*, acrylic on canvas, 91.44 cm × 121.92 cm

SSHRC≡CRSH

Published in collaboration with Borders in Globalization with financial support from the Canadian Federation for the Humanities and Social Sciences.

The University of Ottawa Press gratefully acknowledges the support extended to its publishing list by the Government of Canada, the Canada Council for the Arts, the Ontario Arts Council, the Federation for the Humanities and Social Sciences through the Awards to Scholarly Publications Program and the Social Sciences and Humanities Research Council, and by the University of Ottawa.

ONTARIO ARTS COUNCIL
CONSEIL DES ARTS DE L'ONTARIO
an Ontario government agency
un organisme du gouvernement de l'Ontario

Canada Council   Conseil des arts
for the Arts   du Canada

Canadä

uOttawa

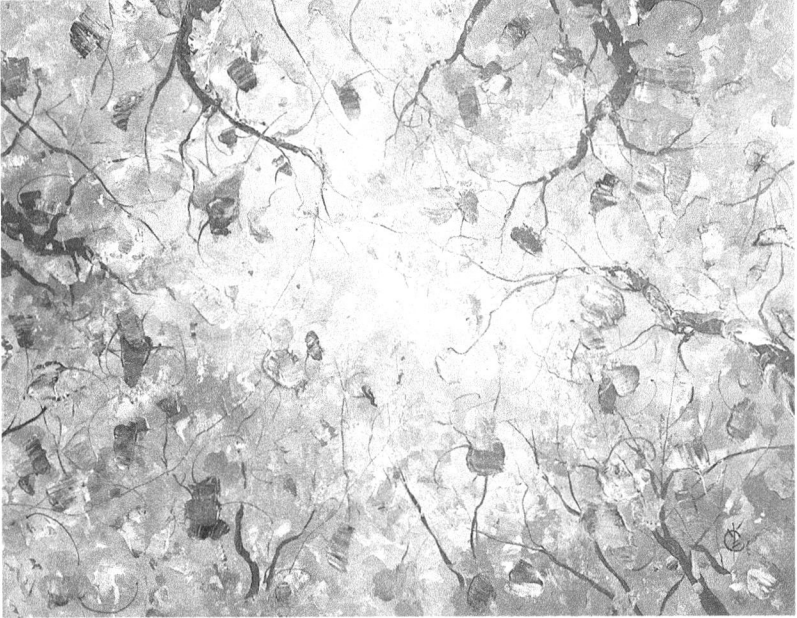

The painting above is entitled *Ce qui est en moi* ("What's Inside Me"), by the Canadian artist Yan-Éric Côté. For the authors, the tree canopy symbolizes the growth that young people in care experience as they discover their inner strength, while the light-blue sky represents the hope they have in realizing their ambitions.

Born in Saint-Jovite, Quebec, on April 9, 1974, Yan-Éric Côté grew up with a manifest passion for drawing and creating. Self-taught, he began painting in 2000, exploring different styles, leading to his "En l'ère Collection," inspired by the changing moods of the sky, the strength and calm of the dancing trees, the vibrant colours of the autumn leaves that swirl in the wind. Always fascinated by the land-scapes that surround him, he lets himself be captured by the beauty of nature, then he gives these landscapes back brightness, colour, and richness.

Table of Contents

CHAPTER 2

CHAPTER 3

CHAPTER 4

CHAPTER 5

CHAPTER 6

CHAPTER 7

CHAPTER 8

CHAPTER 10

Lessons from the Ontario Looking After Children Project
for Improving the Outcomes and Well-Being of Young People
in Care

List of Figures

List of Tables

List of Appendices

Preface

As the principal investigator of the Ontario Looking After Children (OnLAC) Project since it began in the year 2000, following the award of a strategic research grant in late 1999 from the Social Sciences and Humanities Research Council of Canada (SSHRC), I aim to recount the history of the OnLAC Project, in some detail, in this preface. In Chapter 1, my co-authors and I provide further information about the Looking After Children approach, which has been an important contributor to the reform and improvement of child welfare practice, policy, and research in Canada and other countries. We hope that this volume enhances the role of Looking After Children in improving caregiver, staff, and student training, child welfare services, and young people's outcomes and well-being.

In 1993, I travelled to Sudbury to attend a colloquium at Laurentian University. The invited speaker was Professor Roy Parker, from the Department of Social Policy and Social Planning at the University of Bristol, in England. He described a new approach that he and his colleagues were creating in the United Kingdom for assessing outcomes experienced by children and adolescents who were "in care," that is, being looked after away from home. The model considered by Professor Parker was known as "Looking After Children: Good Parenting, Good Outcomes." Based on the best child welfare science available at the time, it was being developed by an independent Working Party on Child Care Outcomes. (In the United

Kingdom, "child care" is the field usually known as "child welfare" in other countries, including Canada [Parker et al., 1991].) The working party had been established in 1987 by the U.K. Department of Health, with Professor Parker as its chairperson and Dr. Harriet Ward (also of Bristol University at the time) as its academic secretary. After an extended period of research and piloting, the Department of Health published in 1995 the key Looking After Children assessment instruments, the Assessment and Action Records (Department of Health, 1995). The work of the working party was closely aligned with new national legislation in the United Kingdom—the Children Act 1989—that was being introduced at this period (Parker et al., 1991).

I was keenly interested in the topic of Professor Parker's colloquium because I had recently begun to collaborate with the Prescott-Russell Children's Aid Society, in a mainly French-speaking region of eastern Ontario, on the evaluation of outcomes experienced by young people in the care of the agency. The executive director, Raymond Lemay, was a personal friend and a well-known innovator in child welfare in Ontario. He and his board of directors wanted to set up a system to evaluate the effectiveness of the services provided to young people in care by their local Society (to refer to both Indigenous and non-Indigenous local child welfare organizations in Ontario).

Following my return from Sudbury, I shared with Raymond Lemay and his senior staff what I had learned from Professor Parker's colloquium. They immediately saw the congruence between the focus of Looking After Children on outcomes and their interest in assessing service effectiveness. After piloting Looking After Children and its main data-collection instrument, the Assessment and Action Record (AAR) in 1994–1995, the Prescott-Russell Society decided to implement the approach and invited Dr. Harriet Ward and Ms. Helen Jones (from the U.K. Department of Health) to come to Canada to provide the needed staff training. In February 1996, Dr. Ward and Ms. Jones came to Ottawa and eastern Ontario and furnished several days of excellent training to the staff of the Prescott-Russell Society on the philosophy and theoretical underpinnings, assessment procedures, evidence base, and implementation to date of Looking After Children. They furnished the training in French, which was greatly appreciated by their audience, as the Society is the only one in Ontario that has French as its working language. (The Indigenous Societies in the province use their Indigenous languages as well as English or French in their day-to-day work.) The previous pilot work, training session, and implementation of Looking After Children in Prescott-Russell marked the launch of the Society's Evaluating Child Welfare Outcomes (ECWO) Project (Flynn & Biro, 1998). This was an important predecessor of our subsequent OnLAC Project.

In the 1990s, Dr. Ward became the director of the International Looking After Children Initiative, professor of social work at Loughborough University, and director of its Centre for Child and Family Research. She also organized a series of memorable summer seminars at the University of Oxford during this period, which people from a number of countries attended who were already piloting or interested in Looking After Children. My PhD students in clinical psychology and I were privileged to have this regular forum in which to present our early Looking After Children research findings and to hear about the experiences and research results of colleagues from the United Kingdom and elsewhere. Professor Ward, now retired, is affiliated with the Rees Centre in the Department of Education at the University of Oxford and remains active in child welfare research.

In 1999, several colleagues and I from the University of Ottawa (Doug Angus, a professor of health economics, Tim Aubry, a professor of clinical and community psychology, and Marie Drolet, a professor of social work), submitted a multi-year research proposal on Looking After Children to the Social Sciences and Humanities Research Council (SSHRC) of Canada (Flynn et al., 1999). Our major partner in this venture was the Ontario Association of Children's Aid Societies (OACAS), located in the provincial capital of Toronto. We also had strong endorsements from the Prescott-Russell Society and several other local Societies in Ontario. Our goal was to produce an Ontario and Canadian adaptation of the AAR and implement it, initially, in local Societies in Ontario. Fortunately, our research proposal was approved for funding as a strategic health grant by SSHRC, in December 1999. At the request of SSHRC, we also obtained secondary funding support from the Ontario social services ministry, known today as the Ministry of Children, Community and Social Services (MCCSS). We spent the year 2000 recruiting local Societies as participants in the OnLAC Project and adapting the U.K. version of the AAR to the Ontario and Canadian contexts. The Looking After Children philosophy and theoretical model, however, required little or no adaptation. From the beginning, we saw OnLAC as a resilience and strength-based approach to promoting the well-being of young people in out-of-home care, based on high-quality substitute parenting or caregiving. We developed this perspective further in an edited book by Flynn, Dudding, and Barber (2006), *Promoting Resilience in Child Welfare.*

The version of the AAR that we adapted for use in the OnLAC Project was approved later by Her Majesty's Stationery Office (HMSO), the U.K. copyright holder of Looking After Children materials), as the only recognized version for Canada, for which OACAS paid a fee and holds the only licence. HSMO established a limit of one official AAR licence per country to avoid a proliferation of different versions within each of the countries that had already begun to pilot Looking After Children or would do so in future. Our Ontario and Canadian version of the AAR was designed for rapid and accurate optical scanning into SPSS or Excel data files, thereby lending itself to ready computer analysis of demographic, service, and outcome data from large numbers of young people in care, their caregivers, and their child welfare workers. Our initial adaptation of the AAR (Flynn et al., 2001) and revised versions in 2006, 2010, and 2016 have thus been more psychometrically and quantitatively oriented than the original, mainly qualitative U.K. model. We believe it is due in no small measure to our ability to optically scan our extensive AAR database each year on large numbers of young people in care and their caregivers and workers into computer-readable data files and then produce timely descriptive or evaluative reports for which our OnLAC Project has received sustained financial support. Annual funding began with the multi-year strategic research grant from SSHRC in late 1999 and has continued from 2004 until today. Annual contracts for the OnLAC Project are negotiated between OACAS and MCCSS and then a contract is signed by OACAS and the University of Ottawa. In Canadian provinces or territories and other countries that adopted mainly qualitative versions of the AAR, the Looking After Children initiative unfortunately did not survive. Without knowing the local, provincial, or national contexts in which Looking after Children was discontinued, we cannot say with certainty why this happened. However, we believe that one probable reason was the widespread reliance on largely qualitative versions of the AAR. That is, in the typical jurisdiction, whether in other Canadian provinces or other countries that adopted Looking After Children, the people who implemented the approach were faced with assessing high numbers (i.e., hundreds or even thousands) of young people in care each year with the AAR. We suspect that the time-consuming tasks of creating databases from AAR qualitative data, and then cleaning, verifying, analyzing, forwarding the data to local Societies, and preparing timely yearly public or confidential outcome-oriented evaluation reports for dissemination to governments and provincial and local child welfare service organizations, were likely to have proven virtually impossible to manage. We also think that many child welfare organizations are not used to storing and analyzing quantitative data such as the AAR, as research in the field tends to be mainly qualitative. Our choice of a primarily psychometric and quantitative version of the AAR, on the other hand, has enabled efficient conversion of the Ontario AAR data into SPSS or Excel data files, making the key tasks of data handling, cleaning, analysis, reporting, and forwarding to local Societies quite feasible, despite relatively modest funding resources for the OnLAC Project relative to the cost of the Ontario in-care system on which it has gathered annual data for 22 years.

In 2000, during an initial year of project planning and instrument development, some 20 Ontario Societies that were members of OACAS agreed to take part in the OnLAC Project on a voluntary and pilot basis. In our first year of data collection, in 2001–2002, we gathered AAR data on approximately 500 young people in care and their caregivers and child welfare workers. In 2022, we are in our 22nd consecutive year of data collection with the AAR in Ontario, with some 85,000 AAR-structured interviews completed with approximately 35,000 young people, their caregivers, and workers. We began to collect data in March 2001 with our initial OnLAC version of the AAR and continued to do so on the basis of voluntary Society participation for the next five years. In 2003, I was invited to the offices of the Ontario social service ministry at Queen's Park in Toronto to present some of our Looking After Children outcome data. A consultant who was undertaking an evaluation of child welfare services in Ontario at the behest of the provincial Cabinet was in the audience. In her subsequent evaluation report to the provincial government, she recommended that Ontario officially adopt Looking After Children and the AAR. The local Societies involved in the OnLAC Project on a voluntary basis were urging the same thing. A couple of years later, I was again invited to the social service ministry's Queen's Park offices in Toronto to give a presentation on OnLAC. This time, there were two deputy ministers and other senior staff responsible for child welfare services in attendance. The audience appreciated the direct relevance of our OnLAC findings on a wide range of outcomes (especially education) to the provincial government's growing emphasis on accountability. In 2006, the Ontario government mandated the adoption of Looking After Children and the OnLAC version of the AAR in local Societies in Ontario. Implementation of this new mandate began in December 2007, and remains in effect today. As previously mentioned, we are now in our 22nd year of continuous data collection, together with data analysis and reporting back to the field. Our annual reports include an annual public (non-confidential) report on the outcomes and well-being of young people in care in Ontario (e.g., Miller, 2021), along with some 44 confidential reports to each of the local Societies that submit AARs on their young people in care. AAR data has been the basis of several books, numerous book chapters, peer-reviewed journal articles, 16 doctoral theses, and hundreds of technical reports produced by our research team and distributed widely to the field. These publications (listed in the OnLAC bibliography; Miller et al., 2022) have covered a wide range of topics directly related to the outcomes and well-being of young people in care: *inter alia,* a book and several articles on resilience in child welfare; a special issue of a journal on improving educational outcomes; guidance on implementing Looking After Children in practice; promoting children's best interests; hope and active coping; the psychological benefits of participation in extracurricular activities; performance measurement in local Societies; benefits of tutoring in reading and math; placement satisfaction; young people's suggestions for improving their placements; protective and risk factors in educational success; transitions from care; positive life experiences in care; mental health and substance-use issues; enhancing the utility of the AAR through systematic use; caregiver parenting practices; early child education; caregiver involvement and educational achievement; developmental and cultural assets and resilience in Indigenous young people; promoting childhood literacy in children in care; training of foster and adoptive resource parents; prosocial and anti-social behaviour in group home care; influence of group home size and neighbourhood location; childhood maltreatment and educational outcomes; improving the use of data in child welfare service planning; using research and outcome data to improve educational services; neglect and educational success; developmental assets and resilience.

Besides our own OnLAC Project, funded by SSHRC, there were other Looking After Children initiatives in Canada at this period (summarized in Legault et al., 2004). In 1997–1999, Kathleen Kufeldt, then affiliated with the University of New Brunswick, and colleagues from Laval University, conducted a project that included pilot projects in each of the six easternmost provinces of Canada: Ontario, Quebec, New Brunswick, Prince Edward Island, Nova Scotia, and Newfoundland and Labrador (Kufeldt et al., 2000). Funded by Human Resources Development Canada (HRDC), this project was seen by some stakeholders as the first phase of what they hoped would evolve into Looking After Children on a national scale in Canada. This hoped-for evolution did not take place. Other pilot efforts were also launched in Canada during this period, most notably the Prescott-Russell project in eastern Ontario that grew from modest roots in 1994–1996 into one of the pillars of our now 22-year-old OnLAC Project. Other pilot initiatives began as well in Alberta, Yukon, the Northwest Territories, and British Columbia. In 1999, the Child Welfare League of Canada (CWLC), with the support of the provincial and territorial directors of child welfare and the collaboration of our OnLAC Project and other local projects, submitted a proposal that was funded by Human Resources Development Canada (HRDC). This project was intended as the second phase of what some had hoped would become Looking After Children on a Canada-wide basis (Legault, 2004). Unfortunately, federal HRDC funding for CWLC's "CanLAC" Project was terminated after only a brief period, ending the initiative. Such has been the all-too-common fate of small-scale, under-resourced pilot projects in Canada. Of the various Looking After Children pilot projects mentioned, our OnLAC Project is the only one in Canada to have survived and become institutionalized, thanks to the substantial SSHRC research grant in 1999 and ongoing Ontario provincial government funding and OACAS support since the beginning in 2000. (The evolutionary model of program development and evaluation of Brown Urban et al., 2014, which we summarize as OnLAC Project lesson No. 3 in Chapter 10 of the present volume, furnishes what we believe is a demanding but promising antidote to the low life expectancy of many pilot projects in Canada.)

A decade later, Quebec carried out an informative pilot project in which the implementation and outcomes of Looking After Children in the provincial *centres jeunesse* (youth centres) were evaluated (Sécurité publique Canada–Public Security Canada, 2012). The *centres jeunesse* were responsible at the time for services for young people in care in each administrative region of Quebec. The implementation evaluation in 2012 studied whether the planned resources and activities were actually put in place and identified factors influencing the implementation process. The outcome evaluation focused on the shorter-term effect of Looking After Children on caregiver and caseworker practices and on the longer-term development and well-being of the young people in care. Despite the favourable findings from the evaluation, the Government of Quebec adopted Looking After Children and the AAR on a voluntary rather than mandated basis, unlike Ontario. Predictably, this decision led to disappointing results, with much more limited project funding for personnel, data collection, and outcomes reporting than in our mandated and more adequately resourced Ontario OnLAC Project.

Despite being another missed opportunity in Canada to improve child welfare services and outcomes, the Quebec project merits a brief summary of results here. The *implementation* evaluation concluded, first of all, that putting in place a new approach such as Looking After Children required careful preparation and adequate resources, before caseworkers or caregivers were recruited. Second, the quality and duration of training and support from the youth centres were also important for caseworker and caregiver skill development, integration of the new approach, and its successful adaptation to programs and practices in the Quebec child welfare system. Third, the evaluators found that the AAR should have been aligned more closely with the other practice tools used in the youth centres.

In the accompanying *outcome* evaluation, about 80% of the caregivers and 90% of the caseworkers stated that the Looking After Children AARs had provided them with better knowledge than they had previously possessed of the needs of the young people in care and had assisted in monitoring the youths' progress. The AARs also helped to consider the personal histories of the young people and made it easier for the latter to talk about taboo subjects and develop closer ties with their caregiving families. In addition, 83% of the caseworkers and 70% of the caregivers stated that the AARs facilitated parental involvement and that the Looking After Children approach offered mental health support that was superior to that available to the general population. The young people's overall health and hospitalization rates were not significantly different from those of the general population (rather than higher). The outcome evaluation also found that more than 95% of the young people in care who were under the age of 16 got needed support to acquire independent living skills, and 75% to 85% of the older youths reported receiving assistance in enhancing their self-care skills. Moreover, the evaluation discovered that the young people experiencing the Looking After Children approach engaged in less property destruction and had many fewer crisis situations (27%) than those in the comparison group (73%).

Overall, Looking After Children and the AAR were evaluated as helping the youth centre caseworkers and caregivers to take better account of the young persons' perspectives and as introducing an improved, albeit sometimes more time consuming, approach to problem solving in caregiving families. The new approach permitted the youth centres to go beyond protecting young people in care to helping promote their development, thanks to a more complete and holistic developmental perspective. The evaluation concluded optimistically that Looking After Children, as of 2009, seemed to be leading to a positive paradigm shift in the practices of Quebec's youth centre staff and caregivers. In retrospect, however, it appears that despite the favourable evaluation findings, Quebec (and Canada) missed yet another opportunity to improve services and outcomes. Major changes to the province's child welfare system, coupled with inadequate provincial government policy and financial support, severely limited the potential impact of Looking After Children in Quebec. Once again, the evolutionary approach of Brown Urban et al. (2014) to program development and evaluation, described briefly in Chapter 10, recommends itself as a more patient, disciplined, and realistic alternative to the recurring Canadian penchant for overly rapid and simple solutions.

Implementation science and its first cousins, program development, fidelity assessment, and program evaluation, have much to say to child welfare in Canada and far beyond, meriting much more systematic research attention and resources to undergird effective practice. Greeson et al. (2020) conducted a "state of the science review" of programs and interventions for youth aging out of foster care (as out-of-home care is called in the United States). The findings of their review are instructive in the present context.

Following U.S. federal legislation on independent living and transition services in 1999, many interventions were initiated to improve the well-being outcomes of young people leaving care, especially in five areas widely considered key "best practice" domains: education, employment, housing, health and mental health, and relationships. Greeson et al. (2020) searched the research and grey literature and found a total of 79 programs and interventions in these 5 domains. However, the authors were able to rate only 10 interventions (13%)

in terms of effectiveness, based on peer-reviewed scientific articles and evaluation reports and using the Scientific Rating Scale of the California Evidence-Based Clearinghouse (CEBC) for Child Welfare. On this scale, a rating of 1 = Well supported by research evidence; 2 = Supported by research evidence; 3 = Promising research evidence; 4 = Failure to demonstrate effect; and 5 = Concerning practice (i.e., negative; risk of harm). Greeson et al. (2020) were not able to rate 69 of the 79 interventions due to a lack of research evidence on effectiveness.

The authors concluded that only 10 of the 79 programs and interventions could be rated due to several reasons. (Moreover, none of the 10 rated programs achieved a rating of 1, the top of the scale.) Some interventions may have been evaluated in community agencies, but the results had not been disseminated. This suggests the need for research-practice partnerships (of which we consider the OnLAC Project an excellent example), to promote knowledge creation and information sharing. Another contributing factor according to Greeson et al. (2020) was the limited integration within child welfare of implementation science as a crucial area of research and practice. Programs cannot be rated in terms of effectiveness unless they have first been implemented with fidelity (an issue, along with adequate training, to which we turn in Chapter 10). Finally, Greeson et al. (2020) recommended that given the large number of programs that have been developed in the last 20 years or so, it would make eminent sense to focus on implementing and evaluating those that already exist, rather than developing new ones for youth transitioning from care. The same principle obviously applies to other areas of child welfare research and practice.

The chapters herein describe selected findings that reflect the strengths and resilience as well as the challenges of young people in care in Ontario and the interventions used by local Societies to serve them. Chapter 1 examines the convergence of the developmental domains covered by the Looking After Children approach, of U.K. origin, and the Child Well-Being model, as articulated in the United States. The chapter also describes the 20 guiding principles and values at the heart of Looking After Children's enduring contribution to child welfare service quality and reform. In addition, the chapter includes examples of the many contributions that the OnLAC Project has made to knowledge, practice, and policy in Ontario through its numerous reports to the field and, as a result of its numerous peer-reviewed publications and presentations at national and international conferences. It concludes with some reflections on the future of the OnLAC Project, in light of international trends in child welfare.

Chapter 2 describes a significant contribution of the OnLAC Project to Looking After Children theory and practice, namely, the idea and measurement of developmental assets as an eighth domain of child and youth development. The concept was not ours; rather, we borrowed it from the Search Institute (SI) in Minneapolis, whose vigorous dissemination has made developmental assets into a positive and widely embraced staple of child and youth development theory in community organizations in the United States, Canada, and internationally. Incorporating developmental assets into the AAR has thus built an important bridge between child welfare and other youth-serving fields, such as mental health. The OnLAC Project measurement of developmental assets has differed from that of the SI. Instead of the SI's lengthy youth self-report version, our measurement approach asked the young person's child welfare worker to rate the young person's current assets. That is, having participated in the detailed AAR conversational interview with the young person and caregiver, the child welfare worker rates the young person's possession of each of the 40 developmental assets as a "Yes" (present), "No" (absent), or "Uncertain" (not sure). We count only the number of "Yes" responses made by the worker. As Chapter 2 describes, the number of developmental assets possessed by the young person, based on the worker's assessment, has proven to be a highly reliable and valid predictor of a wide range of resilience-related outcomes in the OnLAC Project. Helping the young person add a small number of specific assets has also emerged as a concrete clinical strategy for use in the next year's plan of care.

Chapter 3 examines the health status of specific groups of children and young people in care in Ontario, with comparisons made between Indigenous and non-Indigenous females, Indigenous and non-Indigenous males, and combined samples of females and males, within each of four age groups: 0–5 years, 6–9 years, 10–15 years, and 16 years and over. We present results for several health inputs: completion of annual medical and dental exams, immunizations, and possession of valid health cards. We also present findings for a range of health outcomes: general health status; learning-related health conditions (fetal alcohol spectrum disorder, developmental disability, learning disability, attention deficit hyperactivity disorder, and emotional, psychological, or nervous disorder); frequency of "soft" drug use—tobacco, alcohol, or marijuana—and "hard" (illicit) drug use—cocaine, glue, non-prescribed drugs, hallucinogens, etc.; use of prescribed psychotropic drugs; and, in an appendix, physical health conditions.

Chapter 4 describes OnLAC results regarding the education of young people in care, from young children to older adolescents and young adults, as well as from other research. We begin by sketching the impact of pre-K programs and the situation in Ontario of early child education, and then describe the motor, social, and cognitive development of an OnLAC sample of more than 500 young children aged 12 to 47 months. The children, on average, were 0.76 standard deviations behind their general-population age peers. It was encouraging, however, to find that caregivers' literacy-promoting activities during daily interactions with the children were associated with a higher level of development.

As well, we present results for young children from the OnLAC database who were assessed with the two Ages and Stages Questionnaires (ASQ) that we embedded within the 2016 version of the AAR: the Ages and Stages Questionnaire, Third Edition (ASQ-3; $N = 834$), a measure of general child development, and the (ASQ:SE; $N = 910$), a measure of social-emotional functioning. The results suggest that a substantial minority of children seen in the OnLAC Project should be referred immediately to community intervention programs or at least followed up in future for further screening and possible referral. The ASQ results we present here, however, should be seen as preliminary, as we are currently working with other Canadian ASQ researchers to establish more rigorous ASQ norms for young children in care.

Chapter 4 next provides data on the educational outcomes of Ontario children in care who were of primary, secondary, and post-secondary school age. The proportion of girls and boys in primary and secondary school who were rated by their child welfare workers as performing at only a "fair" or "poor" level in reading and math was concerning, even though the girls outperformed the boys. Moreover, data from the Ontario Ministry of Education strongly suggests that many young people in care in primary and secondary schools in the province are clearly in need of evidence-based interventions such as high-impact tutoring. This conclusion was also consistent with OnLAC results that we present for young people in care of post-secondary age (18–21 years). The last section of Chapter 4 provides information aimed at child welfare personnel, caregivers, and policy-makers who would like to take concrete action to improve the currently weak educational outcomes of many young people in care in Ontario.

Chapter 5 describes an "educational snapshot," created from information drawn from the AAR, which child welfare workers and caregivers can use as a planning tool to promote the educational success of young persons in care. (We hope to create other snapshots in future, also based on AAR data, in developmental domains such as mental health, life skills, or transition planning.) The educational snapshot in Chapter 5 was produced by Professor Elisa Romano of the School of Psychology at the University of Ottawa, one of her PhD students, Lauren Stenason, and two members of the OnLAC Project team, Erik Michael and Meagan Miller. It is intended to provide child welfare workers with information from variables in the young person's AAR known to influence educational outcomes, within a social-ecological conceptual framework, and in a way and at a time that would facilitate preparation of an effective plan of care for the young person. We look forward to workers' adoption of educational (and eventually other) snapshots as a means of using the very rich information in the AAR in a more focused and efficient manner.

The social-ecological conceptual framework employed in the educational snapshot is, of course, applicable to many other aspects of the lives of young people in care, beyond the realm of education. We therefore provide further comment on the ecological perspective here. In general, people closest to the young person in care (e.g., birth parents, caregivers, or young people who share the same placement setting) are likely to have a relatively direct and potentially powerful impact on young people's immediate outcomes and well-being. However, intermediate organizational systems and individuals working therein (e.g., child welfare workers, supervisors, or managers in local Societies, teachers in schools, or personnel in local hospitals) are also likely to have an important influence on the experiences of young people in care. Finally, at the societal level (e.g., provincial decision makers and policies, including the proportion of funding allocated to child welfare, educational, health, or mental health) will affect outcomes and well-being by shaping the accessibility, quality, and effectiveness of the programs and interventions offered by local Societies, schools, health, mental health, or other public or voluntary organizations.

Berger and Slack (2014) provided an illuminating discussion of how these different levels of influence operate together to affect child protection systems and young people's well-being. According to Berger and Slack (2014), the ecological models used to explain the causes of child abuse or neglect suggest that there is no single cause nor are there any necessary or sufficient causes. Instead, these ecological models point to joint causation by multiple risk factors, including characteristics of the child and parents, family interactions, parenting knowledge and behaviour, socioeconomic status, economic difficulties, and the broader social and environmental context of the family. The sheer complexity of the causation of child maltreatment is shown clearly in a thorough review and meta-analysis of 155 studies by Stith et al. (2009), who identified no fewer than 39 risk factors for child abuse and 22 for child neglect.

Chapter 6 explores the development of the cultural and personal identity of members of racial or ethnic groups of particular importance within Canadian society and the OnLAC Project. The chapter describes, first of all, the lengthy abusive history of the residential schools in Canada in the nineteenth and twentieth centuries and their long-term negative impact on the identity and well-being of Indigenous children and their families, including the continuing overrepresentation of Indigenous young people in care in Ontario's and Canada's child welfare services. Besides recounting some of the findings from our OnLAC Project research involving young people from Indigenous backgrounds, the chapter cites groundbreaking Canadian research that has found that individual identity formation, community control of resources and services, and cultural autonomy are characteristic of Indigenous communities that are healthier, with lower rates of suicide and self-harm. Chapter 6 also examines the growing concern in Ontario and other jurisdictions in Canada with the overrepresentation in care of children of colour, especially from Black but also from Latin and Asian communities. In Toronto, in 2013, almost 41% of children in care were reported to be Black. Recent anti-racism initiatives by OACAS, the Ontario government, and the Ontario Human Rights Commission are reviewed, and the chapter concludes with consideration of young Francophones in care, noting that they come from by far the largest linguistic minority in the province and, like other groups, require culturally appropriate child welfare services.

Chapter 7 is concerned with a topic at the heart of child welfare, namely, young people's relationships with other people, including members of their families of origin, friends, caregivers, teachers, child welfare workers, and others, and the influence of these relationships on the young people's acceptance and well-being. The chapter has a secondary focus on how young people in care present themselves socially, with regard to cleanliness, hygiene, dress, speech, and politeness. After reviewing the literature briefly on these topics, the chapter presents selected findings from the OnLAC Project on the confidants of young people in care, that is, people with whom they could talk about their concerns or problems. Female caregivers and child welfare workers emerged as particularly important confidants for all young people in care, as did male caregivers for boys. The quality of the young person's relationship with the caregiver, as perceived by the young person, was an especially important predictor of the young person's satisfaction with his or her current placement. The chapter concludes with a brief consideration of new theory and research from the Search Institute on the significance of developmental relationships, a perspective from which child welfare research and practice is likely to benefit in future as the perspective becomes more widely known.

Chapter 8 provides a simple and rapid tool that will permit child welfare workers or caregivers to use data from the OnLAC AAR to assess quickly the mental health status of young people in care, especially those whom they may not know well. To use the tool, the worker or caregiver has to answer just two questions. First, does the young person's AAR score on Keyes' (2006) 14-item measure of well-being fall within the highest, middle, or lowest tertile (i.e., third) of the distribution of OnLAC Project scores? Second, does the young person currently reside in a kinship care or foster care home (likely to have, on average, a relatively higher level of well-being) or in an independent living or group home (likely to have, on average, a relatively lower average level of well-being)? The chapter reviews the literature on the mental health of young people in care and on Keyes' measure of well-being, and then shows in a large OnLAC Project sample that answers to the two questions mentioned are good guides to the young person's status on multiple positive and negative indicators of youth mental health.

Chapter 9 provides detailed OnLAC Project norms for the new Canadian version of the Casey Life Skills Assessment, which was incorporated into the 2016 revision of the AAR. Several redundant items from the U.S. version of the Casey have been eliminated from the Canadian version, which consists of eight scales: Permanency (20 items), Daily Living (15), Self-Care (15), Relationships and Communication

(11), Housing and Money Management (19), Work and Study (18), Career and Education Planning (6), and Looking Forward (8). A young person's scores on these scales can be summed to form a total Casey score (also equal to the sum of the 112 individual Casey items). We hope the Casey norms, presented at both the item and scale levels, for the sample as a whole and for sub-groups based on sex (females vs. males), age (16-year-olds vs. 17-year-olds), type of residential placement (independent living vs. kinship, foster, and group homes), and well-being (highest vs. middle vs. lowest tertiles), will be useful for young people planning to leave care, their caregivers, and child care workers. The Casey items, scales, and norms can be used in transition planning both with individual young people and with groups. We also hope that quality assurance or other local society personnel charged with evaluating the effectiveness of local programs in preparing young people for transition from care will find the Casey item and scale norms useful. We also encourage applied research (including undergraduate, master's, or doctoral theses) on the predictive validity of the Casey scales, in relation to various transition outcomes, such as young people's success in post-secondary education, housing, mental health, or employment. Such research has unfortunately been surprisingly rare, even in the United States where the Casey has been widely used clinically in transition programs.

Chapter 9 also provides summaries of three recent Canadian research projects on transitions from care. The first, by researchers from McGill University (Gunawardena & Stich, 2021), was an informative systematic review of 30 scientific studies of transition-related interventions, the first of its kind, according to the authors. The interventions included 12 with a focus on readiness for independent living, 4 on policy changes allowing young people to remain in care after the age of majority, 3 on mentoring, 3 on art or mindfulness interventions, 2 on post-secondary education, 2 on employment, 2 on self-empowerment or self-determination, and 2 on extracurricular activities. According to Gunawardena and Stich (2021), independent-living programs emerged as especially promising in their ability to provide support to care leavers. More such studies are certainly needed in Canada and other countries, for which the Casey items, scales, and norms should prove particularly useful.

The second recent Canadian research study on transitions was a report on the needs of care leavers by Jane Kovarikova (2017) for the Ontario Provincial Advocate for Children and Youth. Kovarikova, a former young person in care who is currently pursuing a PhD in political science at Western University in London, Ontario, is the founder of the influential Child Welfare Political Action Committee Canada (Child Welfare PAC). Her report was based on the peer-reviewed and "grey" literature as well as 17 interviews with staff from Ontario organizations serving young people in care. She catalogues the problems frequently encountered by care leavers: often-poor academic outcomes, unemployment and underemployment, housing insecurity, early pregnancy or parenthood, health and mental health issues, and loneliness, isolation, and stigma. Kovarikova made a number of recommendations to improve the effectiveness of child welfare services in the face of these issues.

The third study was a needs-assessment and pilot-intervention study by Lamborn and Aubry (2021), conducted at the University of Ottawa in conjunction with the Children's Aid Society of Ottawa and the Children's Aid Foundation of Ottawa. The authors sought to determine whether a tuition-support program would help students who had a care background and were enrolled as undergraduate students at the University of Ottawa. Interviews were carried out with 12 individuals: 6 current University of Ottawa students with experience of care, 3 University of Ottawa alumni with care backgrounds, 2 Ottawa Society informants, and 1 University ofOttawa informant. Lamborn and Aubry (2021) described financial, academic, social, and other obstacles mentioned by their interviewees and made several recommendations aimed at improving the situation. These covered financial, navigational/human, and accessible support, tracking of educational outcomes of student recipients of bursaries, and funding of psychoeducational assessments that would enable students to document disabilities and procure academic accommodations when needed.

Chapter 10 analyzes eight major lessons that, somewhat arbitrarily, we have identified as deserving of special mention from our 22 years of experience to date of the OnLAC Project. These lessons are, in order, the need for the following:

- high-quality and accessible OnLAC and AAR training for caregivers and child welfare personnel;
- the routine use of OnLAC information and AAR data for clinical service planning, outcome-monitoring, and program evaluation by local Societies, OACAS, and MCCSS;

- adequate knowledge and capacity on the part of local Societies, OACAS, and MCCSS to be able to construct and evaluate effective programs;
- local application of an exemplary case study that shows Societies can use their AAR data to improve service delivery;
- provision by Ontario of universal access to high-quality early childhood education and care for young children in out-of-home care;
- a new Ontario project ("OnLAC-2"), funded by MCCSS and OACAS, that will follow up an annual sample of care leavers to know how they are faring in terms of permanency, health, education, employment, mental health, and other important outcomes;
- a special Ontario child welfare research fund that will permit sustained applied research to be carried out in partnership between local or provincial child welfare organizations and university researchers; and
- an updating of the OnLAC Project partnership by the University of Ottawa, OACAS, and MCCSS.

In conclusion, my co-authors and I believe that in its 22 years of operation to date, our OnLAC Project has contributed to a needed shift in child welfare in Ontario from a primary focus on psychosocial and educational risks to a more central and balanced concern with high expectations, positive outcomes, and resilience. Our project has also helped to create a clearer and more widespread appreciation in government and service delivery agencies that child welfare is a knowledge-intensive and intellectually demanding field. It is now obvious to any informed and critical observer that high-quality data on services and outcomes, procured through more systematic, longitudinal, and excellent social science research, will be essential if MCCSS, in collaboration with OACAS, is to be successful in its current redesign of provincial child welfare services and its quest for dramatically improved outcomes. The attention and resources that the Ministry of Health and, to a lesser extent, the Ministry of Education devote to applied science and research have to become the norm in child welfare services. Much more remains to be accomplished in the years ahead, but we must not lose sight of the significant conceptual, practice, and research progress made in the last two decades, thanks in part to the pioneering accomplishments of the OnLAC Project.

I wish to conclude by thanking the young people in care, their caregivers, and the Societies and staff members that support them for their long-term collaboration. It has been a privilege for us as applied researchers to have had the opportunity to contribute to an improved child welfare system. I want to also thank my co-authors for their many contributions to this book, which have gone well beyond the call of their usual duties, and for their sustained devotion to the success of the OnLAC Project itself. Three co-authors are long-time members of the OnLAC Project research team: Meagan Miller, Cynthia Vincent, and Barbara Greenberg, with whom it has been a pleasure to collaborate. I also want to thank our other co-author, Tessa Bell, a developmental psychologist who conducted her doctoral research on resilience among young people in care, with OnLAC data. She has chosen to make her career in child welfare as an applied researcher and quality-assurance leader in the Ottawa Society. Thanks also to the authors of Chapter 5—Professor Elisa Romano, Lauren Stenason, Erik Michael, and Meagan Miller—for their educational snapshot, which promises to make AAR data on education easier to use in case planning. Finally, I speak for my co-authors in thanking our OnLAC Project partner, the Ontario Association of Children's Aid Societies (OACAS), for its ongoing support since we launched the project together in 2000. We are also grateful to the Social Sciences and Humanities Research Council (SSHRC) of Canada, without whose strategic research grant in 1999 the OnLAC Project would not have begun. We also thank Ontario Ministry of Children, Community, and Social Services (MCCSS) for its financial support of the OnLAC Project in 2000 and annually since 2004, which has enabled the project to continue without interruption. Finally, we want to thank the many administrative colleagues at the University of Ottawa who have helped us so often during the last two decades with contract negotiations and related matters. They work in Innovation Support Services, the Faculty of Social Sciences, the Centre for Research on Educational and Community Services (CRECS), and the School of Psychology. You are too numerous to mention by name, but you and we know who you are, and we thank you!

ROBERT FLYNN

References

Berger, L. M., & Slack, K. S. (2014). Child protection and child well-being. In A. F. Ben-Arieh, F. Casas, I. Frones, & J. E. Korbin (Eds.), *Handbook* of child well-being (pp. 2965–2992). Springer Science + Business Media Dordrecht. https://doi.org/10.1007/978-90-481-9063-8_120

Brown Urban, J., Hargraves, M., & Trochim, W. M. (2014). Evolutionary evaluation: Implications for evaluators, researchers, practitioners, funders, and the evidence-based program mandate. *Evaluation and Program Planning, 45,* 127–139.

Child Welfare League of Canada (CWLC). (1999, September). *Project proposal – Looking After Children in Canada. Phase II.* [Report submitted to Human Resources Development Canada].

Department of Health. (1995, May). *Looking After Children: Assessment and Action Records,* London, U.K.

Farris-Manning, C., & Zandstra, M. (2003). *Children in Care in Canada: A summary of current issues and trends with recommendations for future research.* Foster LIFE Inc.

Flynn, R. J., Angus, D., Aubry, T., & Drolet, M. (1999). *Improving child protection practice through the introduction of Looking After Children into the 54 local Children's Aid Societies in Ontario: An implementation and outcome evaluation.* [SSHRC Strategies Grant No. 828-1999-1008]. Centre for Research on Community Services, University of Ottawa.

Flynn, R. J., & Biro, C. (1998). Comparing developmental outcomes for children in care with those of other children in Canada. *Children & Society, 12,* 228–233.

Flynn, R. J., Dudding, P. M., & Barber, J. G. (2006). *Promoting resilience in child welfare.* University of Ottawa Press.

Flynn, R. J., Ghazal, H., Moshenko, S., & Westlake, L. (2001). Main features and advantages of a new, "Canadianized" version of the Assessment and Action Record from Looking After Children. *Ontario Association of Children's Aid Societies Journal, 45*(2), 3–6.

Greeson, J. K. P, Garcia, A. R., Tan, K., Chacon, A., & Ortiz, A. J. (2020). Interventions for youth aging out of foster care: A state of the science review. *Children and Youth Services Review, 113,* 1–11. https://doi.org/10.1016/j.childyouth.2020.105005

Gunawardena, N., & Stich, C. (2021). Interventions for young people aging out of the child welfare system: A systematic literature review. *Children and Youth Services Review, 127,* Article 106076.

Keyes, C. L. M. (2006). Mental health in adolescence: Is America's youth flourishing? *American Journal of Orthopsychiatry, 76*(3), 395–402. https://doi.org/10.1037/0002-9432.76.3.395

Kovarikova, J. (2017). *Exploring youth outcomes after aging-out of care.* Provincial Advocate for Children & Youth, Toronto, Ont.

Kufeldt, K., Simard, M., & Vachon, J. (2000). *Looking After Children in Canada final report.* Submitted to Social Development Partnerships of Human Resources Development Canada.

Lamborn, P. & Aubry, T. (2021). *Assessment of the needs of University of Ottawa students with extended society care status – final report.* Centre for Research on Educational and Community Services (CRECS), University of Ottawa.

Legault, L., Flynn, R., Artz, S., Balla, P., Dudding, P., Norgaard, V., Cole, S., Ghazal, H., Lemay, R., Petrick, S., Vandermeulen, G., Poirier, M. A., & Simard, M. C. (2004). Looking After Children: Implementation and outcomes in Canada. *Journal of Child and Youth Care Work* 19, 159–169.

Miller, M. (2021, June). *2020 Ontario Looking After Children provincial report.* Centre for Research on Educational and Community Services (CRECS), University of Ottawa.

Miller, M., Vincent, C., & Flynn, R. (2022). *Bibliography of papers, chapters, and conference presentations from the Ontario Looking After Children (OnLAC) Project.* Centre for Research on Educational and Community Services (CRECS), University of Ottawa.

Ministry of Education and Ministry of Children and Family Development. (2008, August). *Joint educational planning and support for children and youth in care: Cross-ministry guidelines.* Government of British Columbia.

Parker, R., Ward, H., Jackson, S., Aldgate, J., & Wedge, P. (1991). *Looking After Children: Assessing outcomes in child care.* The report of an independent working party established by the Department of Health. HSMO.

Sécurité publique Canada—Public Safety Canada. (2012). *Projet pilote d'implantation de l'approche S'occuper des enfants (SOCEN) dans les centres jeunesse du Québec.* (Pilot project to implement the Looking After Children [LAC] approach in Quebec). National Crime Prevention Centre.

Stith, S. M., Liu, T., Cavies, L. C., Boykin, E. L., Alder, M. C., Harris, J. M., Som, A., McPherson, M., & Dees, J. (2009). Risk factors in child maltreatment: A meta-analytic review of the literature. *Aggression and Violent Behavior* 14(1), 13–29.

Chapter 1

The Convergence of Two Developmental Frameworks in Services to Young People in Out-of-Home Care

A s the basic conceptual framework for this volume, we have drawn on two converging developmental frameworks that have inspired recent attempts in the United Kingdom, Europe, and North America to promote more positive outcomes and resilience for young people who have typically entered out-of-home care (i.e., are "in care") because of neglect or abuse in their families of origin. By *developmental framework*, we mean a perspective that aims at the healthy development of young people in the physical, social, psychological, emotional, cognitive, and behavioural domains, beyond attempts merely to prevent or remediate specific problems (Biglan, 2014). This ambitious objective is consistent with evidence that effective preventive interventions work precisely because they foster pro-social behaviours and values that run counter to the emergence of problems (Biglan et al., 2012).

The two perspectives to which we refer are, respectively, Looking After Children, an international initiative that originated in the United Kingdom (Parker et al., 1991) and Child Well-Being, formulated by the U.S. Administration of Children, Youth, and Families (2012) and further elaborated on by Biglan (2014). The two frameworks have much in common: the creation of nurturing environments, the prevention of risk, and the overarching goal of positive child and youth development and resilience.

1. Developmental Framework No. 1: Looking After Children— Good Parenting, Good Outcomes

The preface provided an overview of the history and approach of Looking After Children in the United Kingdom and Canada. This framework strives to achieve good outcomes for young people in care through high-quality substitute parenting (Parker et al., 1991). Contextual factors in the United Kingdom in the 1980s and 1990s were an important influence on the working group in the United Kingdom that first formulated Looking After Children in the 1980s and 1990s. These factors included poor quality and inappropriateness in out-of-home care services; a growing emphasis on preventing young people's entry into care or, if this could not be prevented, on returning them to their families as quickly as feasible; and a series of investigations into serious situations within the care system, including several deaths of young people (Parker et al., 1991). Also, the increasing cost of out-of-home care raised the issue of "value for money" and, more broadly, of service effectiveness. All these elements led to a heightened concern in the United Kingdom with *outcomes* (especially the benefits—or disbenefits—actually experienced by young people in care and their families, and not merely with *outputs*, or the services provided to them). This concern with outcomes extended to measuring and improving them with a new sense of urgency. Many of the same contextual factors in the countries—including Canada—that very quickly displayed serious interest in Looking After Children explain why there was piloting of the approach in a dozen or so countries.

In 1989, the U.K. Parliament passed the Children Act, the most far-reaching legislation affecting children and adolescents ever enacted (Parker et al., 1991). The act was the product of a fundamental reconceptualization of children's well-being, and its implementation in 1991 was marked by several innovations: an emphasis on setting goals, reviewing progress, and monitoring outcomes; the inclusion of the views of young people in care and their families and caregivers; and a focus on care services as supportive rather than punitive of families.

1.1. Guiding Principles of Looking After Children

Another major reason for the international enthusiasm that greeted the introduction of the Looking After Children framework in the

United Kingdom was the set of guiding principles that the working party clearly articulated to prepare the way for implementation of the Children Act 1989 and the reform of child welfare services. We believe they are as relevant now in Canada and elsewhere as they were 30 years ago, and thus present them here.

1. The welfare of the young person is paramount.
2. Agencies should aim for standards equivalent to those of a well-informed parent with adequate resources.
3. Agencies require a formal system to plan and record what good parents do daily.
4. Agencies with care of and responsibility for young people must work in partnership with birth parents, current care-givers, and other relevant professionals.
5. Young people must be consulted and listened to as soon as they are old enough.
6. Each young person is an individual with unique needs.
7. A young person with a disability is firstly a young person who has additional needs.
8. Access should only happen if it is meaningful and beneficial to the young person and does not prevent the permanency of placement.
9. Young people have a right to keep in touch with their birth family's cultural traditions.
10. The aim of Looking After Children is to promote children and youth well-being and success, not just to prevent harm.
11. Young people in care may have needs that are more difficult to meet than their peers, but outcome targets should not be set at a lower standard than those for their equals; child welfare workers should act on behalf of the young person to organize resources.
12. Looking After Children focuses on daily experiences that improve young people's prospects for adult life.
13. Looking After Children is a youth-centred developmental way of working, not a bureaucratic system.
14. Assessments should take account of the perspectives of all those involved, paying particular attention to the young person's interests and feelings.
15. Positive action will improve a young person's health and educational performance.

16. Achievable objectives should be the focus of collaboration for all developmental dimensions.
17. All plans of care make it clear who is responsible for what and by when.
18. Positive work is possible even in less-than-ideal circumstances.
19. In implementing these principles, Looking After Children has insisted that effective partnerships must be established between people of unequal power.
20. Such partnerships require listening to users and carers, anti-discriminatory practices, agreements about and recording of progress, adequate information, honesty and openness, and genuine participation.

1.2. Developmental Domains of Looking After Children

Looking After Children sought to improve young people's outcomes in seven major areas of development, reflected in many of the chapters of this volume: health, education, identity, family and social relationships, social presentation, emotional and behavioural development, and self-care skills. In our Ontario Looking After Children (OnLAC) Project, we have added an eighth outcome dimension—developmental assets (see Chapter 2). These assets are either external supports or internal strengths that have been shown by the Search Institute of Minneapolis (Lerner & Benson, 2012) to underlie positive youth development. We added the developmental assets (with our own method of measuring them) to our OnLAC Project version of the AAR) because of their demonstrable conceptual and operational compatibility with the Looking After Children developmental perspective, with its emphasis on achieving good outcomes and resilience through high-quality substitute parenting.

After the Children Act 1989 became law in the United Kingdom and had been implemented, Ward (1998) pointed out that Looking After Children makes use of a child and adolescent development model to meet children's unmet needs and contributes to their long-term well-being. The approach does so by asking to what extent young people in care (a) are making progress towards recognized developmental objectives and (b) are being provided the services or experiences needed to attain these objectives. In adherence to these core themes, the current standardized version of the AAR, used since January 1, 2016 (and known as the AAR-C2-2016), asks, for example, whether 6-to-9-year-old children in care are acquiring many (versus only some, few, or no) special educational skills and interests. The AAR also describes the wide range of services and experiences that most children will need to achieve these special educational skills and interests. These include being enrolled in school, experiencing no or few unplanned changes in schools, having an actually implemented individual education plan (IEP), as needed, exhibiting excellent or good rather than only fair or poor basic skills in reading and math, being involved in engaging extracurricular clubs or activities, or being read to by a caregiver on a daily basis. The same approach—a combination of high-expectancy developmental objectives and age-appropriate and effective experiences and services—is applied throughout the other OnLAC development domains.

2. Developmental Framework No. 2: Child Well-Being

The second developmental approach, the structure of which we have integrated in the present chapter with that of Looking After Children, is the Child Well-Being framework formulated by the U.S. Administration on Children, Youth and Families (ACYF, 2012). The ACYF model promotes the social and emotional well-being of young people in out-of-home care, despite the serious abuse or neglect most have experienced in their families of origin. This developmental framework, which originated in research by Lou et al. (2008), includes four key domains of well-being: physical development; cognitive development; psychological, emotional, and behavioural development; and social development. Adaptive functioning within each domain is conceptualized as varying according to the child's chronological age, developmental status, and contextual factors, such as caregiver background or child temperament (see Table 1.1).

To elaborate and refine the ACFY framework, the U.S. Children's Bureau commissioned a series of papers that were published as the *Integrating Safety, Permanency and Well-Being Series* (Wilson, 2014). For present purposes, one of these papers is particularly relevant: Biglan's (2014) *Comprehensive Framework for Nurturing the Well-Being of Children and Adolescents*. Biglan (2014; see also Biglan, 2015) identified the principal domains and indicators of children's well-being, described children's and adolescents' normal developmental trajectories, and provided examples of evidence-based interventions capable of raising the developmental trajectories of children whose growth has been impeded by abuse or neglect.

Table 1.1. Key outcomes in the Child Well-Being developmental framework, by outcome domain and developmental phase

Outcome Domains of Child Well-Being Developmental Framework				
Developmental Phase	Physical Development	Cognitive Development	Psychological, Emotional & Behavioural Development	Social Development
Prenatal-infancy (birth to age 2)	Birth weight; physical & motor skill development; injuries	Language development; executive functioning	Self-awareness develops; emotional & behavioural development	Social development; attachment
Early childhood (3–5 years)	Physical development; injuries; illness; diet; physical activity; height/weight percentiles; oral health	Language & early literacy development (e.g., picture naming, rhyming, letter naming); executive functioning	Self-concept develops; emotional & behavioural development; attentional & hyperactivity difficulties; conduct problems	Self-regulation; social relations; prosocial behaviour, skills, attitudes
Childhood (6–11 years)	Same as above; plus: strength and athletic skills improve	Reading & math proficiency; executive functioning	Same as above, plus: more complex self-concept; aggressive behaviour; depressive symptoms	Same as above, plus: gradual shift in control from parents to child; peers assume a more central role
Early adolescence (12–14 years	Same as above, plus: more rapid physical growth & changes; puberty & reproductive maturity; self-inflicted injuries; type 2 diabetes;	Same as above, plus: intellectual development, abstract thinking	Same as above, plus: violent behaviours; drug use; risky sexual behaviour	Same as above, plus: central role of peer group; identity formation
Adolescence (15–19 years)	Same as above, plus: STDs; BMI*; unplanned pregnancy; diet; physical activity	Executive functioning; critical & rational thinking	Same as above	Same as above, plus: moral development; intimacy development

Source: Adapted from Biglan, 2014, p. 5.
*STI = sexually transmitted disease; BMI = body mass index

2.1. Crucial Role of Nurturing Environments

Biglan et al. (2012) describe the kinds of environments that nurture successful child and adolescent development and prevent psychological or behavioural problems. Such environments exhibit four key characteristics: they minimize toxic biological or psychological events, they teach and reward prosocial and self-regulatory behaviour, they monitor and limit opportunities for problem behaviour, and they promote the psychological flexibility of being aware of one's thoughts and feelings and acting in a way aligned with one's values. Biglan et al. (2012, p. 258) proposed the following succinct and straightforward principle of action for a field such as child welfare: *"If we want to prevent multiple problems and increase the prevalence of young people who develop successfully, we must increase the prevalence of nurturing environments"* (italics in the original).

Regarding the ill effects of toxic environments, the Royal Society of Canada (RSC; Boivin & Hertzman, 2012, p. 118) concluded that child maltreatment is "perhaps the most severe early childhood adversity" that children and young people experience, with chronic exposure to poor quality parenting and maltreatment especially damaging. Like both the Looking After Children and Child Well-Being developmental frameworks just described, the RSC analysis indicated that a service model focused on developing a nurturing environment of protective factors is most likely to promote healthy child development.

3. Integrating Looking After Children and Child Well-Being

The Looking After Children and Child Well-Being developmental frameworks converge in two complementary ways. First, as Table 1.2 illustrates, their respective outcome domains are clearly congruent: the eight specific outcome dimensions of Looking After Children dovetail nicely with the four broad Child Well-Being outcome domains, which provide the organizing skeleton of this volume. Like introductory Chapter 1 and concluding Chapter 10, Chapter 2 (OnLAC developmental assets) is relevant to all four Child Well-Being outcome domains. Chapter 3 (OnLAC health) corresponds closely to the physical development aspect of Child Well-Being. Chapter 4 (OnLAC education) is directly related to the cognitive development dimension of Child Well-Being. Chapter 5 (OnLAC cultural and personal identity), Chapter 7 (OnLAC emotional and behavioural development), and Chapter 8

Table 1.2. Convergence of the outcome domains of the Looking After Children and Child Well-Being developmental frameworks for promoting positive development and resilience among children and youth in out-of-home care

	Four Outcome Domains of the Child Well-Being Framework			
	Physical Development	Cognitive Development	Psychological, Emotional & Behavioural Development	Social Development
Eight Outcome Domains of the Ontario Looking After Children (OnLAC) Framework	Chapter 1: Introduction			
1. Developmental Assets	Chapter 2: Developmental Assets			
2. Health	Chapter 3: Physical Development and Health			
3. Education		Chapter 4: Education Chapter 5: Educational Snapshot		
4. Identity			Chapter 6: Cultural & Personal Identity	
5. Family & Social Relationships **6. Social Presentation**				Chapter 7: Family, Social Relationships, & Social Presentation
7. Emotional & Behavioural Development			Chapter 8: Emotional & Behavioural Development	
8. Self-Care Skills			Chapter 9: Self-Care Skills & Transitions	
	Chapter 10: Implications & lessons from the OnLAC Project			

Source: Adapted from Biglan, 2014, p. 2-5.

(OnLAC self-care skills) overlap substantially with the psychological, emotional, and behavioural development domain of Child Well-Being. Finally, Chapter 6 (OnLAC family and social relationships, together with OnLAC social presentation) fits well with the social development aspect of Child Well-Being.

We are not the first to have seen this parallel between the aims of Looking After Children and Child Well-Being. A decade and a half ago, Scott and Ward (2005) used well-being as a basic theme to tie together the findings of an international group of researchers concerned with vulnerable children, families, and communities. In a similar way, we have drawn on the ACYF Child Well-Being framework, as further elaborated by Biglan (2014, 2015), because of its clarity and congruence with the OnLAC perspective.

There is a second sense in which the Looking After Children and Child Well-Being frameworks fit together well. As shown in Table 1.1, Biglan's (2014) formulation of the Child Well-Being model proceeds in successive developmental phases, from prenatal infancy (birth to age 2) and early childhood (6–11 years) through early adolescence (12–14 years) and adolescence (15–19). At each phase, specific milestones need to be mastered and risks avoided, in the physical, cognitive, psychological-emotional-behavioural, and social domains. The Looking After Children framework proceeds in exactly the same fashion. Our OnLAC version of the approach has the considerable advantage of having created and refined the AAR since the year 2000 as a set of needs-assessment, care-planning, and outcome-monitoring instruments of good psychometric quality. The current AAR-C2-2016 grew out of two previous standardized versions, employed initially in 2006 and 2010, respectively. These, in turn, had grown out of earlier, experimental versions, used on a pilot basis between 2001 and 2006, which had been adapted from the original U.K. version of the AAR.

4. Current Version of the Assessment and Action Record (AAR-C2-2016)

The AAR-C2-2016 consists of nine age-appropriate forms, available in English and French, for use, respectively, with infants aged 0–11 months; young children aged 12–23 months or 24–35 months; young children aged 3–5; primary-school children aged 6–9 or 10–12; adolescents aged 13–15 or 16–17; and late adolescents or young adults aged 18+. This comprehensive set of instruments provides the age-related precision needed to implement the broad goals and specific developmental objectives that unite the OnLAC and Child Well-Being frameworks.

The AAR tracks a child's progress in eight outcome domains: health, education, identity, family and social relationships, social presentation, emotional and behavioural development, self-care skills, and developmental assets. The tool is completed annually in a conversational interview in which the child welfare worker, the young person (if aged 10 or over), and the caregiver participate. If the young person is Indigenous (i.e., First Nations, Métis, or Inuit), an effort is made to have an Elder, Cultural Teacher, Band or community representative present to assist.

Like its predecessors, the AAR-C2-2016 has three complementary purposes, on three interrelated levels. On the level of the individual young person, the AAR has the clinical function of helping child welfare professionals and caregivers to assess the young person's needs comprehensively, to prepare and implement high-quality, collaborative plans of care, and to monitor the young person's progress from year to year. On the level of the local Society, the aggregated data generated by the AAR has the managerial function of enabling middle and senior managers and board members to monitor the progress of whole groups of young people each year. The AAR data allow comparisons between actual and targeted developmental outcomes and more evidence-based decisions to improve the relevance of services and the quality of the young people's lives, on an ongoing basis. On the level of the provincial child welfare system, the aggregated Society data from the AAR have the policy function of encouraging decision makers to monitor young people's outcomes on a system-wide basis, to evaluate these outcomes in light of targeted progress, and to formulate improved policies and practices.

The language used in the AAR has evolved to become more inclusive over the 22 years (and counting) of the OnLAC Project, and this is reflected in the present volume. For example, the 2016 version of the AAR records the child's or young person's biological sex as female, male, or intersex, and the adult caregivers and child welfare workers can choose among several options to identify themselves: "male," "female," "non-binary," "trans," or "prefer not to answer." We have also endeavoured herein to avoid using terms such as "minority groups," preferring instead to refer to "racial or ethnic groups," for example. Similarly, we have used the pronouns "they," "their," and "them" instead of "he/she," "his/her," and "himself/ herself." The American Psychological Association has published an excellent resource on these questions of inclusive language, https:// www.apa.org/about/apa/equity-diversity-inclusion/language-guidelines.

5. Evolution of Looking After Children in Canada and Ontario

The first training event in Canada was held in February 1996, at the Prescott-Russell Children's Aid Society (now known as Valoris), in Plantagenet, Ontario. As mentioned in the preface, the training was conducted by two leaders of the International Looking After Children Initiative, Harriet Ward and Helen Jones. Early Looking After Children pilot projects in Canada that preceded the current OnLAC Project included the Evaluating Child Welfare Outcomes (ECWO) Project at the Prescott-Russell Children's Aid Society; a Canadian project led by Kathleen Kufeldt that spanned six Canadian provinces (from east to west: Newfoundland and Labrador, Nova Scotia, Prince Edward Island, New Brunswick, Quebec, and Ontario; Kufeldt, Vachon, and Simard, 2000; and a project in British Columbia). All these initiatives contributed to the early development of Looking After Children in Canada. However, only sustained collaboration among various bodies that has lasted for more than 20 years (i.e., 2000–present) has enabled the OnLAC Project to endure over time. This collaboration has included the OnLAC Project team, located at the Centre for Research on Educational and Community Services (CRECS) in the Faculty of Social Sciences at the University of Ottawa; the Ontario Association of Children's Aid Societies (OACAS); and some 44 local Societies in Ontario. Moreover, the launching of the OnLAC Project in 2000 was made possible only by an initial strategic health research grant from the Social Sciences and Humanities Research Council of Canada (SSHRC; Flynn et al., 1999) and subsequent annual funding (2004–present) from the Ontario Ministry of Children, Communities and Social Services (MCCSS) and its predecessors. These financial resources have enabled the OnLAC Project to build large and still-growing data sets, consisting of approximately 85,000 annual AAR interviews with some 35,000 young people in out-of-home care in Ontario. This collaboration and funding have also allowed us to create and refine a set of detailed needs assessment and outcome-monitoring instruments, in English and French, publish or assist in the publication of approximately 100 books, book chapters, peer-reviewed papers, and doctoral theses; as well as produce hundreds of technical reports and numerous conference presentations (see Miller, Vincent, & Flynn, 2021).

The number of children and adolescents assessed each year in the OnLAC Project since data collection began in 2001 is shown in Figure 1.1. The data displayed in the figure consist of an annual series of cross-sectional samples. That is, the number of young people assessed with the AAR in any given year consists of (a) those already enrolled in the OnLAC Project in one or more previous years and (b) those who were new to the project in that particular year. Figure 1.1 shows that the total annual number of young people evaluated in the project was modest during years 1–5, in which participation by local Societies was voluntary. The number began to rise in year 6, when the Government of Ontario stated that it planned to make use of the AAR mandatory in the province's Societies. The number then more than doubled in year 7, when the province actually implemented the mandated use of the AAR to assess service needs, help prepare plans of care, and monitor outcomes. The annual number remained high for the next six years (2008–2013), remaining close to or above 7,000 young people assessed each year. Since 2014, the annual number has declined, due to a change in provincial policy that now emphasized that coming into care was a last resort. Since 2020, COVID-19 also rendered face-to-face AAR interviews and assessments more difficult.

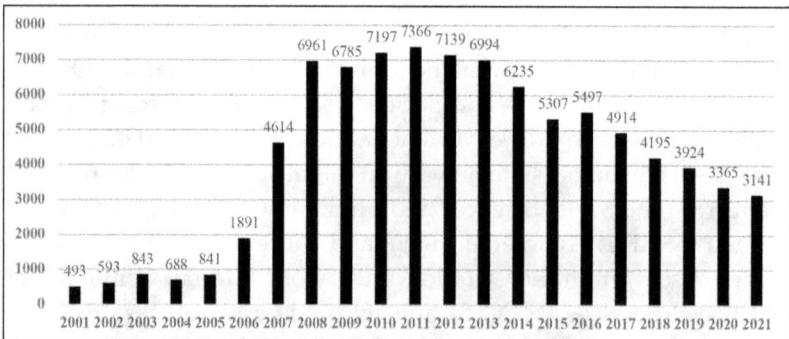

Figure 1.1. Number of Assessment and Action Records completed with and on young people in care in Ontario between 2001 and 2021.
Source: Ontario Looking After Children Project data from 2001 to 2021.

6. OnLAC Project Data Collection, Verification, and Preparation at the University of Ottawa

Once child welfare workers have completed an AAR for a young person in their charge, Ontario Societies submit the file to the OnLAC team at the University of Ottawa for processing. The primary method of submission from 2010 to 2022 was the Web Capture Network, which used secure, web-based software to digitally transfer AAR-image data to a secure server at the University of Ottawa. Since June 2022, the primary method of submission of AARs is via upload to secure SharePoint folders. Each Society has identified authorized users for the SharePoint AAR submission system, and those users are granted access to their Society's secure SharePoint folder within the system. Once uploaded for submission, AARs are downloaded by OnLAC research staff and rigorously verified using TeleForm character recognition software, and are then exported into SPSS files in .sav file format. (A review of the reliability and validity of AAR data [especially its construct, concurrent, and predictive validity] in the context of its use in performance indicators and accountability for local Ontario Societies, is available in a technical report by Flynn and Miller, 2017.) The OACAS has also invested in an electronic vehicle for administration of the AAR. Currently, some Ontario Societies are using this web-based software to complete AARs with young people in their care. Once a supervisor has signed off on the completed electronic AAR, it becomes available for download in SPSS .sav format from the software website by the OnLAC team at the University of Ottawa.

Individual SPSS .sav files are merged into the Ontario provincial OnLAC database. Upon the completion of their first AAR, each young person in care is assigned an OnLAC identification number by the OnLAC Project team. This enables accurate year-to-year tracking of young persons' exits or re-entries to care or moves between Societies. Smaller age-group databases can be merged into larger ones, with the most common groupings being 0–5 years, 6–9 years, 10–15 years, and 16 years and over. The final steps in OnLAC data preparation include filling in gaps in information, whenever possible (e.g., a young person's missing age or sex) and data cleaning, which includes identifying and eliminating any out-of-range values. Agency-specific databases are provided to Societies in SPSS .sav format and, if requested, in Microsoft Excel .xlsx format. The Ontario provincial database is held on a secure server at the University of Ottawa. A policy has been and remains in effect (OACAS, 2009) that has enabled external researchers, including PhD students at the Universities of Ottawa, Guelph, Windsor, Oxford, and Loma Linda, to gain access to the OnLAC database by presenting an acceptable research proposal to a committee at OACAS.

7. Contributions of the OnLAC Project to Knowledge, Policy and Practice in Child Welfare

The comprehensive bibliography mentioned above, comprising books, chapters, peer-reviewed papers, technical reports, and PhD theses (Miller, Vincent, & Flynn, 2021) stemming from the OnLAC Project includes a large number of contributions to child welfare knowledge, policy, and practice. Now we provide a sampling of the topics addressed by this research over the years.

7.1. Satisfaction of Young People in Care with their Current Placements

Flynn, Robitaille, and Ghazal (2006) examined young people's satisfaction with their current placements and related their satisfaction to a number of predictors. The participants were 414 young people in out-of-home care with whom an early version of the AAR had been completed; 52% were male, 48% female, ranging in age from 10 to 17 years (M = 13.46, SD = 2.17), and 89% were living in foster homes versus 11% in group homes. Placement satisfaction was measured with a 9-item scale. Those living in foster homes were highly satisfied with their placements, considerably more so than those residing in group homes. The strongest predictor of placement satisfaction by far was the quality of the relationship of the young person (as rated by the young person themselves) with the foster mother or female group home worker, followed by living in a foster rather than a group home and the quality of the young person's relationship with friends.

7.2. Suggestions by Young People in Care for Improving their Placements

Robitaille, Flynn, and Ghazal (2004) classified the responses made by young people in care in Ontario to an open-ended question in the AAR about how their current living situations could be improved. Of the 294 young people, aged 10–21, who participated, 23% indicated that they felt no improvements in their placements were needed; 25% said they wanted more flexible rules and privacy; 15% wanted their own room or a larger room; 10% said they would like to move to a different type of placement setting or location; 9% desired a better relationship with their caregivers or other children in care; 7% wanted improvements in their own school performance or interpersonal relationships; and 6% wanted better relationships with their birth families, including more frequent contact with their birth mothers.

7.3. Positive Experiences Reported by Young People in Care

Legault and Moffat (2006) carried out a qualitative analysis of positive life events that young people in care aged 10 and over had identified in response to two open-ended questions in the AAR, namely, "What, to the best of the knowledge and in the joint opinion of the child/youth, the caregiver, and the child welfare worker, is/are the most positive life experience(s) that [the young person] has experienced in terms of promoting their positive development? (a) In the last 12 months? (b) Since birth but more than 12 months ago?" Of the 641 participants, 78% reported that a positive life event had occurred in their lives during the past 12 months, and 63% said that a positive life event had taken place more than 12 months ago. In all, 1,530 responses were analyzed and categorized. Approximately 24% of the young people aged 10 and over nominated positive events that consisted of activities or events (e.g., playing a sport, participating in clubs, and going to camp or on trips) while 23% named a relationship with a birth family (11%) or foster family member (5%), and 18% flagged living in a foster home as a positive experience. Approximately 13% identified education, such as attending or graduating from school or receiving an award for good grades. Another 8% nominated events that reflected personal growth, such as good health, a life-changing experience, or belonging to a religion or possessing a sense of spirituality. "Coming of age" experiences, such as a transition to adulthood, becoming employed, or acquiring personal possessions such as a bicycle or a stereo, were identified by 6% of participants.

7.4. Participation in Structured Voluntary Activities and Psychological Outcomes among Young People in Care

Many studies of young people in the general population have indicated that more frequent involvement in structured voluntary activities (SVAs), that is, in healthy extracurricular or community-based activities, is related to a wide range of positive outcomes, including better mental health and improved school performance. This issue, however, has rarely been examined among young people in care. Gilligan (2000), one of the few child welfare researchers to have done so, has urged that SVAs be made accessible to youths in care as an important vehicle of resilient development. Flynn, Beaulac, and Vinograd (2006) investigated the role of participation in SVAs in the psychological adaptation of young people in care. Of the OnLAC sample of 442 participants, 50% were male and 50% female. Ranging in age from 10–17 years (M = 13.55, SD = 2.20), they resided mainly in foster homes (82%), with another 9% in group homes, 3% in kinship care, 2% in independent living, 3% in institutional settings (e.g., psychiatric or young offenders' facilities), and 1% in unknown settings. The young people had experienced serious adversity in their families of origin, including parental incapacity, physical, sexual, or psychological abuse, neglect, or abandonment. With controls for sex and age, the risk factor of substance use, and the protective factor of the youth's perception of the quality of their relationship with the female caregiver, Flynn et al. (2006) tested the hypothesis that more frequent participation in SVAs would be associated with higher levels of three positive outcomes: self-esteem, pro-social behaviour, and happiness in the present as well as optimism about the future. The results indicated that playing sports or carrying out physical activities without a coach or instructor was easily the most common activity, with 47% of the young people reporting a frequency of four or more times a week and 78% a frequency of at least once a week. On the other hand, half or more of the young people said that outside of gym or other classes at school, they never took part in three of the six types of activities studied: art, drama or music groups, clubs or lessons (66% said "never"); dance, gymnastics, karate, or other similar groups or lessons (61% "never"); and Guides or Scouts, 4-H club, community, church or other religious groups (50% "never"). Regression analyses supported the study hypothesis: the frequency of participation in SVAs was a statistically significant and positive (albeit modest) predictor of higher self-esteem, more pro-social behaviour, and greater happiness/ optimism. The young person's relationship with the female caregiver was an even stronger and positive predictor of all three psychological outcomes. Finally, for pro-social behaviour and self-esteem, the benefits of participation in SVAs were greatest among youth with low levels of substance use (cigarettes, alcohol, or marijuana) but virtually absent among frequent users of these substances.

7.5. Resilient Outcomes among Young People in Care

Flynn et al. (2004) investigated the proportion of young people in care who experienced resilience, defined as "positive patterns of functioning or development during or following exposure to adversity, or, more simply, as good adaptation in a context of risk" (Masten, 2006, p. 4), on selected outcomes. The sample included 340 young people aged 10–15 and 132 children aged 5–9; most resided in foster care. Each age group was compared on selected variables (as measured by the AAR) with a larger sample of the same age from the general population (as assessed on the same variables in the National Longitudinal Survey of Children and Youth [NLSCY; Statistics Canada & Human Resources Development Canada, 1995]). Resilience in the young people in care was operationally defined as average or above average functioning, relative to that of the general population sample of the same age. A relatively high proportion of the OnLAC sample was currently experiencing resilient outcomes in health, self-esteem, and pro-social behaviour, compared with only a moderate number on relationships with friends and anxiety/emotional distress and a relatively low proportion on educational outcomes. This study provided a differentiated picture of adaptation in the young people in care and highlighted the need for concerted action to improve educational outcomes.

7.6. Educational Resilience among Young Children in Care

Children who experience early academic success are more likely to pursue their education, and the early school performance of children in care is especially important. Although many young people in care experience difficulties in school, some are successful despite the severe adversity they face. Legault, Lebel, and Flynn (2003) explored the relative importance of protective and risk factors for educational resilience in an OnLAC sample of 5-to-9-year-olds in care. In a regression model that accounted for 47% of the variance, better academic performance was associated with children who had less hyperactivity, better problem-solving skills, and greater placement stability. Better educational resilience was also associated with caregivers who had higher academic expectations of the children in their care and stimulated their literacy by encouraging them to read for pleasure or by reading to them.

Tessier, O'Higgins, and Flynn (2018) also studied educational resilience and its predictors, but among older Ontario young people in care. In a cross-sectional OnLAC sample, composed of 3,659 young people (56.1% male, 43.9% female, 11.5–18.0 years of age [M = 15.1, SD = 1.6], and residing in foster or kinship homes [80.1%] or group homes [19.8%], Tessier et al., 2018) assessed educational resilience with a 7-item rating scale of educational success that combined 2 AAR ratings by the young person's child welfare worker, 4 AAR ratings by the young person's caregiver, and 1 AAR rating by the young person themselves. The predictive model tested by Tessier et al. (2018) was based on a systematic review of risk and protective factors of educational outcomes by O'Higgins, Sebba, and Gardner (2017). Of the 20 conceptual categories of factors identified by O'Higgins et al. (2017), Tessier et al. (2018) were able to operationalize 15 contained in the AAR, with a total of 19 variables: 5 contextual risk, 7 individual risk, 3 contextual protective, and 4 individual protective factors. At the final step of a hierarchical regression model, a total of 12 of the 19 predictor variables had a statistically significant relationship with the outcome variable of educational success: 2 contextual risk factors (neglect as a reason for entry of the young person into care and grade retention), 4 individual risk factors (special educational needs, racial minority status: Black, behavioural problems, and soft drug use), 2 contextual protective factors (caregiver educational aspirations for the young person in care and placement stability), and 4 individual protective factors (internal developmental assets, female sex, positive mental health, and young person's educational aspirations). In a longitudinal sub-sample of 962 young people who had data on educational success three years later, time-1 educational success, soft drug use, internal developmental assets, female sex, and positive mental health had a statistically significant relationship with time-2 educational success at the final step of a hierarchical regression model. These cross-sectional and longitudinal findings are relevant to a more precise understanding of why some young people in care experience educational resilience and also to the construction of more effective evidence-based interventions.

7.7. Caregiving Practices and Young People's Mental Health

Despite the importance of caregiving in out-of-home care, there has been relatively little research on the actual parenting practices that caregivers use. To help fill this gap, Perkins-Mangulabnan and Flynn (2006) analyzed AAR data on a sample of 432 young people living in Ontario foster homes (85%), group homes (11%), or kinship care (3%). Of this sample, 52% were male and 48% female, virtually all were 10–17 years of age (M = 13.51, SD = 2.22), and they had been in care for an average (median) of two years. As hypothesized, caregiver–parenting variables (parental nurturance, caregiver-youth conflict, and caregiver-youth shared activities), as a set, accounted for a statistically significant increment in the variance explained in each of four youth-in-care mental health outcomes (i.e., the frequency of prosocial behaviour, emotional disorder, conduct disorder, and indirect aggression), beyond that accounted for by the young person's sex, age, and years in the current placement. Also, as hypothesized, greater parental nurturance predicted more frequent prosocial behaviour and less frequent emotional disorder, conduct disorder, and indirect aggression, and higher levels of parent–child conflict predicted more frequent conduct disorder and physical aggression on the part of the youths in care. However, contrary to what had been hypothesized, more frequent parent–child conflict was not related to the frequency of the youth's pro-social behaviour or indirect aggression, nor was more frequent participation by caregivers in shared activities with the youths in their care related to any of the youth outcomes.

7.8. Internalizing and Externalizing Mental Health Adjustment in Adolescents in Care

Few studies have examined contextual and personal factors in the psychological adjustment of young people in out-of-home care, and even fewer have tested formal models of their adaptation. Legault, Anawati, and Flynn (2006) formulated and tested a predictive model of psychological adjustment (i.e., anxiety and physical aggression) in an OnLAC sample of 220 young people, aged 14–17. Regression analyses showed that lower anxiety was associated with a higher-quality relationship (as perceived by the young person in care) with the female caregiver, a greater number of close friends, and higher self-esteem. Less frequent physically aggressive behaviour was associated with having had fewer primary caregivers in the past, a higher-quality relationship with the female caregiver, a greater number of close friendships, higher self-esteem, greater use of approach coping strategies and less frequent use of avoidance coping. Overall, the results suggested the importance for better psychological adjustment among young people in care of rewarding relationships with caregivers and friends, placement stability, and approach rather than avoidance coping.

7.9. Hope in Adolescents in Care

Dumoulin and Flynn (2006) conducted what seems to have been one of the first studies of hope and its predictors among young people in care. The importance of hope derives from its links to numerous aspects of positive adaptation, including goal-oriented action, optimism, effective coping, academic and athletic achievement, adjustment, self-esteem, and problem-solving. Snyder et al. (1997) define hope in terms of two main components, pathways and agency thinking. *Pathways thinking* is the self-perceived ability to generate feasible routes to desired goals and is manifested in internal thoughts such as "I'll find a way to get this done!" *Agency thinking*, the motivational aspect of hope, is the self-perceived capacity to use the pathways one has generated to pursue one's goals. Identifying a pathway without the motivation to follow through will not lead to optimal purposeful action, as both pathways and agency thinking are necessary. The OnLAC sample used by Dumoulin and Flynn (2006) was composed of 374 young people in care, 51% male and 49% female, aged 10–17, and living in foster or group homes in Ontario. Their average level of hope was similar to that observed in the norm groups described by Snyder et al. (1997). Regression analysis indicated that higher individual hope scores were reported by young people in care who were male, younger, less physically aggressive, residing in foster rather than group homes, experiencing a more positive relationship with the female caregiver, and engaged in higher levels of active as opposed to avoidant coping. The predictive model accounted for 43% of the variance in the young people's hope scores.

7.10. Enhancing the Utility of the Assessment and Action Record in Implementing OnLAC

Pantin, Flynn, and Runnels (2006) conducted a survey of 146 child welfare workers or supervisors in local Societies involved in the OnLAC Project, with a response rate of 64%. The purpose was to determine the degree to which practitioners perceived the AAR as useful in their direct service or supervisory work with young people in care and their caregivers. Pantin et al. (2006) assumed that a more favourable perception of the utility of the AAR would encourage its use in practice and facilitate implementation of the OnLAC approach as a whole. Of the child welfare workers or supervisors who had received at least some OnLAC training and had made at least some use of the AAR in practice, a clear majority saw the tool as useful in their work. The AAR was rated as "very useful" or "useful" in helping them better understand the needs of the young person in care by 77%, 73% said that the AAR helped them collaborate more effectively with caregivers in implementing young persons' plans of care, and 70% reported that the AAR helped them contribute to preparing more useful plans of care. Regression analysis showed that four implementation-process variables—the amount of OnLAC training that respondents had received, the perceived quality of this training, the number of respondents' cases in using the AAR, and the frequency of their discussion of AAR information in supervision—each made an independent and positive contribution to the ability of the predictive model to account for more favourable evaluations of the utility of the AAR. The most important predictor was the frequency of discussion of AAR information in supervision. Workers and supervisors who discussed AAR information regularly in supervision had a very favourable perception of the utility of the AAR, more favourable than those who discussed this information only occasionally in supervision and much more favourable than those who virtually never discussed it.

7.11. Outcome Monitoring and Feedback to Local Societies

Every year, OnLAC Project staff produce a confidential report on a large number of outcome indicators for each local Society in Ontario that provides data from its AAR interviews. OnLAC staff also produce an annual non-confidential, public report (see, for example, Miller, 2020) on the outcomes of children in care in the province as a whole,

for use by Societies, OACAS, MCCSS, and other interested stakeholders. Together, the annual local reports and the provincial public report
enable Societies to compare the outcomes of the young people in their
care in a given year with those in Ontario as a whole. Societies can
thus establish an organizational baseline and see whether their outcomes are improving over time. Societies can also compare their own
results with those of Societies in Ontario as a whole and, on some
variables, with the general population in Ontario or Canada.

7.12. OnLAC-Based Performance Indicators of Youth Well-Being in Ontario Societies

OnLAC AAR data on young people in care currently serve as the source
of three well-being performance indicators (PIs) in Ontario's accountability system for local Societies: average educational performance in
reading and math (for young people aged 5–17), average quality of the
caregiver-youth relationship (as perceived by the young person, for
young people aged 10–17), and average level of developmental assets
(for young people aged 0–17). Only the second PI, the quality of the
caregiver–youth relationship, is made public each year through publication on the MCCSS website (see http://www.children.gov.on.ca/
htdocs/English/professionals/childwelfare/societies/publicreporting/
well-being.aspx). The average provincial and individual Society scores
on the caregiver–youth relationship have been quite stable over time.
In 2018, the mean (average) score was 6.6, out of a maximum of 8.0, for
young people aged 10–15 (n = 1,303), and 6.2 (out of 8.0) for those aged
16–17 (n = 596; Miller 2019, p. 10). However, when analyzed by placement setting, these PI scores show greater differentiation. The mean
score of young people living in kinship care homes (7.1 for those aged
10–15, vs. 6.7 for those aged 16–17) were the highest of all, followed by
the mean scores of young people residing in foster homes (6.7 vs. 6.5)
and in group homes (5.9 vs. 5.3). In future, AAR data from the OnLAC
Project may become the source of a wider range of well-being PIs, and
a larger number of PIs from MCCSS's accountability system for local
Societies may be made public each year.

8. Concluding Thoughts on Enhancing the AAR and on the International Relevance of the OnLAC Project

Beyond the major revisions that we make to the AAR every five to ten years, two immediate changes would enhance its use and utility. First, it would help for planning and evaluating transitions from care if MCCSS were to extend the present mandated use of the AAR with young people aged 0–17 to those aged 18 and over. An age-appropriate AAR form already exists, in both English and French, for the 18+ age group. Currently, upon turning 18, young adults in Ontario are legally (de jure) no longer in care, even though many continue to be served by caregivers and Society staff and thus de facto are still in care. Because the AAR is currently not mandated for use with young people aged 18 and older (because the latter are technically not in care), we have much less knowledge about their objective and subjective outcomes than for 0-to-17-year-olds. Second, systematic integration of the rich outcome data from the AAR with the extensive output (i.e., service-process) data from Ontario's Child Protection Information Network (CPIN) system would permit major advances in our knowledge of whether in-care services are indeed contributing to desirable outcomes.

As the AAR and the OnLAC Project continue to evolve, we believe that the assessment approach and outcome findings that they make possible are likely to have considerable relevance for other jurisdictions on the international level. Fernandez and Delfabbro (2020) recently summarized international trends in child welfare, including out-of-home care, and we use their discussion as a convenient guide on which to hang our concluding thoughts. First, the Assessment and Action Record (AAR) has shown its ability to illuminate differences in the relative quality of outcomes associated with each of the key service forms that comprise the child welfare continuum: family foster care, kinship care, customary care (for Indigenous children and youth), group care, and residential care. These differences should guide policies favouring higher-scoring over lower-scoring services. Second, the AAR has successfully measured different forms of child maltreatment, including neglect and physical, sexual, and emotional abuse, and their respective associations with developmental outcomes in education, physical health, mental health, substance use, well-being, and resilience. The tool is thus likely to be useful in improving resilience and mitigating risk over time. Third, the AAR has recently been improved for the task of collecting identity-based data, making possible better analyses of the consequences of today's overrepresentation of Indigenous and Black young people in child welfare. We hope that a better understanding of this overrepresentation will also lead to its reduction. Fourth, the success of the OnLAC Project over more than two decades in helping to promote child welfare reform in Ontario may furnish a useful model for other jurisdictions. Sustaining reform movements over an extended period is challenging but necessary for institutionalizing their success. Fifth, the AAR facilitates a public health-oriented risk-and-resilience approach to prevention in child welfare. The tool incorporates a range of standardized instruments for evaluating risk and resilience-related developmental outcomes. Sixth, in the domain of out-of-home care, the OnLAC Project and AAR have promoted a needed extension of the purview of child welfare in many countries. The field is increasingly mandated to ensure not only the traditional outcomes of safety, stability, and permanence but also to achieve the broader goal of well-being, with its educational, health, mental health, relational, and other dimensions. Seventh, the OnLAC Project and the AAR have gathered much useful information on how to help young people still in care to prepare for successful transitions to life in the community. This information, however, has made only too clear that we also need an "OnLAC-2" Project that will provide data on young people's outcomes after they have left care. Eighth, the AAR takes the form of a yearly face-to-face "conversational interview" in which participate young people in care (if aged 10 or over), their caregivers, and their child welfare workers. This format ensures and operationalizes today's insistence in many countries that young people contribute actively in discussions that affect them and their futures.

Each of the following chapters will discuss the eight developmental domains of the AAR (developmental assets, physical development and health, education, cultural and personal identity, family and social relationships, and social presentation, emotional and behavioural development, and self-care skills and transitions), presents their findings and suggests recommendations to foster positive outcomes for young people in the child welfare system relevant to the domain discussed. The final chapter considers implications and lessons for improving the outcomes and well-being of young people in care.

References

Administration for Children and Families. (2012). *Promoting social and emotional well-being for children and youth receiving child welfare services.* (Information memorandum ACYF-CB-IM-12-04). U.S. Department of Health and Human Services.

Biglan, A. (2014). *A comprehensive framework for nurturing the well-being of children and adolescents.* (Integrating safety, permanency and well-being series, 1–27). Administration for Children and Families, U.S. Department of Health and Human Services.

Biglan, A. (2015). *The nurture effect: How the science of human behavior can improve our lives & our world.* New Harbinger Publications.

Biglan, A., Flay, B. R., Embry, D. D., & Sandler, I. (2012). Nurturing environments and the next generation of prevention research and practice. *American Psychologist, 67*(4), 257–271. https://doi.org/10.1037/a0026796

Boivin, M., & Hertzman, C. (Eds.). (2012). *Early childhood development: Adverse experiences and developmental health.* Royal Society of Canada – Canadian Academy of Health Sciences Expert Panel.

Carroll, A., Vincent, C., & Flynn, R. J. (2007). Suggestions made by the young people in care for improving their placements. *Ontario Association of Children's Aid Societies Journal, 51*(2), 2–5.

Courtney, M. E., Dworsky, A., Brown, A., Cary, C., Love, K., & Vorhies, V. (2011). *Midwest evaluation of the adult functioning of former foster youth: Outcomes at age 26.* Chapin Hall at the University of Chicago.

Courtney, M. E., Hook, J. L., and Lee, J. S. (2010). *Distinct groups of former foster youth during the transition to adulthood: Implications for policy and practice.* Chapin Hall at the University of Chicago.

Courtney, M. E., Okpych, N. J., Park, K., Harty, J., Feng, H., Torres-García, A., & Sayed, S. (2018). *Findings from the California Youth Transitions to Adulthood Study (CalYOUTH): Conditions of youth at age 21.* Chapin Hall at the University of Chicago.

Dumoulin, A., & Flynn, R. J. (2006). Hope in young people in care: Role of active coping and other predictors. In R. J. Flynn, P. M. Dudding, and J. G. Barber (Eds.), *Promoting Resilience in Child Welfare* (pp. 206–215). University of Ottawa Press.

Fernandez, E., & Delfabbro, P. (2020). Policy and trends in child welfare in Australia and the global context. In E. Fernandez & P. Delfabbro (Eds.), *Child protection and the care continuum* (pp. 3–26). Routledge.

Flynn, R. J., Aubry, T., Drolet, M., and Angus, D. (1999). *Improving child protection practice through the introduction of Looking After Children into local Children's Aid Societies in Ontario: An implementation and outcome evaluation.* (SSHRC Strategic Grant # 828-1999-1008). Centre for Research on Educational and Community Services, University of Ottawa.

Flynn, R. J., Beaulac, J., & Vinograd, J. (2006). Participation in structured voluntary activities, substance use, and psychological outcomes in out-of-home care. In R. J. Flynn, P. M. Dudding, & J. G. Barber (Eds.), *Promoting resilience in child welfare* (pp. 16–230). University of Ottawa Press.

Flynn, R. J., Ghazal, H., Legault, L., Vandermeulen, G., & Petrick, S. (2004). Use of population measures and norms to identify resilient outcomes in young people in care: An exploratory study. *Child and Family Social Work, 9*(1), 65–79. https://doi.org/10.1111/j.1365-2206.2004.00322.x

Flynn, R. J., & Miller, M. (2017). *Review of the reliability and validity of current and potential performance indicators derived from OnLAC for Ontario's children's aid societies.* Centre for Research on Educational and Community Services, University of Ottawa.

Flynn, R. J., Robitaille, A., & Ghazal, H. (2006). Placement satisfaction of young people living in foster or group homes. In R. J. Flynn, P. M. Dudding, and J. G. Barber (Eds.), *Promoting resilience in child welfare* (pp. 191–205). University of Ottawa Press.

Gilligan, R. (2000). Adversity, resilience and young people: The protective value of positive school and spare time activities. *Children and Society, 14*(1), 37–47. https://doi.org/10.1111/j.1099-0860.2000.tb00149.x

Goyette, M., Bellot, C., Blanchet, A., & Silva-Ramirez, R. (2019). *Youth leaving care, residential stability and instability and homelessness.* Étude longitudinale sur le devenir des jeunelacesés. École nationale d'administration publique.

Greeson, J. K. P, Garcia, A. R., Tan, K., Chacon, A., & Ortiz, A. J. (2020). Interventions for youth aging out of foster care: A state of the science review. *Children and Youth Services Review, 113*, 1–11. https://doi.org/10.1016/j.childyouth.2020.105005

Kufeldt, K., Vachon, J., & Simard, M. (2000). *Looking After Children in Canada.* (Final report). University of New Brunswick & Université Laval.

Legault, L., Anawati, M.,& Flynn, R. J. (2006). Factors favoring psychological resilience among fostered young people. *Children and Youth Services Review, 28*(9), 1024–1038. https://doi.org/10.1016/j.childyouth.2005.10.006

Legault, L., Lebel, M., & Flynn, R. J. (2003. *Children in care: Education and protective factors.* (Poster presented at the annual meeting of the Canadian Psychological Association, Hamilton, June).

Legault, L., & Moffat, S. (2006). Positive life experiences that promote resilience in young people in care. In R. J. Flynn, P. M. Dudding, and J. G. Barber (Eds.), *Promoting resilience in child welfare* (pp. 206–215). University of Ottawa Press.

Lerner, R., & Benson, P. (Eds.). (2012). *Developmental assets and asset-building communities: Implications for research, policy, and practice.* Search Institute.

Lou, C., Anthony, E. K., Stone, S., Vu, C. M., & Austin, M. J. (2008). Assessing child and youth well-being: Implications for child welfare practice. *Journal of Evidence-Based Social Work,* 5(1–2), 91–133. https://doi.org/10.1300/J394v05n01_05

Masten, A. S. (2006). Promoting resilience in development: A general framework for systems of care. In R. J. Flynn, P. M. Dudding, and J. G. Barber (Eds.), *Promoting resilience in child welfare* (pp. 3–17). University of Ottawa Press.

Miller, M. (2019). *Ontario Looking After Children (OnLAC) 2018 provincial report.* Centre for Research on Educational and Community Services, University of Ottawa.

Miller, M., Vincent, C., & Flynn, R. J. 2021. *Bibliography of papers, chapters, and conference presentations from the Ontario Looking After Children (OnLAC) Project.* Centre for Research on Educational and Community Services, University of Ottawa.

Montgomery, P., Donkoh, C., & Underhill, K. (2006). Independent living programs for young people leaving the care system. *Children and Youth Services Review,* 28(12), 1435–1448. https://doi.org/10.1016/j.childyouth.2006.03.002

O'Higgins, A., Sebba, J., & Gardner, F. (2017). What are the factors associated with educational achievement for children in kinship or foster care: A systematic review. *Children and Youth Services Review,* 79, 198–220. https://doi.org/10.1016/j.childyouth.2017.06.004

Pantin, S., Flynn, R. J., & Runnels, V. (2006). Training, experience, and supervision: Keys to enhancing the utility of the Assessment and Action Record in implementing Looking After Children. In R. J. Flynn, P. M. Dudding, and J. G. Barber (Eds.), *Promoting resilience in child welfare* (pp. 281–296). University of Ottawa Press.

Parker, R. A., Ward, H., Jackson, S., Aldgate, J., & Wedge, P. (Eds.). (1991). *Looking After Children: Assessing outcomes in child care.* HMSO.

Perkins-Mangulabnan, J., & Flynn, R. J. (2006) Foster parenting practices and foster youth outcomes. In R. J. Flynn, P. M. Dudding, and J. G. Barber (Eds.), *Promoting resilience in child welfare* (pp. 231–247). University of Ottawa Press.

Robitaille, A., Flynn, R. J., & Ghazal, H. (2004). Satisfaction with Out-of-Home Care Placements: Suggestions for improvements from young people in foster or group homes. [Conference paper]. 6th International Looking After Children Conference, Ottawa, Ontario.

Scott, J., & Ward, H. (2005). *Safeguarding and promoting the well-being of children, families and communities.* Jessica Kingsley Publishers.

Snyder, C. R., Hoza, B., Pelham, W. E., Rapoff, M., Ware, L., Danovsky, M., Highberger, L., Ribinstein, H., & Stahl, K. J. (1997). The development and validation of the Children's Hope Scale. *Journal of Pediatric Psychology,* 22(3), 399–421. https://doi.org/10.1093/jpepsy/22.3.399

Statistics Canada & Human Resources Development Canada. (1995). *National Longitudinal Survey of Children and Youth: Overview of survey instruments for 1994-95, data collection cycle 1.*

Tessier, N. G., O'Higgins, A., & Flynn, R. J. (2018). Neglect, educational success, and young people in out-of-home: Cross-sectional and longitudinal analyses. *Child Abuse & Neglect, 75,* 115–129. https://doi.org/10.1016/j.chiabu.2017.06.005

Ward, H. (1998). Using a child development model to assess the outcomes of social work interventions with families. *Children & Society, 12*(3), 202–211. https://doi.org/10.1111/j.1099-0860.1998.tb00067.x

Wilson, C. (2014). *Integrating safety, permanency and well-being: A view from the field.* (Integrating safety, permanency and well-being series, pp. 1–4). Administration for Children and Families, U.S. Department of Health and Human Services.

Chapter 2

Developmental Assets

The theoretical and research foundation of the developmental assets frameworks holds that young people require a range of opportunities and supports that will enable them to experience widely desired outcomes such as greater school success, pro-social behaviour, resilience, and lower levels of risk behaviours (Benson, Scales, & Syvertsen, 2011). Developed at the Search Institute (or SI) in Minneapolis, Minnesota, beginning in 1990, the approach has become one of the most frequently employed and cited perspectives for conceptualizing and promoting positive youth development (PYD), in fields such as education, social work, community psychology, youth development, prevention, or counselling. According to Benson et al. (2011), within two decades, developmental assets became a very influential PYD framework. By 2010, citations to developmental assets/SI had already numbered 12,567 in Google Scholar, Academic Search Premier, and PsycInfo, far more than to other PYD models, including Communities That Care/social development (2,282 citations), the Five Promises (149), or the Five Cs (97). Today, the developmental assets framework is now a foundation of program development and implementation in national organizations such as the Y USA, Y Canada, Boys and Girls Clubs, The Salvation Army, and others. By 2010, over 300,000 leaders had been trained in the assets perspective, and some 10,000 schools and youth programs were using Search Institute books and other resources (Benson et al., 2011).

Development assets are internal or external resources that contribute to a child or young person's ability to thrive and have been linked in research to protective factors that mitigate risk and promote positive outcomes and resilience (Benson, 2002; Sesma Jr., Mannes, & Scales, 2013; Scales et al., 2006a). The 20 *external* assets are environmental actions or factors that promote positive development. They are reinforced through positive interactions with a range of individuals with whom children and young people interact, including parents, caregivers, teachers, neighbours, and others in the community (VanderVen, 2008). The external assets are divided into four categories: support, empowerment, boundaries and expectations, and constructive use of time (Benson et al., 2011). *Support* includes a range of contexts through which a child or young person may experience affirmation, approval, and acceptance, and comprises six specific assets: caregiver support, positive communication, other adult relationships, caring neighbourhood, caring school environment, and caregiver involvement. *Empowerment* subsumes assets or resources that lead to a child or young person's participation in the community: community values youth, youth as resources, service to others, and safety. *Boundaries and expectations* underline the importance of consistent messages across contexts and the presence of positive role models and includes the assets of caregiver boundaries, school boundaries, neighbourhood boundaries, adult role models, positive peer observations, and high expectations. Finally, *constructive use of time* includes assets that provide important opportunities to children and young people, namely creative activities, youth programs, religious or spiritual community, and time at home.

The 20 *internal* assets represent psychological and developmental capacities that develop over time. They are also divided into four categories: commitment to learning, positive values, social competencies, and positive identity. *Commitment to learning,* comprising personal beliefs, values, and skills, includes the assets of achievement motivation, school engagement, homework, bonding to school, and reading for pleasure, all linked with better academic performance. *Positive values* consist of prosocial ideals and personal character and encompass the assets of caring, equality and social justice, integrity, honesty, responsibility, and self-regulation. *Social competencies* enable a young person to face a variety of challenges and choices in a complex society and include the assets of planning and decision-making, interpersonal competence, cultural competence, resistance skills, and peaceful conflict resolution. Finally, *positive identity development* is a crucial component of desirable adolescent development and comprises the assets of personal power, self-esteem, sense of purpose, and a positive view of one's personal future (Benson, 2002; Mannes, Roehlkepartain, & Benson, 2005; VanderVen, 2008).

Originally, the developmental assets framework consisted of 30 assets (Benson, 1990), which were based on empirical research described in reports that drew on data gathered in 460 school districts (Leffert et al., 1998). Expanded to 40 assets in 1996, the framework also adopted a broader lifespan perspective, to include infancy, childhood, and young adulthood (Benson et al., 2011). In 1998, Scales and Leffert published a review and synthesis of the findings from more than 1,200 articles and reports from many fields of child and adolescent development. They linked these research results with each of the 40 developmental assets and the 8 asset categories. Leffert et al. (1998) concluded that at that period, there was already much empirical research that supported the conceptualization of 4 of the 8 asset categories (support, boundaries and expectations, constructive use of time, and commitment to learning), a moderate amount of research grounding the social competencies and positive identity categories, but only a smaller body of research on the empowerment and positive values categories.

The adoption of the developmental assets framework in many communities and organizations in the United States and, increasingly, in other countries, enabled a good deal of empirical research work of a measurement and validation nature to be carried out, often with very large samples. Theokas et al. (2005), for example, employed a sample of 229,596 young people in grades 6–12 from across the United States to study the first-order and second-order factor structure of the 92 developmental assets items used by the Search Institute to assess the 40 developmental assets. These items were part of a larger instrument of 156 items, the Profiles of Student Life: Attitudes and Behavior Scale (PSL-AB; Leffert et al., 1998), with which the Search Institute assessed a range of other PYD outcomes, including aspects of thriving.

The factor analyses by Theokas et al. (2005), including cross-validation on large sub-samples, yielded 14 interpretable and interrelated first-order factors. A second-order factor analysis, in turn, yielded two correlated factors ($r = .64$), individual assets and ecological assets (corresponding to the two dimensions usually referred to as internal and external assets). Both second-order factors contributed significantly to the prediction of a composite thriving index. Of theoretical and practical interest was the finding that, in accord with the hypothesized cumulative nature of assets, young people with a relatively high number of assets in either the individual or the ecological domain were found to have a higher degree of thriving behaviour. Those with a high number of assets in both domains had the highest level of thriving, and those with a low number of assets in both domains had the lowest level of thriving. No doubt because of the cumulative nature of assets and the substantial correlation between the two second-order asset dimensions, much of the Search Institute's published research uses the total number of assets (out of 40) to predict outcomes rather than the number of internal or external assets separately (out of 20). Benson et al. (2011), for example, found that young people in grades 4–12 who were asset-rich (i.e., had 31–40 assets), compared with those who were, respectively, above average (21–30 assets), average (11–20 assets), or asset poor (0–10 assets), had a stepwise advantage in terms of outcomes. Thus, in relation to problematic alcohol use, the asset-rich young people, compared with the above-average, average, and asset-poor young people, respectively, had a stepwise advantage in the relative size of their positive effects (Cohen's ds): .29, .56, and 1.0. Similarly, on the outcome of not engaging in violence, the asset-rich young people had effect sizes that were .31, .69, and 1.31 larger than the outcomes of the three other asset groups. Regarding the obtaining of high grades in school, the asset-rich youths had effect sizes that were .43, .95, and 1.70 larger and, in relation to the outcome of feeling physically healthy, they experienced effect sizes that were .43, 1.17, and 1.49 larger. Similarly, Scales et al. (2000) reported similar stepwise differences among younger students, in grades 4–6, on a wide range of indicators of the outcome of thriving. The greater the number of assets, the more positive were the outcomes: obtaining high grades, helping others, valuing diversity, delaying gratification, sharing in self-regulation with parents, displaying coping skills, and experiencing life satisfaction.

Other cross-sectional research in the general population has similarly suggested the cumulative nature of assets. Assets have been found to combine to promote receptive and expressive language development in preschool children (Weigel, Lowman, & Martin, 2007) and leadership abilities, prosocial behaviour, delayed gratification, affirmation of diversity, and academic achievement in adolescents (Benson, 2002; Scales, Benson, & Mannes, 2006a; Scales et al., 2006b; Scales & Taccogna, 2000; Theokas & Lerner, 2006). A greater number of developmental assets has been associated with more positive developmental trajectories among gang members (Taylor et al., 2002), nonuse of drugs and alcohol (Oman et al., 2004), thriving behaviours (Scales et al., 2000), and a lower risk of engaging in violence (Aspy et al., 2004) or early sexual activity (Doss et al., 2006; Harris et al., 2006; Vesely et al., 2004). In a community sample of 95,396 young people in grades 6 to 12, a greater number of internal assets was associated with a more positive identity (as indicated by a greater sense of purpose and personal power, higher self-esteem, and a more positive view of the future) and, among girls, was also a protective factor vis-à-vis unhealthy eating behaviour (French et al., 2001).

There have been relatively few longitudinal studies of increases in assets or the relationship of assets with subsequent outcomes. In one such study, Scales et al. (2006b) investigated whether developmental assets were related to higher grade point averages (GPAs) over time. A sample of 370 students was followed from 1998, when they were in grades 7–9, to 2001, when they were in grades 10–12. The greater the number of assets that students reported in 1998, the higher their actual GPA was in 2001. Furthermore, those who had remained stable or had increased their assets by at least 0.5 standard deviations (SDs) between 1998 and 2001 had significantly higher mean GPAs in 2001, compared with students who had declined at least 0.5 SDs in their number of assets.

In an international project conducted between 2006 and 2010, Scales et al. (2013) studied the health, education, economic opportunity, and social well-being of adolescent girls living in rural Bangladesh villages. Villages with at least 40 adolescent girls, who were 10–19 years of age, were invited to participate. Two cohorts of villages, assessed in 2009 and 2010, were randomly assigned to intervention or control conditions. The intervention was comprised of an intensive peer-education program involving two-hour sessions five or six days a week for a six-month period. The Developmental Assets Profile was completed on the first and last days of the intervention. In the combined cohorts, there was a mean asset improvement of 22%, net of contamination and control group effects, and a large mean net effect size of 0.80. This research supported the feasibility of using the developmental assets framework validly in a culture very different from that of the United States, and also with a randomized study design. The research also suggested that a peer-education intervention could be used to increase developmental assets.

1. Research on Developmental Assets in the Ontario Looking After Children Project

1.1. The OnLAC Measure of Developmental Assets

The measure of developmental assets used in the OnLAC Project is different from the two instruments used by the Search Institute (SI). The more frequently used of the two main SI tools is the *Attitudes and Behaviors Profile of Student Life* (A & B) survey (Benson et al., 2011), consisting of 160 self-report items and used in more than 80% of the asset surveys conducted by the Search Institute, according to Benson et al. (2011). The tool includes 92 items that measure the 40 individual assets, with the other items assessing a range of risk-taking and positive behaviours. The second, shorter SI measure is the 58-item *Developmental Assets Profile* (Search Institute, 2005; Benson et al., 2011), which measures the 8 developmental asset *categories* (mentioned earlier) but not the 40 individual assets.

In incorporating a measure of assets into the OnLAC Assessment and Action Record (AAR), we wanted an instrument that would assess the 40 individual assets (which could thus serve as specific intervention targets), would be relatively brief, and would make the child welfare worker the source of the ratings rather than the young person or the caregiver. We chose the simple expedient of adopting the well-known 40-item Search Institute form that lists each of the assets. For each asset, we asked the child welfare worker to rate whether the young person possessed the asset in question ("yes," "uncertain," or "no"), with "yes" to be answered only if the worker was absolutely certain that the young person truly possessed the asset. The total developmental assets score is thus the number of "yes" responses (out of 40), as are the internal and external assets scores (each out of 20).

The 40-item total Developmental Asset Profiles for the various age groups of young people in care, whom we assess each year with the AAR, have shown acceptable to excellent internal consistency coefficients (alphas), in the .70s, .80s and .90s. The shorter 20-item external and internal assets scales for the different age groups have also displayed internal consistencies in the acceptable to excellent range, in the .60s, .70s, .80s, and .90s (see Miller et al., 2017). Also, like the Search Institute asset measures, our AAR version has proven to be a very good and consistent predictor of positive outcomes. In addition, as we will show here, we find that with our AAR assets measure, as with those of the Search Institute, developmental assets have a cumulative impact on outcomes, older youths typically have fewer assets than those who are younger, and girls usually have more assets than boys.

1.2. Prevalence of Developmental Assets among Young People in Care

Based on data gathered between 2010 and 2011 and between 2014 and 2015 in the OnLAC Project, the mean number of total developmental assets was examined for three age groups: 0–4, 5–11, and 12–17 (Figure 2.1). These age groups capture developmentally specific periods, namely, preschool, elementary school, and high school. The cross-sectional results displayed an inverse relationship with age, with 12-to-17-year-olds reporting the lowest mean number of assets. To investigate this further, the total developmental assets score for each age group was divided into three categories: young people with 0–20 assets formed the *Low-Assets* category, those with 21–30 assets the *Medium-Assets* category, and those with 31–40 assets the *High-Assets* category. Interestingly, the majority of children 0–4 (94.8%) and 5–11 (76.9%) years of age fell into the high assets category, whereas young people aged 12–17 were more evenly distributed across the low, medium, and high-asset categories (Figure 2.2).

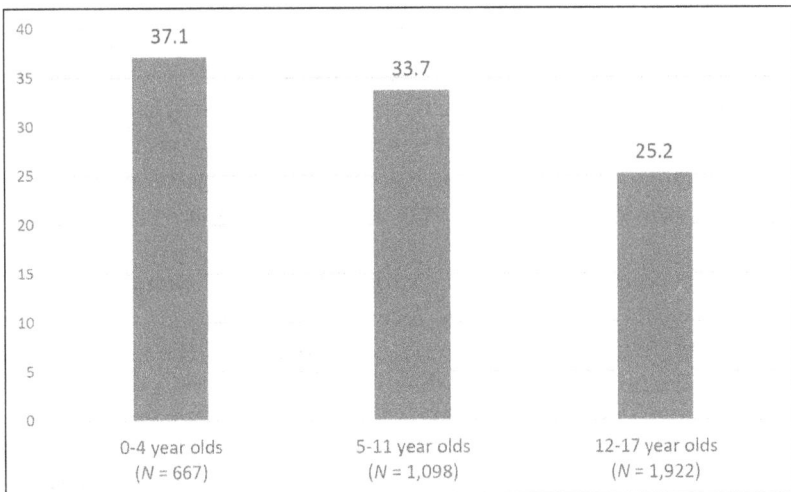

Figure 2.1. Average total developmental assets by age group.

Source: Ontario Looking After Children Project data.

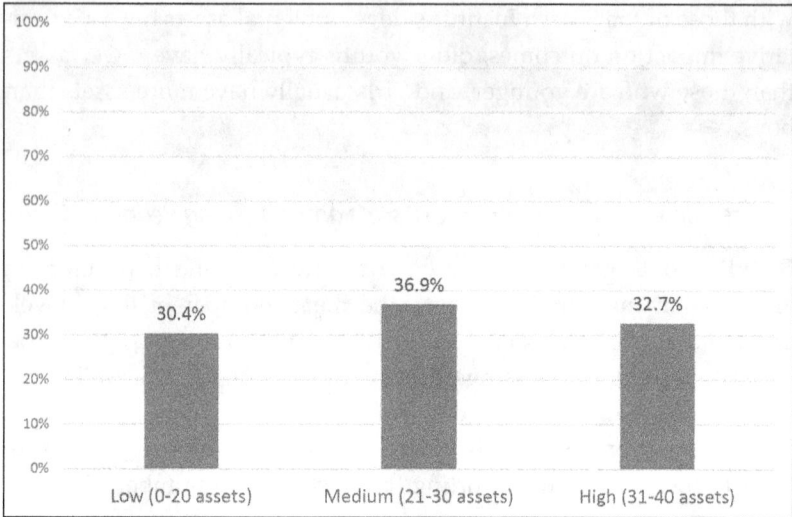

Figure 2.2. Low, medium, and high developmental assets for
12-to-17-year-olds (*N* = 1,922).
Source: Ontario Looking After Children Project data.

When internal and external assets were examined separately, we
found the same cross-sectional relationship with age, in which older
children or youth had, on average, fewer developmental assets. Those
aged 0–4 were rated by their caregivers as having an average of 18.1
external and 19.5 internal assets (out of 20); those aged 5–11 had a
mean of 16.7 external and 17.4 internal assets; and those aged 12–17
had a mean of 13.1 external and 12.2 internal assets. This effect, seen in
both OnLAC samples of young people in care and in SI samples from
the general population, is likely due partly to older youths' exposure
to riskier environments and their greater propensity to take risks, as
well as to caregivers' more benign assessments of assets in younger
children.

Given the relative lack of variability in assets among the 0–4
and 5–11 years age groups, the focus, in this chapter, will be on the
young people in care who were 12–17 years of age. The internal consistency (Cronbach's alpha) of the total developmental assets scale in
this group was .93 (excellent). We examined the relationship between
low, medium, and high assets and several outcomes, placement satisfaction, educational success, and total difficulties (Figure 2.3). Higher
scores indicated higher levels of the construct in question. The placement satisfaction scale (alpha = .89), answered by the youth, comprised

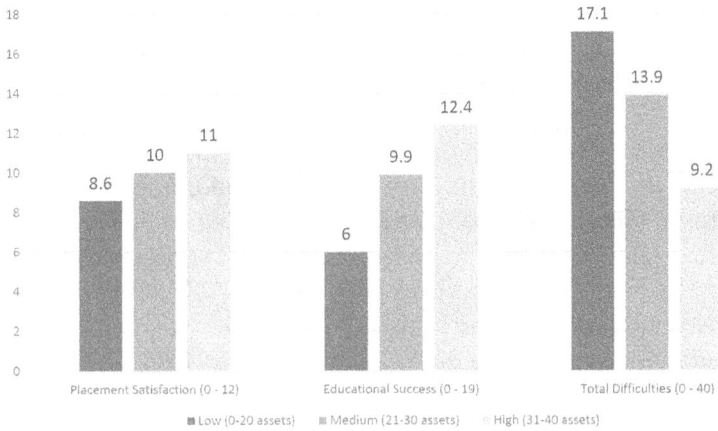

Figure 2.3. Low, medium, and high developmental assets and average scores on placement satisfaction, educational success, and total difficulties for 12-to-17-year-olds (*N* = 1,922).

Source: Ontario Looking After Children Project data.

six items, with total scores ranging from 0 to 12. The educational success scale (alpha = .83), answered by the youth, caregiver, and child welfare worker, included eight items assessing how the young person was doing in school, with total scores ranging from 0 to 19. The total difficulties scale (alpha = .86), answered by the young person's caregiver, included 20 items assessing the young person's emotional and behavioural difficulties, with total scores ranging from 0 to 40.

The findings showed that young people in the high-assets category experienced greater placement satisfaction, greater educational success, and fewer behavioural difficulties than those in the medium-assets and low-assets groups. As already noted, this OnLAC result agrees well with the Search Institute's hypothesis that developmental assets are cumulative in nature, such that young people who possess a greater number of developmental assets also enjoy better outcomes in multiple domains of functioning.

1.3. Outcomes Associated with Developmental Assets among Young People in Care

The OnLAC Project has been one of the first to show that among young people in out-of-home care, developmental assets predict more positive outcomes in the behavioural and emotional (Bell et al., 2013;

Cheung et al., 2011) and educational domains (Romano et al., 2014). An important conclusion from our OnLAC research has been that assets provide critical support that buffers and reduces the negative effects of early adversity. Bell et al. (2013) found, for example, that a greater number of internal assets predicted a lower frequency of conduct problems in a sample of 531 Canadian children, aged 5–9, living in foster family or kinship care placements. This finding remained significant after controlling for several child-level variables (e.g., sex, age, and maltreatment exposure), family-level variables (e.g., caregiver parenting practices and household size), and worker-level variables (e.g., education, years of experience, and caseload). This result indicated that developmental assets have a robust ability to predict well-being. Furthermore, internal assets had a statistically significant negative correlation with emotional problems, while both internal and external assets had significant positive correlations with prosocial behaviour and academic performance (Bell et al., 2013).

Flynn et al. (2013) found in an OnLAC sample of 1,106 young people, aged 12–17, residing in out-of-home care that a greater number of internal developmental assets was associated with higher average marks, after controlling for the young person's demographics (i.e., sex, age, and placement type) and several risk factors (i.e., repeated a grade, cognitive impairments, and total behavioural difficulties). These findings remained significant in both cross-sectional and longitudinal analyses. Other significant predictors of educational success included female sex and fewer behavioural difficulties. Filbert and Flynn (2010), Flynn et al. (2012), and Flynn and Tessier (2011) used the total number of developmental assets with OnLAC samples. These studies suggested that, with young people in out-of-home care, as in the Search Institute research in the general population, the total number of developmental assets is associated with greater prosocial behaviour and self-esteem, fewer behavioural difficulties, higher school grades, educational aspirations, and academic achievement. On the reasonable theory-based assumption that at least some of this consistent association is likely to be causal in nature, developmental assets provide an important source of leverage for intervening to improve resilience among young people in care, with broad implications for further child welfare research, policy, and practice.

1.4. Trajectories of Developmental Assets over Time

Besides examining developmental assets cross-sectionally (i.e., in participants assessed on a single occasion, at the same time point), we also conducted longitudinal analyses to investigate asset trajectories over a 5-year period. We used OnLAC data from 2010–2011 to 2014–2015 to investigate changes in the total number of developmental assets possessed by a sample of 1,031 young people in care. They were 12–13 years of age at time 1, in 2010–2011, and 16–17 five years later in 2014–2015. Over half were boys (58.1%), and most (75.1%) in 2010–2011 were living in foster family homes. They had been admitted to care for one or more reasons: neglect (70.1%), emotional harm (39.1%), physical harm (29%), domestic violence (24.1%), problematic behaviour (14.9%), abandonment/separation (14.8%), and sexual harm (8.8%).

Developmental assets were modelled across the 5-year period using growth mixture modeling (GMM) in Mplus 7 (Muthén & Muthén, 2012). This method identifies classes of individuals who follow a similar developmental pathway on an outcome of interest, which here was the young people's total number of assets. Multiple models are tested to determine the best number of classes to fit the data. In the current analyses, we tested 1-class to 4-class models. There are several statistical indices used to establish the best fitting model, including the Bayesian Information Criterion (BIC) and the Lo, Mendell, and Rubin likelihood ratio test (LMR-LRT; Geiser, 2013; Jung & Wickrama, 2008; Ram & Grimm, 2009; see Appendix Table A).

The best number of classes is determined by a combination of factors, including the statistical indices, the research question, one's theoretical understanding of the research topic, and the interpretability of the findings (Jung & Wickrama, 2008). Given these considerations, the best-fitting model for our sample was a 4-class model (Figure 2.4).

The *High, stable* group comprised 68.7% (*n* = 708) of the sample. These young people exhibited a consistently high number of developmental assets over the 5-year period. The *Descending* group included 10.6% (*n* = 109) of the sample and exhibited a consistent decrease in the number of developmental assets over the 5-year period. The *Ascending* group included the fewest number of young people, 7.0% (*n* = 72) of the sample, and exhibited a consistent increase in the number of developmental assets over the 5-year period. Finally, the *Low-moderate, stable* group, 13.8% (*n* = 142) of the sample, exhibited in a

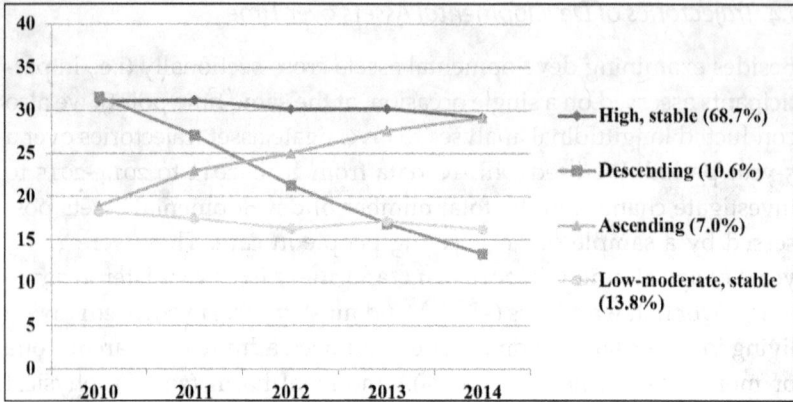

Figure 2.4. Total developmental asset classes from 2010 to 2014.
Source: Ontario Looking After Children Project data.

stable fashion the fewest number of developmental assets over the 5-year period. To know which variables (e.g., sex, age at first place-ment) might characterize membership in each of the identified classes, we conducted bivariate analyses to examine the frequency of each of these variables, by class (Table 2.1).

Regarding class membership, there were no significant differ-ences between boys and girls, in the number of placements, or in adverse life experiences. However, we did find a statistically signifi-cant difference by age at first placement: young people in the *High, stable* assets class were significantly younger at their first placement in comparison with those in the *Descending* assets class. This suggests that a greater length of time in care may lead to greater stability, and, in turn, to an increase in developmental assets. Similarly, the length of the current placement was statistically significant, such that those in the *High, stable* assets class had been living with their current caregiv-ers for a significantly longer period of time in comparison with those in the *Ascending* and *Low-moderate, stable* classes. Furthermore, we also found significant differences by placement type. In 2010–2011, in the *High, stable* assets class, there were *more* young people in foster family and kinship home placements and *fewer* in group-home placements than would be expected. There were also *fewer* than expected in foster family and kinship homes and *more* in group homes than would be predicted in the *Low-moderate, stable class*. This finding indicates that family-based placements (i.e., foster family and kinship homes) may contribute to a greater number of developmental assets, with young

Table 2.1. Bivariate associations between variables
and developmental asset classes (N = 1,031)

Correlates	Developmental asset classes				F	χ^2
	Low-moderate, stable %	Ascending %	Descending %	High, stable %		
Sex						6.40
Boys	66.9	58.3	61.5	55.9		
Girls	33.1	41.7	38.5	44.1		
Age at first placement[a]	6.53	6.05	6.82	5.83	3.19*	
Current placement length (years)[a]	3.01	2.82	3.78	4.08	6.15***	
Number of placements[a]	5.13	5.48	5.68	4.99	1.46	
Placement type						61.82***
Foster family	62.7	75.0	74.3	78.0		
Kinship	4.2	6.9	11.0	12.6		
Group home	33.1	18.1	14.7	9.4		
Adverse life experiences[a]	1.56	1.32	1.36	1.17	1.55	

Note. An analysis of variance (ANOVA) was conducted for continuous variables while a chi-square analysis was used for dichotomous and categorical variables.
[a] Mean scores
* $p < .05$ ** $p < .01$ *** $p < .001$
Source: Ontario Looking After Children Project data.

people in these placements experiencing greater caregiver stability and, in turn, more opportunities to develop a support network. (See also chapter 8 for differences in well-being between types of placements that mirror the present findings.)

While our longitudinal findings provide insight into these classes of young people in out-of-home care, it is important to note that additional factors outside the scope of our analysis may also have had an impact on the number of developmental assets, such as the foster family home environment or relationships among family members. One way to address this in future research would be through application of the Search Institute's more recent developmental relationships framework (Roehlkepartain et al., 2017). Building upon the developmental assets model, the developmental relationships framework focuses on the young person's key relationships, encompassing five key elements: express care, challenge growth, provide support, share power, and expand possibilities. These elements, in turn, are expressed through 20 actions, such as listen, encourage, and inspire. Assessing young people's developmental relationships in child welfare would no doubt also provide additional insight into their internal and external developmental assets, given that connections are so crucial for the well-being and thriving of young people, including those in out-of-home care (Search Institute, 2017).

2. Practical Implications

Our findings have several implications for child welfare practice. The developmental assets that a young person has are important to view as an ongoing process, in light of our longitudinal analyses that showed that assets are not necessarily stable over time. One way to encourage the continuing growth of assets would be to target specific assets as part of a child or young person's annual plan of care. This may be accomplished through involvement in extracurricular activities or other opportunities to succeed within the home or school. Moreover, our findings indicate that ensuring stability for children and young people living in out-of-home care is of paramount importance. Such findings are in line with previous research and support the international responsibility of child welfare systems to ensure the safety, permanency, and well-being of children and young people in their care. For practice, this would suggest a continued focus on family-based placements (e.g., foster family and kinship homes) and keeping placement disruptions to a minimum.

References

Aspy, C. B., Oman, R. F., Vesely, S. K., McLeroy, K., Rodine, S., & Marshall, L. (2004). Adolescent violence: The protective effects of youth assets. *Journal of Counseling & Development, 82*(3), 268–276. https://doi.org/10.1002/j.1556-6678.2004.tb00310.x

Bell, T., Romano, E., & Flynn, R. J. (2013). Multilevel correlates of behavioural resilience among children in child welfare. *Child Abuse & Neglect, 37*(11), 1007–1020. https://doi.org/10.1016/j.chiabu.2013.07.005

Benson, P. L. (1990). *The troubled journey: A portrait of 6th-12th grade youth.* Search Institute.

Benson, P. L. (2002). Adolescent development in social and community context: A program of research. *New Directions for Youth Development, 95,* 123–148. https://doi.org/10.1002/yd.19

Benson, P. L., Scales, P. C., & Syvertsen. (2011). The contribution of the developmental assets framework to positive youth development theory and practice. *Advances in Child Development and Behavior*, 41, 197–230. https://doi.org/10.1016/B978-0-12-386492-5.00008-7

Cheung, C., Goodman, D., Leckie, G., & Jenkins, J. (2011). Understanding contextual effects on externalizing behaviours in children in out-of-home care: Influence of workers and foster families. *Children and Youth Services Review*, 33(10), 2050–2060. https://doi.org/10.1016/j.childyouth.2011.05.036

Doss, J. R., Vesely, S. K., Oman, R. F., Aspy, C. B., Tolma, E., Rodine, S., & Marshall, L. (2006). A matched case-control study: Investigating the relationship between youth assets and sexual intercourse among 13- to 14-year-olds. *Child: Care, Health and Development*, 33(1), 40–44. https://doi.org/10.1111/j.1365-2214.2006.00639.x

Filbert, K. M., & Flynn, R. J. (2010). Developmental and cultural assets and resilient outcomes in First Nations young people in care: An initial test of an exploratory model. *Children and Youth Services Review*, 32(4), 560–564. https://doi.org/10.1016/j.childyouth.2009.12.002

Flynn, R. J., & Tessier, N. G. (2011). Promotive and risk factors as concurrent predictors of educational outcomes in supported transitional living: Extended care and maintenance in Ontario, Canada. *Children and Youth Services Review*, 33(12), 2498–2503. https://doi.org/10.1016/j.childyouth.2011.08.014

Flynn, R. J., Tessier, N. G., & Coulombe, D. (2013). Placement, protective and risk factors in the educational success of young people in care: Cross-sectional and longitudinal analyses. *European Journal of Social Work*, 16(1), 70–87. https://doi.org/10.1080/13691457.2012.722985

French, S. A., Leffert, N., Story, M., Neumark-Sztainer, D., Hannan, P., & Benson, P. L. (2001). Adolescent binge/purge and weight loss behaviours: Associations with developmental assets. *Journal of Adolescent Health*, 28(3), 211–221. https://doi.org/10.1016/S1054-139X(00)00166-X

Geiser, C. (2012). *Data analysis with Mplus*. Guilford Press.

Harris, L., Oman, R. F., Vesely, S. K., Tolma, E. L., Aspy, C. B., Rodine, S., Marshall, L., & Fluhr, J. (2006). Associations between youth assets and sexual activity: Does adult supervision play a role? *Child: Care, Health and Development*, 33(4), 448–454. https://doi.org/10.1111/j.1365-2214.2006.00695.x

Jung, T., & Wickrama, K. A. S. (2008). An introduction to latent class growth analysis and growth mixture modeling. *Social and Personality Psychology Compass*, 2(1), 302–317. https://doi.org/10.1111/j.1751-9004.2007.00054.x

Leffert, N., Benson, P. L., Scales, P. C., Sharma, A. R., Drake, D. R., & Blyth, D. A. (1998). Developmental assets: Measurement and prediction of risk behaviors among adolescents. *Applied Developmental Science*, 2(4), 209–230. https://doi.org/10.1207/s1532480xads0204_4

Mannes, M., Roehlkepartain, E. C., & Benson, P. L. (2005). Unleashing the power of community to strengthen the well-being of children, youth, and families: An asset-building approach. *Child Welfare*, 84(2), 233–250.

Miller, M., Vincent, C., & Flynn R. (2017). *User's manual for the AAR-C2-2016.* Centre for Research on Educational and Community Services, University of Ottawa.

Muthén, L. K. & Muthén, B. O. (1998–2012). *Mplus user's guide.* (7th ed.) Muthén and Muthén.

Oman, R. F., Vesely, S., Aspy, C. B., McLeroy, K. R., Rodine, S., & Marshall, L. (2004). The potential protective effect of youth assets on adolescent alcohol and drug use. *American Journal of Public Health*, 94(8), 1425–1430. https://doi.org/10.2105/AJPH.94.8.1425

Ram, N., & Grimm, K. J. (2009). Growth mixture modeling: A method for identifying differences in longitudinal change among unobserved groups. *International Journal of Behavioural Development*, 33(6), 565–576. https://doi.org/10.1177/0165025409343765

Roehlkepartain, E., Pekel, K., Syvertsen, A., Sethi, J., Sullivan, T., & Scales, P. (2017). *Relationships first: Creating connections that help young people thrive.* Search Institute.

Romano, E., Babchishin, L., Marquis, R., & Fréchette, S. (2014). Childhood maltreatment and educational outcomes. *Trauma, Violence, and Abuse*, 16(4), 418–437. https://doi.org/10.1177/1524838014537908

Scales, P. C., Benson, P. L., Fraher, K., Syvertsen, A. K., Dershem, L., Fraher, K., Makonnen, R., Nazneen, S., Syvertsen, A. K., & Titus, S. (2013). Building developmental assets to empower adolescent girls in rural Bangladesh: Evaluation of project *Kishoree Kontha. Journal of Research on Adolescence*, 23(1), 171–184. https://doi.org/10.1111/j.1532-7795.2012.00805.x

Scales, P. C., Benson, P. L., Leffert, N., & Blyth, D. A. (2000). Contribution of developmental assets to the prediction of thriving among adolescents. *Applied Developmental Science*, 4(1), 27–46. https://doi.org/10.1207/S1532480XADS0401_3

Scales, P. C., Benson, P. L., & Mannes, M. (2006a). The contribution to adolescent well-being made by nonfamily adults: An examination of developmental assets as contexts and processes. *Journal of Community Psychology*, 34(4), 401–413. https://doi.org/10.1002/jcop.20106

Scales, P. C., Benson, P. L., Roehlkepartain, E. C., Sesma Jr., A., & van Dulmen, M. (2006b). The role of developmental assets in predicting academic achievement: A longitudinal study. *Journal of Adolescence*, 29(5), 691–708. https://doi.org/10.1016/jadolescence.2005. 09.001

Scales, P. C., & Leffert, N. (1998). *Developmental assets: A synthesis of the scientific research on adolescent development.* Search Institute.

Scales, P. C., & Taccogna, J. (2000). Caring to try: How building students' developmental assets can promote school engagement and success. *NASSP Bulletin*, 84(619), 69–78. https://doi.org/10.1177/019263650008461908

Search Institute. (2005). *Developmental Assets Profile: User manual.* Search Institute.

Sesma Jr., A., Mannes, M., & Scales, P. C. (2013). Positive adaptation, resilience, and the developmental asset framework. In S. Goldstein and R. Brooks (Eds.), *Handbook of Resilience in Children* (pp. 427–442). Springer. https://doi.org/10.1007/978-1-4614-3661-4_25

Taylor, C. S., Lerner, R. M., von Eye, A., Balsano, A. B., Dowling, E. M., Anderson, P. M., Bobek, D. L., & Bjelobrk, D. (2002). Individual and ecological assets and positive developmental trajectories among gang and community-based organization youth. *New Directions for Youth Development, 95,* 57–72. https://doi.org/10.1002/yd.16

Theokas, C., Almerigi, J. B., Lerner, R. M., Dowling, E. M., Benson, P. L., Scales, P. C., & von Eye, A. (2005). Conceptualizing and modeling individual and ecological asset components of thriving in early adolescence. *Journal of Early Adolescence, 25*(1), 113–143. https://doi.org/10.1177/0272431604272460

Theokas, C., & Lerner, R. M. (2006). Observed ecological assets in families, schools, and neighborhoods: Conceptualization, measurement, and relations with positive and negative developmental outcomes. *Applied Developmental Science, 10*(2), 61–74. https://doi.org/10.1207/s1532480xads1002_2

VanderVen, K. (2008). *Promoting positive development in early childhood.* Springer.

Vesely, S. K., Wyatt, V. H., Oman, R. F., Aspy, C. B., Kegler, M. C., Rodine, S., Marshall, L., & McLeroy, K. R. (2004). The potential protective effects of youth assets from adolescent sexual risk behaviours. *Journal of Adolescent Health, 34*(5), 356–365. https://doi.org/10.1016/j.jadohealth.2003.08.008

Weigel, D. J., Lowman, J. L., & Martin, S. S. (2007). Language development in the years before school: A comparison of developmental assets in home and child care settings. *Early Child Development and Care, 177*(6 & 7), 719–734. https://doi.org/10.1080/03004430701379173

Health Conditions, Substance Use, and Psychotropic Medications among Children and Young People in Care in Ontario, by Indigenous or non-Indigenous Background, Sex, and Age

Health during childhood and adolescence is foundational for lifelong health and well-being (Ontario Government Annual Report, 2016). Research, both Canadian (Rothwell et al., 2015; Boivin & Hertzman, 2012) and international (Mensah et al., 2019; Björkenstam et al., 2013), indicates that adverse childhood experiences can have long-term negative consequences for health and social outcomes. Young people in out-of-home care often experience greater acute and chronic health problems, including those undiagnosed and untreated, than their age peers in the general population (Vinnerljung, 2014; Martin et al., 2014; Fortin, 2011). Between 45% and 87% of American children in care have at least one chronic illness, which, in combination with other health issues, may jeopardize their placement stability. Woods et al. (2013), for example, found that young people with a chronic illness had significantly greater internalizing and externalizing difficulties and more delinquent acts, with depression a significant mediator of the effects of health on delinquency. The stress of placement instability, in turn, poses a greater risk of poor physical or psychological development (Kools et al., 2013), low educational achievement, low self-esteem, homelessness, substance use, and social network disruption in young people in the child welfare system (Cullen, 2020; Courtney et al., 2005; Pecora et al., 2005; Perry, 2006).

Studies have generally found that physical and mental health issues can increase and often worsen with short lengths of stay and number of placements (Hébert et al., 2018; Villodas et al., 2016; Maliszewski & Brown, 2014; Newton, Litrownik, & Landsverk, 2000), such that children and young people with health problems are more likely to experience placement instability (Woods et al., 2012), which, in turn, jeopardizes the consistent medical and mental health care that would mitigate the effects of abuse and neglect as well as the detection of new medical issues (Hébert & MacDonald, 2009). While research has established the bidirectional relationship between placement disruptions and elevated physical and mental health issues, Villodas et al. (2016, p. 77) have noted that "the mechanisms that link these disruptions to youth's physical and mental health have not been previously investigated." Their findings suggested that, in addition to the adversity and trauma experienced by children and young people prior to entry into the child welfare system, the traumatic stress induced by unstable placements and repeated separation from caregivers that disrupted caregiver–youth attachments contributed to further adverse childhood experiences (ACE) and cumulative posttraumatic stress (PTS) reactions. Villodas and colleagues noted the importance of long-term permanency planning, and recommended trauma-focused assessments and intervention strategies in addressing the needs of the child welfare population.

Epidemiological and neuroscience studies have determined that early adversity, whether from poverty, abuse, neglect, maltreatment, chronic stress, or family dysfunction, may significantly impair early childhood development, with cumulative and lasting effects on adult physical and mental health (Boivin & Hertzman, 2012; Afifi et al., 2016). Additionally, children from low-socioeconomic-status (SES) families have more frequent difficulties in language processing, executive function, selective attention, filtering out distractions, and emotion regulation (Boivin & Hertzman, 2012). Moreover, epigenetic studies have shown that early experiences may affect gene expression and brain development (Rothwell et al., 2015), with environmental factors interacting with the development of neurological and biological systems to influence genetic characteristics (Boivin & Hertzman, 2012).

The Indigenous population (First Nations, Métis, and Inuit) in Canada has been found to be especially vulnerable to chronic health concerns, physical disabilities, and mental health and behavioural issues. These negative health outcomes are associated with social determinants of health, such as inequality, poverty, racism, or colonialism (Nelson & Wilson, 2017; Di Pietro & Illes, 2014; Tait, Henry, &

Loewen-Walker, 2013). Research has found a robust correlation between ineffective government policies, elevated rates of Indigenous children in out-of-home care, and "the vast and generational effects of resulting poor health and social outcomes for these children" (Tait et al., 2013, p. 50). Health disparities between Indigenous and non-Indigenous people in Canada have been linked to cultural discontinuity and socioeconomic and environmental factors, such that Indigenous children "represent the poorest and most vulnerable population in this country" (Di Pietro & Illes, 2014, p. 74).

On most measures of child health and well-being, Indigenous children rank well below Canadian national averages. It is thus imperative that research on health and well-being pay particular attention to Indigenous young people in care, as they face the "double jeopardy" of being Indigenous and in care. In 2019, the Canadian government passed into law Bill C-92, An Act Respecting First Nations, Inuit and Métis Children, Youth and Families. C-92 recognizes the right of Indigenous Peoples to exercise jurisdiction over Indigenous child welfare services, marking the first time that the federal government has used its power to legislate in the domain of Indigenous child welfare (Yellowhead Institute, 2019). C-92 thus represents an important opportunity to improve the health and well-being of Indigenous young people in care across Canada. Researchers at the Yellowhead Institute identified five areas in which the interpretation of the new law by judicial bodies and decision-makers will be crucial. First, it will be essential that the new national standards be interpreted in a way that is genuinely consistent with the best interests of the Indigenous young person. That is, not merely reasonable but also active efforts will be needed to preserve the young person's ongoing relationships and community and cultural ties, including maintaining the young person in the home of the family or extended family, before any apprehension decision is made. Second, the issue of jurisdiction is potentially problematic, with Canadian courts possibly interpreting the best interests of the young person in ways that challenge or overturn Indigenous legislative jurisdiction. The potential for continued jurisdictional squabbles between the federal and provincial governments also exists, including who pays for which services. Third, the Yellowhead Institute asserted that C-92 does not adequately address the funding of existing child welfare services, with the possibility that past federal-provincial disagreements over funding will continue. In instances of disagreement, funding should proceed, with dispute-settlement negotiations following, rather than the other way around. Fourth, in the interests of accountability, an independent dispute-resolution mechanism needs to be created. And fifth, mandatory data collection needs to be implemented.

1. Ethical Principles of Indigenous Ownership, Control, Access, and Possession of Research Data and Their Interpretation

Of particular relevance to the present chapter on health, in which we compare selected health indicators among Indigenous and non-Indigenous youths in care in Ontario, and to Chapter 6, on cultural and personal identity and the residential schools, is the important ethical question of Ownership, Control, Access, and Possession (OCAP) by First Nations communities of research data and their interpretation, which we address at this point.

In September 2020, the Office of Research Ethics and Integrity at the University of Ottawa approved our ethics proposal to write this book, to be based on secondary analyses of data originally collected in fulfillment of our mandate from the Ontario government (Ministry of Children, Community and Social Services) to collect data on young people in out-of-home care for service-planning and outcome-monitoring purposes. The Ethics Office subsequently approved two one-year extensions to the project in 2021 and 2022, after we had submitted the required annual reports on the project.

Approximately 20% of each year's Ontario Looking After Children (OnLAC)/Assessment and Action Record (AAR) sample throughout most of the project has been composed of Indigenous young people in out-of-home care (the proportion has increased somewhat recently, perhaps related to COVID-19). At the suggestion of an external reviewer of our manuscript, we asked an Indigenous scholar located at a Canadian university to review, from an OCAP perspective, the preface and two chapters that dealt especially with Indigenous young people in care: Chapter 3, on health, and Chapter 6, on personal and cultural identity and the residential schools, as well as this OCAP section. We also approached two Indigenous organizations to do the OCAP consultation, but they were not able to do so. The Indigenous scholar, who agreed to carry out the consultation, was very familiar with the overriding objective of OCAP principles, namely, ensuring that the process of gathering and interpreting research data promotes the well-being of Indigenous Peoples and communities and causes them no harm. The Indigenous scholar informed us, after a lengthy telephone conversation and a careful review of the manuscript, that, in their opinion, the manuscript was clearly in conformity with OCAP principles, such that they had no revisions to suggest.

Like our scholar/consultant, we believe that our manuscript adheres to OCAP principles in a number of ways. First, the OnLAC Project and Ontario Association of Children's Aid Societies (OACAS) have always taken the position that local Societies—the 38 local Societies and the 13 Indigenous child and family well-being agencies in Ontario—decide whether they will participate in the OnLAC Project and also own their data. The 38 CASs and 7 of the 13 Indigenous Societies currently do participate in the OnLAC Project and forward their AAR data each year, on their young people in care, to the project at the University of Ottawa. However, on the advice of a lawyer hired by OACAS some 20 years ago, the copyright to the amalgamated OnLAC provincial data set, managed on an ongoing basis by the OnLAC Project, is owned by OACAS. This arrangement was intended to ensure that the OnLAC Project would continue in the future after Robert Flynn (the project's principal investigator since its founding in 2000) had retired or was otherwise unavailable.

Second, the manager of the OnLAC data set, Meagan Miller, has always provided each local Society with its own confidential, up-to-date data within two weeks of a request. In fact, all local Societies now receive a complete, confidential, and aggregated data package annually, without having to ask for it. This enables the Society to conduct its own analyses and answer its own informational or evaluation questions.

Third, every year, Miller sends each Society a confidential report on the progress of its own young people in care, based on the data submitted during the previous year by the Society. Each Society also receives each year a public (non-confidential) report on the same variables and questions but based on the amalgamated provincial OnLAC data set. This provides a provincial context within which the Society can more easily interpret the results of its own young people.

Fourth, during the most recent major revision of the AAR, used since January 2016, the 15-member committee convened by OACAS that worked throughout 2014 on the revision included two Indigenous masters of social work (MSWs) who had field positions with two Indigenous local Societies. The revisions process benefited greatly from their contributions.

Fifth, all new studies (e.g., peer-reviewed articles, book chapters, books, or PhD theses) proposed by OnLAC Project staff, graduate students, or collaborators must first be approved by the Office of Research Ethics and Integrity at the University of Ottawa, for which adherence to OCAP principles is important. Also, requests for access to the OnLAC data by researchers affiliated with other universities require submission and approval by an OACAS committee of a completed research protocol and ethics approval from their home university.

Sixth, in the Identity section of the current version of the AAR, young people (if aged 10 or over, or their caregivers if younger than 10) are asked the following OCAP-relevant questions:

- Do you have enough opportunities to practice your religion or spiritual affiliation (including traditions, religious services, festivals and holidays, prayers, clothing, diet, fasting, traditional sweat lodge, pow-wow, drumming)?

If the young person is a First Nations, Métis, or Inuit (FNMI) young person:

- Did your ancestors belong to a First Nation Band, Community, or Nation?
  - o (If yes, to which Band, Community, or Nation did they belong?)
- Do you belong to a clan or have a clan affiliation?
- Do you visit or meet with people from your own FNMI community?
- Do you have a relationship to the land or landmarks in your community (e.g., lake, rock, trees)?
- Do you learn about traditional teachings, customs, or ceremonies?
- Do you participate in your own FNMI community events, activities, traditional meals/foods, and ceremonies?
- How often do you speak your own First Nations or Inuit language?
- Do you have a personal connection with an Elder, Healer, and/or Cultural Teacher?
- Do you have a native Spirit Name?

2. Basic Health-Care Indicators: Health Cards, Annual Medical and Dental Exams, and Immunizations

In the present chapter, we present AAR data from the OnLAC Project on children and young people who were in care during calendar year 2019. Our focus is on comparisons between broad categories of young people in care, based on their Indigenous versus non-Indigenous status, sex, and age. Such information, important for practice and policy, is uniquely available in the OnLAC data set.

Among young people in care aged 16 or older in Ontario in 2019, 97% of females and males reported having a valid health card. Their child welfare workers observed whether they had received the annual medical and dental exams required by provincial health-care regulations and whether their immunizations were up to date. In the event, 98% or more of the young people aged 0–15, whether male or female, had had a medical exam within the past 12 months. For those 16 and older, however, a higher proportion of females than males (97% vs. 93%; p = .04) had had a medical exam within the past year.

Regarding dental exams, 99% of the young people aged 6–15, whether female or male, had had such an exam within the past year, with the proportion slightly lower among those 16 or older. On the other hand, among children in care aged 0–5, only 57% of males and females had visited a dentist within the past year, even though the Canadian Dental Association and the Canadian Paediatric Society (Rowan-Legg, 2013) recommend that a first dental visit takes place before a child's first birthday.

The immunizations of most of the children and young people were up to date. The rates for females aged 0–5 were 96% and for males 97%; for females aged 6–9, 98%, and for males, 99%; for females aged 10–15, 99%, and for males, 98%; and for females and males aged 16 or older, 97%.

3. General Health Status of Ontario's Children and Young People in Care

Table 3.1 displays the general health status of children and adolescents whose AAR data for calendar year 2019 had been forwarded by their respective local Societies to the OnLAC Project. We compared Indigenous and non-Indigenous children or adolescents in care, within four age groups (0–5, 6–9, 10–15, and 16+ years) and within

Table 3.1. General health of children and young people in care in Ontario, by Indigenous versus non-Indigenous background and age (within sex), and by sex and age

Age Group	General Health	Females			Males			Sex		
		Indigenous (n = 119) %	non-Indigenous (n = 305) %	p	Indigenous (n = 149) %	non-Indigenous (n = 344) %	p	Females (n = 424) %	Males (n = 493) %	p
0–5	Excellent	48.7	51.1		40.9	39.2		50.5	39.8	
	Very good	38.7	33.8	ns	43.6	39.8	ns	35.1	41.0	.001
	Good	10.9	12.5		10.7	17.2		12.0	15.2	
	Fair/poor	1.7	2.6		4.7	3.8		2.4	4.1	
		(n = 79) %	(n = 179) %		(n = 100) %	(n = 243) %		(n = 258) %	(n = 343) %	
6–9	Excellent	46.8	49.2		45.0	44.4		48.4	44.6	
	Very good	35.4	35.2	ns	40.0	40.3	ns	35.3	40.2	ns
	Good	16.5	14.0		13.0	11.5		14.7	12.0	
	Fair/poor	1.3	1.7		2.0	3.7		1.6	3.2	
		(n = 174) %	(n = 456) %		(n = 159) %	(n = 604) %		(n = 630) %	(n = 763) %	
10–15	Excellent	33.9	42.8		49.1	37.1		40.3	39.6	
	Very good	41.4	36.0	ns	33.3	43.2	.05	37.5	41.2	ns
	Good	20.1	19.5		15.1	17.1		19.7	16.6	
	Fair/poor	4.6	1.8		2.5	2.6		2.5	2.6	
		(n = 69) %	(n = 276) %		(n = 59) %	(n = 303) %		(n = 345) %	(n = 362) %	
16+	Excellent	18.8	23.2		25.4	27.7		22.3	27.3	
	Very good	39.1	38.0	ns	32.2	38.3	ns	38.3	37.3	ns
	Good	36.2	31.2		37.3	30.0		32.2	31.2	
	Fair/poor	5.8	7.6		5.1	4.0		7.2	4.1	

Note. For children in care aged 0–12, the child's *caregiver* provided the health rating. For those aged 13–16+, the *young person* provided the rating; ns = not significant. Statistical significance and *p*-levels were determined with the chi-square test. In the tables that follow in this chapter, statistical significance in fourfold (2 × 2) tables was determined with the continuity correction, as recommended by Fleiss et al., 2003, p. 58. Percentages may not sum to 100 due to rounding in this and other tables in the chapter.
Source: Ontario Looking After Children Project data in 2019.

categories defined by sex. We also directly compared females and males within the same age groups. We made comparisons in our cross-sectional analyses with crosstabs and tested them via chi-square in our 2 × 4 tables, or, in our fourfold (2 × 2) tables, via the continuity correction (as recommended by Fleiss et al., 2003, p. 58).

As Table 3.1 shows, there were no statistically significant differences in general health status between Indigenous and non-Indigenous females, in any age group. It is noteworthy, however, that the proportion of females whose general health was rated by their caregivers (ages 0–5 and 6–9) or by themselves (10–15 and 16+ years) as either excellent or very good declined with age, such that in the oldest age group, roughly 40% self-rated their health status as only good or fair/poor. Among the Indigenous and non-Indigenous males, only one of the four comparisons was statistically significant: in the 10-to-15-year-old age group, the Indigenous young people rated their health status as somewhat better than their non-Indigenous age peers did ($p < .05$). Additionally, the same tendency of declining ratings of excellent or very good overall health, as seen among the females, was also in evidence among the males. This appears consistent with Canadian research (Kwak & Rudmin, 2014) that has found a more pronounced effect of social factors such as socioeconomic status (SES) on health among older children or adolescents than among younger ones.

Finally, direct female–male comparisons revealed only one statistically significant difference by age, namely, among the youngest children, aged 0–5 ($p < .001$). The caregivers rated the health of the very young girls as somewhat better than that of the very young boys.

4. Learning-Related Health Conditions in Children and Young People in Care in Ontario

Canadian and international studies have found that the prevalence in young people in care of learning-related health conditions (on which we present OnLAC data in Table 3.2) is higher than in the general population. This is the case for attention deficit hyperactivity disorder (ADHD; Villegas & Pecora, 2012), developmental disabilities (Trocmé et al., 2008), and prenatal alcohol exposure and fetal alcohol spectrum disorder (FASD; Goodman et al., 2014). The *Canadian Incidence Study of Reported Child Abuse and Neglect* (Trocmé et al., 2008) noted a higher rate of diagnosis and treatment of ADHD and developmental disability in the child welfare population compared with the general population. Klein et al. (2014) reported that maltreated children are more likely to have ADHD, a developmental delay in language or learning, post-traumatic stress disorder (PTSD), or an attachment, mood, or anxiety disorder.

The lifelong negative effects of prenatal exposure to alcohol on the developing brain and body are well established (Burns et al., 2021; Kambeitz et al., 2019). Canadian research has identified FASD as a preventable health condition that has considerable social, health, and economic costs (Goodman et al., 2014; Millar et al., 2014). Although the severity of the impact of FASD on individuals varies considerably (Kambeitz et al., 2019; Popova et al., 2014), ongoing targeted support is often necessary to address problems or skill deficits in many areas, including physical health, daily living, and motor functioning; learning, memory, and attention; and communication, emotion regulation, and social functioning (Burns et al., 2021, p. 78). FASD and its associated physical, mental, behavioural, and learning disabilities are directly related to children's placement and overrepresentation in out-of-home care (Popova et al., 2014; Kambeitz et al., 2019; Millar et al., 2014).

Regarding the prevalence of FASD in Canada, Burns et al. (2021), based on data from the Canadian National FASD Database, estimated that the prevalence of FASD in the Canadian population was approximately 4%, with a higher prevalence in the child welfare population. Also, a meta-analysis of 33 international studies investigating FASD in children and young people in care found that although prevalence rates varied across countries, the overall rate of FASD was very high (Lange et al., 2013). On the other hand, Health Canada estimated in 2006 that FASD affected only 1% of the Canadian population, but this was considered an underestimate, as many individuals had not been adequately assessed or diagnosed (Millar et al., 2014). Overall, it appears that precise Canadian prevalence estimates of FASD in high-risk groups such as the in-care population are not yet available. Prevalence estimates have ranged widely, between less than 1% to 23% according to Goodman et al. (2014, p. 9), between 17% and 50% in the child welfare population in Manitoba (Fuchs et al., 2010), and at 23% among young people admitted for psychiatric assessment in British Columbia (Jonsson et al., 2009).

In the OnLAC Project, the current AAR (AAR-C2-2016) requires the child welfare worker, with assistance as needed from the young person (if aged 10 or older) or from the caregiver, to indicate whether the young person or child has one or more of 16 listed long-term health conditions ("none" or "any other" are also possible responses). The AAR defines "a long-term health condition" as one that has lasted or is expected to last six months or more and has been diagnosed by a health professional.

In Table 3.2, we present OnLAC data from 2019 on five learning-related long-term health conditions. Of the 16 long-term health conditions diagnosed by a health professional that are listed in the AAR, we consider these five to be especially likely to have a direct effect on the young person's ability to learn: FASD, developmental disability, learning disability, attention deficit disorder, and emotional/psychological/nervous difficulties. They are listed in Table 3.2 within the same four age groups as in the other tables in this chapter: 0–5, 6–9, 10–15, and 16+ years. (To anticipate, we also provide OnLAC data from 2019 in Table 3.3 on the use of tobacco, alcohol and marijuana; in Tables 3.4.1 and 3.4.2, on the use of illicit drugs; in Table 3.5, on the prescribed use of psychotropic drugs; and in Appendix Tables B to E, on 11 long-term physical health conditions.)

Table 3.2 shows the long-term learning-related health conditions, as reported by child welfare workers, with assistance from the caregiver as needed. Within each of the four age groups, for each of the five learning-related long-term health conditions, and within the female, male, and combined female–male sub-samples, we carried out a series of 2 × 2 cross-tab analyses (i.e., the young person's health condition [present/absent] by their ethno-cultural background [Indigenous/non-Indigenous]). With each fourfold (2 × 2) table, we used the continuity correction for purposes of statistical testing (Fleiss et al., 2003, p. 58).

As Table 3.2 indicates, among the young children aged 0–5, there were no statistically significant differences between the percentages of Indigenous and non-Indigenous girls or boys who had been diagnosed by a health professional as having any of the five learning-related health conditions (as reported by the child welfare workers, with assistance as needed from the caregivers). Similarly, there were no significant differences between females and males in the combined Indigenous/non-Indigenous sample in the diagnostic prevalence of any of the learning-related conditions.

Among the 6-to-9-year-old children, the picture was rather different. In general, the diagnosed frequency of all five learning-related conditions was considerably higher than among the 0-to-5-year-olds,

Table 3.2. Long-term learning-related health conditions of children and young people in care in Ontario, by Indigenous versus non-Indigenous background and age (within sex), and by sex and age

Age Group	Long-term Learning-Related Health Conditions	Females		p	Males		p	Sex		p
		Indigenous (n = 126) %	non-Indigenous (n = 310) %		Indigenous (n = 157) %	non-Indigenous (n = 356) %		Females (n = 436) %	Males (n = 513) %	
0–5	FASD	0.8	2.9	ns	1.3	2.8	ns	2.3	2.3	ns
	Developmental Disability	7.9	10.6	ns	12.1	12.4	ns	9.9	12.3	ns
	Learning Disability	3.2	4.2	ns	4.5	7.0	ns	3.9	6.2	ns
	Attention Deficit Disorder	1.6	1.3	ns	2.5	3.4	ns	1.4	3.1	ns
	Emot/psych/nerv Diff.	3.2	2.6	ns	5.1	2.0	ns	2.8	2.9	ns
		(n = 83) %	(n = 181) %		(n = 104) %	(n = 249) %		(n = 264) %	(n = 333) %	
6–9	FASD	2.4	6.6	ns	11.5	4.8	.04	5.3	6.8	ns
	Developmental Disability	4.8	17.7	.01	17.3	23.3	ns	13.6	21.5	.02
	Learning Disability	9.6	26.5	.01	19.2	28.1	ns	21.2	25.5	ns
	Attention Deficit Disorder	10.8	21.5	.06	26.9	36.5	ns	18.2	33.7	.001
	Emot/psych/nerv Diff.	10.8	20.4	.08	15.4	24.9	.07	17.4	22.1	ns

	(n = 181) %	(n = 496) %		(n = 165) %	(n = 666) %		(n = 677) %	(n = 831) %	
10–15									
FASD	7.7	4.4	ns	10.9	6.2	.05	5.3	7.1	ns
Developmental Disability	10.5	15.7	ns	15.2	23.9	.02	14.3	22.1	.001
Learning Disability	24.9	29.8	ns	27.3	36.9	.03	28.5	35.0	.01
Attention Deficit Disorder	19.3	28.4	.02	44.2	47.3	ns	26.0	46.7	.001
Emot/psych/nerv Diff.	24.3	32.7	.05	21.8	33.9	.01	30.4	31.5	ns
	(n = 73) %	(n = 326) %		(n = 67) %	(n = 382) %		(n = 399) %	(n = 499) %	
16+									
FASD	9.6	4.9	ns	9.0	7.1	ns	5.8	7.3	ns
Developmental Disability	13.7	13.5	ns	9.0	26.2	.01	13.5	23.6	.001
Learning Disability	23.3	31.9	ns	26.9	37.4	ns	30.3	35.9	ns
Attention Deficit Disorder	20.5	24.5	ns	35.8	36.9	ns	23.8	36.7	.001
Emot/psych/nerv Diff.	34.2	39.0	ns	25.4	29.1	ns	38.1	28.5	.01

Note. ns = not significant, using continuity correction for fourfold tables; p-levels are 2-tailed.
FASD = Fetal Alcohol Spectrum Disorder. Emot/psych/nerv Diff = Emotional/psychological/nervous difficulties.
Source: Ontario Looking After Children Project data in 2019.

for all five conditions and in all three sub-samples. On four of the five conditions (namely, developmental disability, learning disability, attention deficit disorder, and emotional/psychological/nervous difficulties), a significantly higher proportion of the non-Indigenous than the Indigenous females had been diagnosed with the condition. In the male sub-sample, however, the Indigenous males aged 6–9 were more likely than the non-Indigenous to have been diagnosed with FASD, with a trend in the opposite direction for emotional/psychological/nervous difficulties. Finally, the 6-to-9-year-old males were significantly more likely than the females of the same age to have been diagnosed with developmental disability and attention deficit disorder, with no significant differences on the other three conditions.

In the female sub-sample of 10-to-15-year-old young people, the non-Indigenous young people had a significantly higher likelihood of a diagnosis of attention deficit disorder or emotional/psychological/nervous difficulties. In the male 10-to-15-year-old sub-sample, the non-Indigenous young people had a significantly higher prevalence of developmental disability, learning disability, and emotional/psychological/nervous difficulties, with the opposite result on FASD. In the combined Indigenous/non-Indigenous sub-sample, a higher proportion of male than female young people had been diagnosed with developmental disability, learning disability, and attention deficit disorder.

Finally, in the oldest group (16+, of whom most were 16 or 17 years of age), the non-Indigenous males were more likely than their Indigenous peers to have received a diagnosis of developmental disability. In the combined sub-sample, however, the males were significantly more likely than the females to have had a diagnosis of developmental disability or attention deficit disorder but were less likely to have been diagnosed as experiencing emotional/psychological/nervous difficulties.

Overall, our findings suggest that Ontario needs to focus much greater attention and resources on the early assessment and prevention of learning-related health conditions among young people in care. The educational consequences of the high prevalence rates of learning-related problems displayed in Table 3.2 (and of the challenges shown in the other tables in this chapter) can be seen in chapter 4 (on education) of this book. Close to half—and sometimes more than half—of the children and young people whose outcomes we monitor each year experience serious difficulties in reading and math. The roots of these enduring problems are traceable, in part, to a preventable lack of developmental opportunities, including high-quality early childhood education (ECE) and high-impact tutoring in the early years of primary school. The federal government's budget of 2021 and the agreements it has signed with the provinces and territories, including Ontario, hold out the promise of more accessible and affordable ECE in Canada. However, Canada's performance to date in this area has been weak, compared with the resources allocated by many European countries (Cameron et al., 2020), and we have no room for complacency regarding program implementation or outcome evaluation. Cleveland (2018) has recommended that the Ontario government should begin by implementing free licenced child care for young children, 30 months to kindergarten age, and then progressively extend capacity to infants and toddlers.

5. Tobacco, Alcohol, and Drug Use among Children and Young People in Care in Ontario

Previous research indicates that young people in care tend to have a higher rate of alcohol and substance use than their age peers in the general population (Braciszewski & Stout, 2012; Popova et al., 2014; Stott, 2012). This increases their risk of not graduating from secondary school and reduces their employment and income prospects (Courtney et al., 2001). Substance abuse is a maladaptive coping strategy that may be used to manage the long-term mental health consequences of childhood maltreatment (Thompson Jr. & Auslander, 2011; Aldao et al., 2010). Female adolescents in care, in particular, are at an increased risk of risky sexual behaviour, delinquency, depression, and suicidality (Hudson, 2012; Robertson, 2013; Thompson Jr. & Auslander, 2011; Kim et al., 2013). Canadian research suggests that females are two to four times more likely than males to encounter sexual abuse in childhood or in their personal relationships. Similarly, Indigenous women are also more likely than Indigenous men to experience child abuse or violence within their marriages or common-law partnerships (The Chief Public Health Officer's Report on the State of Public Health in Canada, 2016).

A Canadian study used OnLAC (AAR) data from 2016 to investigate risk and predictive factors related to alcohol and marijuana use among adolescents in care. The researchers (Cullen et al., 2020) found that the factors most strongly associated with greater marijuana and alcohol consumption were placement instability, placement type, weak attachment to caregivers, peer substance use, and a lower level of self-control. Multiple placement changes, especially at an older age, and later entry into care were associated with a greater risk of serious substance abuse. Instability resulting from the disruption of social networks undermined prosocial attachments that the young people might have developed, such that substance use may have been partly a means of coping with feelings of loss, disconnection, frustration, or hopelessness. Cullen et al. (2020) found that adolescents who had undergone more than one placement change within the last year were significantly more likely to use marijuana and alcohol, with substance use increasing with the number of placement disruptions. Adolescents with placement stability, on the other hand, were significantly more likely to report never using marijuana and were the least likely to use alcohol or marijuana occasionally or daily. Moreover, the young people who had only a low level of attachment to their caregivers were three times more likely to use marijuana and alcohol occasionally or daily, compared to those who reported high attachment to their caregivers. A close relationship between adolescents and their caregivers (as rated by the young people in care) increased the likelihood that the youths would report never using marijuana or alcohol. Also, adolescents with a high degree of self-control were more likely to report not engaging in substance use. Finally, substance use by peers was found to be one of the strongest predictors of alcohol and marijuana use. Young people living in group homes or independent living who spent time with others who used alcohol and marijuana had an increased likelihood of substance use.

In summary, Cullen and colleagues noted that placement instability, placement type, behavioural characteristics, and the relationship with the caregiver were all related to substance use. Consequently, child welfare workers should focus on promoting healthy, prosocial relationships by young people in care to improve transition process and outcomes.

Table 3.3 displays the self-reported use of cigarettes or other tobacco products, alcohol, or marijuana/cannabis (i.e., "soft" drugs) in the last 12 months by young people aged 10–15 and 16+ who participated in the OnLAC Project in 2019. The cross-sectional analyses consisted of cross-tabulations and chi-square. With only one exception (namely, in the lower frequency of use of alcohol by Indigenous compared with non-Indigenous females aged 10–15), there were no statistically significant differences found between Indigenous

Table 3.3. Self-reported use of tobacco, alcohol, and marijuana by young people in care in Ontario aged 10–16+, by Indigenous versus non-Indigenous background and age (within sex), and by sex and age

Age Group	Substances used in last 12 months	Frequency of use	Females Indigenous (n=61) %	Females non-Indigenous (n=111) %	p	Males Indigenous (n=52) %	Males non-Indigenous (n=142) %	p	Sex Females (n=172) %	Sex Males (n=194) %	p
10–15	Cigarettes/Other tobacco products	Not at all	55.7	64.9	ns	71.2	69.7	ns	61.6	70.1	ns
		Tried it	24.6	15.3		11.5	14.1		18.6	13.4	
		Occasionally	8.2	7.2		7.7	5.6		7.6	6.2	
		Daily	11.5	12.6		9.6	10.6		12.2	10.3	
	Alcohol	Not at all	80.3	61.3	.01	82.7	78.2	ns	68.0	79.4	.02
		Tried it	8.2	29.7		9.6	12.7		22.1	11.9	
		Occasionally	11.5	9.0		7.7	9.2		9.9	8.8	
		Daily	0.0	0.0		0.0	0.0		0.0	0.0	
	Marijuana/cannabis	Not at all	62.3	60.4	ns	76.9	69.7	ns	61.0	71.5	.03
		Tried it	23.0	20.7		9.6	14.8		21.5	13.4	
		Occasionally	11.5	16.2		3.8	11.3		14.5	9.3	
		Daily	3.3	2.7		9.6	4.2		2.9	5.7	
			(n=22) %	(n=91) %		(n=26) %	(n=104) %		(n=113) %	(n=130) %	
16+	Cigarettes/Other tobacco products	Not at all	22.7	38.5	ns	26.9	35.6	ns	35.4	33.8	ns
		Tried it	9.1	14.3		15.4	18.3		13.3	17.7	
		Occasionally	22.7	18.7		23.1	20.2		19.5	20.8	
		Daily	45.5	28.6		34.6	26.0		31.9	27.7	
	Alcohol	Not at all	13.6	30.8	ns	26.9	26.9	ns	27.4	26.9	ns
		Tried it	27.3	31.9		30.8	32.7		31.0	32.3	
		Occasionally	54.5	34.1		42.3	38.5		38.1	39.2	
		Daily	4.5	3.3		0.0	1.9		3.5	1.5	
	Marijuana/cannabis	Not at all	18.2	27.5	ns	30.8	19.2	ns	25.7	21.5	ns
		Tried it	13.6	28.6		15.4	34.6		25.7	30.8	
		Occasionally	36.4	17.6		19.2	26.0		21.2	24.6	
		Daily	31.8	26.4		34.6	20.2		27.4	23.1	

Note. ns = not significant; *p*-levels (2-tailed) were determined by chi-square test.
Source: Ontario Looking After Children Project data in 2019.

and non-Indigenous females on any of the substances in question. This was no doubt due in part to the small number of Indigenous females and males in each age group, which limited statistical power. However, in the older age group, compared with their younger peers, the frequency of use, regardless of the substance in question, was dramatically higher in the older (16+) than in the younger (10–15) age group, for both females and males, whether of Indigenous or non-Indigenous background. Regarding the female–male comparisons in the two right-hand-most columns of Table 3.3, in the younger age group the females reported significantly but higher use of alcohol and marijuana/cannabis than did the males. Among the older youths, there was no statistically significant difference between females and males in the frequency of use of any of the three substances. However, the same growth in the frequency of use of all three substances that we noted previously in the older versus the younger youths was again in evidence.

Table 3.4.1 (for the young people in care aged 10–15 in 2019) and Table 3.4.2 (for those aged 16+) present self-reported data on the use of illicit (or "hard") drugs, including whether the young people had ever used these drugs or had done so within the last 12 months. (The relatively small numbers of Indigenous females and males, especially in Table 3.4.2, and the resultant lessened statistical power make caution especially necessary in the interpretation of these findings.) The cross-sectional analyses involved cross-tabulations with Pearson chi-square tests or, for the 2 × 2 ("ever used") tables, with the continuity correction. Among the 10-to-15-year-olds (see Table 3.4.1), the only statistically significant difference suggested that the males in the combined sample were somewhat more likely than the females to report not having used drugs without a prescription in the last year. Overall, about a third of the females and males reported having ever used illicit drugs, with over 90% saying they had not used them in the last 12 months.

Among the young people aged 16 of age and older (see Table 3.4.2), there was again only a single statistically significant difference, with Indigenous males reporting more frequent use of hallucinogens than non-Indigenous males. The issue of limited statistical power, however, due especially to the small number of Indigenous females and males, also applies here. As previously noted with respect to the use of "soft drugs" (cigarettes, alcohol, and marijuana), a higher proportion of the older youths, both females and males, reported having ever

Table 3.4.1. Self-reported use of illicit drugs in the last 12 months, by young people in care in Ontario aged 10–15, by Indigenous versus non-Indigenous background (within sex), and by sex

		Females			Males			Sex		
		Indigenous (n = 61) %	non-Indigenous (n = 111) %	p	Indigenous (n = 52) %	non-Indigenous (n = 142) %	p	Females (n = 172) %	Males (n = 194) %	p
Ever used illicit drugs	No	63.9	64.0	ns	71.2	65.5	ns	64.0	67.0	ns
	Yes	36.1	36.0		28.8	34.5		36.0	33.0	
Substances used in last 12 months	Frequency of use									
Cocaine	Not at all	90.2	86.5	ns	96.2	90.8	ns[a]	87.8	92.3	ns
heroin	Tried it	9.8	11.7		1.9	8.5		11.0	6.7	
speed	Occasionally	0.0	1.8		1.9	0.7		1.2	1.0	
ecstasy	Daily	0.0	0.0		0.0	0.0		0.0	0.0	
Glue	Not at all	96.7	95.5	ns[a]	92.3	97.9	ns[a]	95.9	96.4	ns
gasoline	Tried it	1.6	3.6		5.8	1.4		2.9	2.6	
other	Occasionally	1.6	0.0		1.9	0.7		0.6	1.0	
solvents	Daily	0.0	0.9		0.0	0.0		0.6	0.0	
Drugs without prescription (downers/uppers, tranquilizers, Ritalin)	Not at all	90.2	90.1	ns[a]	98.1	93.7	ns	90.1	94.9	.05
	Tried it	8.2	9.9		0.0	4.2		9.3	3.1	
	Occasionally	1.6	0.0		1.9	0.7		0.6	1.0	
	Daily	0.0	0.0		0.0	1.4		0.0	1.0	
Hallucinogens (LSD, acid, etc.)	Not at all	95.1	90.1	ns[a]	92.3	94.4	ns[a]	91.9	93.8	ns
	Tried it	4.9	8.1		5.8	4.2		7.0	4.6	
	Occasionally	0.0	1.8		1.9	1.4		1.2	1.5	
	Daily	0.0	0.0		0.0	0.0		0.0	0.0	

Note. ns = not significant. [a] Significance test should be interpreted with caution because more than 20% of the cells had expected frequencies of less than 5. The statistical test used was chi-square, except for the 2 × 2 table for "Ever used illicit drugs," where the continuity correction was used.

Source: Ontario Looking After Children Project data in 2019.

Table 3.4.2. Self-reported use of illicit drugs in the last 12 months, by young people in care in Ontario, aged 16+, by Indigenous versus non-Indigenous background (within sex), and by sex

		Females			Males			Sex		
		Indigenous (n = 22) %	non-Indigenous (n = 91) %	p	Indigenous (n = 26) %	non-Indigenous (n = 104) %	p	Females (n = 113) %	Males (n = 130) %	p
Ever used illicit drugs	No	22.7	34.1	ns	38.5	35.6	ns	31.9	36.2	ns
	Yes	77.3	65.9		61.5	64.4		68.1	63.8	
Substances used in last 12 months	Frequency of use									
Cocaine heroin speed ecstasy	Not at all	68.2	67.0	ns[a]	61.5	76.9	ns[a]	67.3	73.8	ns
	Tried it	27.3	20.9		30.8	18.3		22.1	20.8	
	Occasionally	4.5	8.8		7.7	3.8		8.0	4.6	
	Daily	0.0	3.3		0.0	1.0		2.7	0.8	
Glue gasoline other solvents	Not at all	90.9	94.5	ns	92.3	98.1	ns	93.8	96.9	ns
	Tried it	9.1	5.5		7.7	1.9		6.2	3.1	
	Occasionally	0.0	0.0		0.0	0.0		0.0	0.0	
	Daily	0.0	0.0		0.0	0.0		0.0	0.0	
Drugs without prescription (downers/uppers, tranquilizers Ritalin)	Not at all	68.2	73.6	ns[a]	73.1	76.9	ns[a]	72.6	76.2	ns
	Tried it	22.7	17.6		15.4	15.4		18.6	15.4	
	Occasionally	9.1	4.4		11.5	5.8		5.3	6.9	
	Daily	0.0	4.4		0.0	1.9		3.5	1.5	
Hallucinogens (LSD, acid, etc.)	Not at all	68.2	73.6	ns	46.2	76.0	.01	72.6	70.0	ns
	Tried it	27.3	22.0		46.2	16.3		23.0	22.3	
	Occasionally	4.5	4.4		7.7	7.7		4.4	7.7	
	Daily	0.0	0.0		0.0	0.0		0.0	0.0	

Note. ns = not significant. [a] Significance test should be interpreted with caution because more than 20% of the cells had expected frequencies of less than 5. The statistical test used was chi-square, except for the 2 × 2 table for "Ever used illicit drugs," where the continuity correction was used.

Source: Ontario Looking After Children Project data in 2019.

used illicit drugs (Table 3.4.2) than their younger peers (Table 3.4.1). Moreover, the older youths were also more likely to report having used the various types of illicit drugs in the last 12 months, except for glue, gasoline, or other solvents.

6. Use of Prescribed Psychotropic Medications among Young People in Care in Ontario

In a review of international and Canadian research on the use of psychotropic medications in children and adolescents, Garcia-Ortega and Pringsheim (2015) remarked that second-generation antipsychotic medications (SGAs) have been prescribed more frequently in the past decade than previously, especially to males, who have a correspondingly higher rate of use. A number of studies that found a disproportionately high rate of use of psychotropic medication in child welfare have expressed concern regarding the long-term health consequences of this practice and have advocated that more adequate medical monitoring takes place (Garcia-Ortega & Pringsheim, 2015; Warner, Song, & Pottick, 2014; dosReis et al., 2014). Some researchers have even questioned whether these medications are even medically necessary or beneficial (Brenner et al., 2014; Bertram, Narendorf, & McMillan, 2013).

A Canadian study of the use of psychotropic medications with children and adolescents in Canada, Europe, and the United States found increasing prescription rates, with higher use observed among males, young people aged 7 and older, and over longer periods of time (Patten et al., 2012). An American study (Liu et al., 2014) found that White male children and children in care were more likely to receive concomitant multiple psychotropic medications for comorbid ADHD and anxiety disorders.

Table 3.5 shows the percentage of young people in the four age groups who, in 2019, were participants in the OnLAC Project and who used prescribed psychotropic medications, as reported by their child welfare workers. Cross-tabulations were conducted, with statistical significance determined by the continuity correction in each of the 2 × 2 tables. In both the female and male sub-samples, the non-Indigenous young people aged 6–9 and 10–15 were reported as having significantly higher rates of use than their Indigenous peers. In the combined female and male sub-sample, the males had a significantly higher rate of use than the females in the three older age groups. It is

Table 3.5. Prescribed use of psychotropic medications by children and young people in care in Ontario aged 0–16+, by Indigenous versus non-Indigenous background and age (within sex), and sex and age

Age Group	Prescribed Psychotropic Medications	Females			Males			Sex		
		Indigenous	non-Indigenous	p	Indigenous	non-Indigenous	p	Females	Males	p
0–5		(n = 122) %	(n =299) %	ns	(n = 156) %	(n = 349) %	ns	(n = 421) %	(n = 505) %	ns
	No	96.7	96.0		97.4	94.8		96.2	95.6	
	Yes	3.3	4.0		2.6	5.2		3.8	4.4	
6–9		(n = 83) %	(n = 176) %	.01	(n = 99) %	(n = 242) %	.01	(n = 259) %	(n = 341) %	.001
	No	86.7	68.2		70.7	51.7		74.1	57.2	
	Yes	13.3	31.8		29.3	48.3		25.9	42.8	
10–15		(n = 177) %	(n = 482) %	.01	(n = 160) %	(n = 644) %	.001	(n = 659) %	(n = 804) %	.001
	No	67.8	56.4		51.1	36.2		59.5	39.2	
	Yes	32.2	43.6		48.8	63.8		40.5	60.8	
16+		(n = 67) %	(n = 301) %	ns	(n = 65) %	(n = 352) %	ns	(n = 386) %	(n = 417) %	.03
	No	64.2	57.8		60.0	49.4		59.0	51.1	
	Yes	35.8	42.2		40.0	50.6		41.0	48.9	

Note. ns = not significant; p-levels (2-tailed) were determined by continuity correction.

Source: Ontario Looking After Children Project data in 2019.

worth noting that the reported rate of prescribed medication use was in the 40–60% range among the males aged 6–9 and among both the females and males in the 10–15 and 16+ age groups.

7. Appendix: Long-Term Physical Health Conditions in Children and Young People in Care in Ontario

Appendix Tables B–E show the prevalence of long-term physical health conditions in children or youths in care in Ontario aged 0–5, 6–9, 10–15, and 16+, respectively. These data complete the picture of long-term health conditions, begun in Table 3.2 by displaying the prevalence of long-term learning-related conditions. In Appendix Tables B–E, in each successive age group, we compare the prevalence of the various conditions first in the Indigenous and non-Indigenous females, second in the Indigenous and non-Indigenous males, and third in the combined sample of female and male participants. (See the Appendix section of the book for Appendix Tables B–E.)

Among the young children aged 0–5, the most noteworthy difference was related to sex: the females were significantly more likely than the males to have no reported long-term physical health conditions. The males also had higher reported rates of food/digestive allergies and kidney conditions/disease. On the other hand, none of the differences in rates between the Indigenous and non-Indigenous females or males were statistically significant.

Among the 6-to-9-year-old age group, the percentage of the female, male, and combined sub-samples with no reported long-term health conditions was noticeably lower than among the younger children. The Indigenous females seemed in somewhat better overall health than the non-Indigenous females: they were more likely to have no long-term health conditions and less likely to have any other health conditions. The females in the combined sub-sample similarly had reported better overall health than the males, for the same reasons.

In the 10-to-15-year-old age group, there was a further decline in the percentage of young people in each sub-sample with no reported physical health conditions. Among the few statistically significant differences between the Indigenous and non-Indigenous young people were a higher prevalence of diabetes among the Indigenous females, a higher proportion of Indigenous males with no long-term health conditions, and a lower proportion of Indigenous males with any other condition. Regarding sex differences, the females were significantly more likely than the males to have no long-term health conditions and less likely to have any other conditions.

Finally, in the 16+ age group, there were no significant reported differences in prevalence rates between the Indigenous and non-Indigenous young people, except for a higher rate of kidney conditions or disease among the Indigenous females. There were no differences between the females and males.

8. Conclusion

We suggest that local Societies treat the data from 2019 presented in this chapter as normative information for Ontario against which to assess the relative health status of young people of different ages for whom they are responsible. The overall findings imply that while many children and young people in care in the province appear to experience reasonably good physical health, much more prevention-oriented attention is needed to address especially learning-related long-term conditions. The prevalence of FASD, developmental and learning disabilities, attention deficit disorder, and emotional, psychological, and nervous difficulties suggests that early identification of problems and the provision of additional assessment and intervention resources would be beneficial across all age groups for both Indigenous and non-Indigenous children and young people. Moreover, intervening at younger ages may help to reduce the tendency seen across the health conditions examined for the young people's health to become more concerning as they grow older.

References

Afifi, T. O., MacMillan, H. L., Boyle, M., Cheung, K., Taillieu, T., Turner, S., & Sareen, J. (2016). Child abuse and physical health in adulthood. *Health Reports*, 27(3), 10–18, Catalogue no. 82-003-X, Statistics Canada.

Aldao, A., Nolen-Hoeksema, S., & Schweizer, S. (2010). Emotion-regulation strategies across psychopathology: A meta-analytic review. *Clinical Psychology Review*, 30(2), 217–237. https://doi.org/10.1016/j.cpr.2009.11.004

Bertram, J. E., Narendorf, S. C., & McMillan, J. C. (2013). Pioneering the psychiatric nurse role in foster care. *Archives of Psychiatric Nursing*, 27(6), 285–292. https://doi.org/10.1016/j.apnu.2013.09.003

Björkenstam, E., Hjern, A., Mittendorfer-Rutz, E., Vinnerljung, B., Hallqvist, J., & Ljung, R. (2013). Multi-exposure and clustering of adverse childhood experiences, socioeconomic differences and psychotropic medication in young adults. *PLOS ONE, 8*(1), Article e53551. https://doi.org/10.1371/journal.pone.0053551

Braciszewski, J. M., & Stout, R. L. (2012). Substance use among current and former foster youth: A systematic review. *Children and Youth Services Review, 34*(12), 2337–2344. https://doi.org/10.1016/j.childyouth.2012.08.011

Brenner, S. L., Southerland, D. G., Burns, B. J., Wagner, H. R., & Farmer, E. M. Z. (2014). Use of psychotropic medications among youth in treatment foster care. *Journal of Child and Family Studies, 23*, 666–674. https://doi.org/10.1007/s10826-013-9882-3

Boivin, M., & Hertzman, C. (Eds.). (2012). *Early childhood development: Adverse experiences and developmental health.* Royal Society of Canada — Canadian Academy of Health Sciences Expert Panel.

Burns, J., Badry, D., Harding, K. D., Roberts, N., Unsworth, K., & Cook, J. L. (2021). Comparing outcomes of children and youth with fetal alcohol spectrum disorder (FASD) in the child welfare system to those in other living situations in Canada: Results from the Canadian National FASD Database. *Child Care Health Development, 47*, 77–84.

Cameron, C., Höjer, I., Nordenfors, M., & Flynn, R. (2020). Security-first thinking and educational practices for young children in foster care in Sweden and England: A think piece. *Children and Youth Services Review, 119*, 105523. https://doi.org/10.1016/j.childyouth.2020.105523

Cleveland, G. (2018). *Affordable for all: Making licensed child care affordable in Ontario* (Executive Summary). University of Toronto Scarborough.

Courtney, M. E., Dworsky, A., Ruth, G., Keller, T., Havlicek, J., & Bost, N. (2005). *Midwest evaluation of the adult functioning of former foster youth: Outcomes at age 19.* Chapin Hall Center for Children at the University of Chicago.

Courtney, M. E., Piliavin, I., Grogan-Kaylor, A., & Nesmith, A. (2001). Foster youth transitions to adulthood: A longitudinal view of youth leaving care. *Child Welfare, 6*, 685–717.

Cullen, G. J., Walters, D., Yule, C., & O'Grady, W. (2020). Examining the risk and predictive factors for marijuana and alcohol use among adolescent youth in out-of-home care. *Journal of Child & Adolescent Substance Abuse, 29*(1), 88–104. https://doi.org/10.1080/1067828X.2020.1837321

Di Pietro, N. C., & Illes, J. (2014). Disparities in Canadian Indigenous health research on neurodevelopmental disorders. *Journal of Developmental & Behavioural Pediatrics, 35*(1), 74–81. https://doi.org/10.1097/DBP.0000000000000002

dosReis, S., Tai, M.-H., Goffman, D., Lynch, S. E., Reeves, G., & Shaw, T. (2014). Age-related trends in psychotropic medication use among very young children in foster care. *Psychiatric Services, 65*(12), 1452–1457. https://doi.org/10.1176/appi.ps.201300353

Fleiss, J. L., Levin, B., & Paik, M. C. (2003). *Statistical methods for rates and proportions* (3rd edition). John Wiley & Sons.

Fortin, K. (2011). Caring for foster children. In C. Jenney (Ed.), *Child abuse and neglect: Diagnosis, treatment and evidence* (pp. 610–614). Elsevier Saunders.

Fuchs, D., Burnside, L., Marchenski, S., & Mudry, A. (2010). Children with FASD related disabilities receiving services from child welfare agencies in Manitoba. *International Journal of Mental Health and Addiction, 8,* 232–244. https://doi.org/10.1007/s11469-009-9258-5

Garcia-Ortega, I., & Pringsheim, T. (2015). Pharmacoepidemiology of antipsychotic use in Canadian children and adolescents. In N. DiPietro and J. Illes (Eds.), *The Science and ethics of antipsychotic use in children* (pp. 13–25). Science Direct: Academic Press. http://dx.doi.org/10.1016/B978-0-12-800016-8.00002-7

Goodman, D., Badry, D., Fuchs, D., Long, S., & Pelech. W. (2014). *A triprovincial initiative to expand understanding of costs, services & prevention of a public health issue: FASD and children & youth in care.* Child Welfare Institute, Children's Aid Society of Toronto.

Hanlon-Dearman, A., Green, C. R., Andrew, G., LeBlanc, N., & Cook, J. L. (2015). Anticipatory guidance for children and adolescents with fetal alcohol spectrum disorder (FASD): Practice points for primary health providers. *Journal of Population Therapeutics and Clinical Pharmacology,* 22(1), e27–e56.

Hébert, S. T., Esposito, T., & Hélie, S. (2018). How short-term placements affect placement trajectories: A propensity-weighted analysis of re-entry into care. *Children and Youth Services Review, 95,* 117–124. https://doi.org/10.1016/j.childyouth.2018.10.032

Hébert, P. C., & MacDonald, N. (2009). Health care for foster kids: Fix the system, save a child. *Canadian Medical Association Journal, 181*(8), 453. https://doi.org/10.1503/cmaj.091627

Hudson, A. (2012). Where do youth in foster care receive information about preventing unplanned pregnancy and sexually transmitted infections? *Journal of Pediatric Nursing, 27*(5), 443–450. doi:10.1016/j.pedn.2011.06.003

Jonsson, E., Denmitt, L., & Littlejohn, G. (Eds.). (2009). *Fetal alcohol spectrum disorder (FASD) across the lifespan.* Institute of Health Economics. http.//www.ihe.ca/documents/

Kambeitz, C., Klug, M. G., Greenmeyer, J., Popova, S., & Burd, L. (2019). Association of adverse childhood experiences and neurodevelopmental disorders in people with fetal alcohol spectrum disorders (FASD) and non-FASD controls. *BMC Pediatrics, 19,* 498. https://doi.org/10.1186/s12887-019-1878-8

Kim, H. K., Pears, K. C., Leve, L. D., Chamberlain, P., & Smith, D. K. (2013). Intervention effects on health-risking sexual behavior among girls in foster care: the role of placement disruption and tobacco and marijuana use. *Journal of Child and Adolescent Substance Abuse*, 22(5), 370–387. doi:1 0.1080/1067828X.2013.788880

Klein, B., Damiani-Taraba, G., Koster, A., Campbell, J., & Scholz, C. (2014). Diagnosing attention-deficit hyperactivity disorder (ADHD) in children involved with child protection services: are current diagnostic guidelines acceptable for vulnerable populations? *Child: Care, Health and Development*, 41(2), 178–185. https://doi.org/10.1111/cch.12168

Kools, S., Paul, S. M., Jones, R., Monasterio, E., & Norbeck, J. (2013). Health profiles of adolescents in foster care. *Journal of Pediatric Nursing*, 28(3), 213–222. https://doi.org/10.1016/j.pedn.2012.08.010

Kwak, K., & Rudmin, F. (2014). Adolescent health and adaptation in Canada: examination of gender and age aspects of the healthy immigrant effect. *International Journal for Equity in Health*, 13, 103. http://www.equity-healthj.com/content/13/1/103

Lange, S., Shield, K., Rehm, J., & Popova, S. (2013). Prevalence of Fetal Alcohol Spectrum disorders in child care settings: A meta-analysis. *Pediatrics*, 132(4), e980–e995. https://doi.org/10.1542/peds.2013-0066

Liu, X., Kubilis, P., Xu., D., Bussing, R., & Winterstein, A. G. (2014). Psychotropic drug utilization in children with concurrent attention-deficit/hyperactivity disorder and anxiety. *Journal of Anxiety Disorders*, 28(6), 530–536. https://doi.org/10.1016/j.janxdis.2014.06.005

Maliszewski, G., & Brown, C. (2014). Familism, substance abuse, and sexual risk among foster care alumni. *Children and Youth Services Review*, 36, 206–212. https://doi.org/10.1016/j.childyouth.2013.11.021

Martin, A., Ford, T., Goodman, R., Meltzer, H., & Logan, S. (2014). Physical illness in looked after children: a cross-sectional study. *Archives of Disease in Childhood*, 99(2), 103–107. http://dx.doi.org/10.1136/archdischild-2013-303993

Mensah, T., Hjern, A., Håkanson, K., Johansson, P., Jonsson, A. K., Mattsson T., Trænæus, S., Vinnerljung, B., Östlund, P., & Klingberg, G. (2019). Organisational models of health services for children and adolescents in out-of-home care: health technology assessment. *Acta Pædiatrica*, 108(2), 1–8. https://doi.org/10.1111/apa.15002

Millar, J. A., Thompson, J., Schwab, D., Hanlon-Dearman, A., Goodman, D., Koren, G., & Masotti, P. (2014). Educating students with FASD: linking policy, research and practice. *Journal of Research in Special Education Needs*, 17(1), 3–17. https://doi.org/10.1111/1471-3802.12090

Nelson, S. E., & Wilson, K. (2017). The mental health of Indigenous peoples in Canada: A critical review of research. *Social Science & Medicine*, 176, 93–112. https://doi.org/10.1016/j.socscimed.2017.01.021

Newton, R. R., Litrownik, A. J., & Landsverk, J. A. (2000). Children and youth in foster care: disentangling the relationship between problem behaviors and number of placements. *Child Abuse & Neglect*, 24(10), 1363–1374. https://doi.org/10.1016/S0145-2134(00)00189-7

Ontario Government Annual Report. (2016). *Stepping up: A strategic framework to help Ontario's youth succeed.* www.ontario.ca/steppingup.

Patten, S. B., Waheed, W., & Bresee, L. (2012). A review of pharmaco-epidemiologic studies of antipsychotic use in children and adolescents. *The Canadian Journal of Psychiatry, 57*(12), 717–721. https://doi.org/10.1177/070674371205701202

Pecora, P., Kessler, R. C., Williams, J., O'Brien, K., Downs, C., English, D., White, J., Hiripi, E., Roller-White, C., Wiggins, T., & Holmes, K. (2005). *Improving family foster care: Findings from the northwest foster care alumni study.* Casey Family Programs.

Perry, B. L. (2006). Social disruption: The case of youth in foster care. *Social Problems, 53*(3), 371–391. https://doi.org/10.1525/sp.2006.53.3.371

Popova, S., Lange, S., Burd, L., & Rehm, J. (2014). Canadian children and youth in care: The cost of fetal alcohol spectrum disorder. *Child Youth Care Forum, 43*, 83–96. https://doi.org/10.1007/s10566-013-9226-x

Robertson, R. D. (2013). The invisibility of adolescent sexual development in foster care: Seriously addressing sexually transmitted infections and access to services. *Children and Youth Services Review, 35*(3), 493–504. https://doi.org/10.1016/j.childyouth.2012.12.009

Rothwell, D. W., Cherney, K., & Trocmé, N. (2015). Financial strain, child maltreatment and the great recession in Canada (Canadian Child Welfare Research Information Sheet #145E). Centre for Research on Children and Families. Retrieved from Canadian Child Welfare Portal, cwrp.ca.

Rowan-Legg, A. (2013). Oral health care for children — a call for action. *Paediatric Child Health, 18*(1), 37–43. https://doi.org/10.1093/pch/18.1.37

Stott, T. (2012). Placement instability and risky behaviors of youth aging out of foster care. *Child and Adolescent Social Work Journal, 29*(1), 61–83. https://doi.org/10.1007/s10560-011-0247-8

Tait, C. L., Henry, R., & Loewen-Walker, R. (2013). Child welfare: A social determinant of health for Canadian First Nations and Métis children. *Pimatisiwin: A Journal of Aboriginal and Indigenous Community Health, 11*(1), 39–53.

The Chief Public Health Officer's Report on the State of Public Health in Canada. (2016). *A focus on family violence in Canada* (ISSN: 1924–7087 Pub: 160152). Public Health Agency of Canada. Available from: publications@hc-sc.gc.ca.

Thompson, R. G. Jr., & Auslander, W. F. (2011). Substance use and mental health problems as predictors of HIV sexual risk behaviors among adolescents in foster care. *Health and Social Work, 36*(1), 33–43. https://doi.org/10.1093/hsw/36.1.33

Trocmé, N., Fallon, B., MacLaurin, B., Sinha, V., Black, T., Fast, E., Felstiner, C., Hélie, S., Turcotte, D., Weightman, P., Douglas, J., & Holroy, J. (2008). *Canadian incidence study of child abuse and neglect.* Public Health Agency of Canada.

Villegas, J. S. & Pecora, P. J. (2012). Mental health outcomes for adults in family foster care as children: An analysis by ethnicity. *Children and Youth Services Review, 34*(8), 1448–1458. https://doi.org/10.1016/j.childyouth.2012.03.023

Villodas, M. T., Cromer, K. D., Moses, J. O., Litrownik, A. J., Newton, R. R., & David, I. P. (2016). Unstable child welfare permanent placements and early adolescent physical and mental health: The role of adverse childhood experiences and post-traumatic stress. *Child Abuse & Neglect 62,* 76–88. https://doi.org/10.1016/j.chiabu.2016.10.014

Vinnerljung, B. (2014, September 4). *Making a difference? Education and health of children in out-of-home care* [Conference presentation paper]. European Scientific Association on Residential & Family Care for Children and Adolescents (EUSARF) Making a Difference Conference, Copenhagen, Denmark, 26.

Warner, L. A., Song, N. K., & Pottick, K. J. (2014). Outpatient psychotropic medication use in the US: A comparison based on foster care status. *Journal of Child and Family Studies 23,* 652–665. https://doi.org/10.1007/s10826-013-9885-0

Woods, S. B., Farineau, H. M., & McWey, L. M. (2013). Physical health, mental health, and behaviour problems among early adolescents in foster care. *Child: Care, Health and Development, 39*(2), 220–227. https://doi.org/10.1111/j.1365-2214.2011.01357.x

Yellowhead Institute. (2019, July 4). *The promise and pitfalls of C-92: An Act Respecting First Nations, Inuit, and Métis Children, Youth and Families.* Toronto Metropolitan University, Faculty of Arts.

Chapter 4

Education

In this chapter, we present recent findings from the Ontario Looking After Children (OnLAC) Project on the educational development and outcomes of young people in care in the province. We begin with the motor, social, and cognitive development of very young children, go on to describe the academic performance of children and adolescents of primary- and secondary-school ages, and end with the progress of young people of post–secondary school age. Our findings make it clear that Ontario needs to improve the educational outcomes of young people in care at all levels, as is also the case in other provinces and countries. The science enabling substantial and rapid improvement in young people's educational outcomes now exists, and one of our aims is to make this science more widely known and applied in child welfare organizations and schools serving young people in care. In examining here the educational outcomes of four age groups of young people in care in Ontario—pre-school (12–47 months), primary school (6–13 years), secondary school (14–17 years), and post-secondary (18–21 years)—it is apparent that many roots of educational achievement or underachievement lie in children's early lives. It is equally apparent that effective educational interventions have to begin in the care settings and schools that mark early childhood and must continue throughout primary, secondary, and post-secondary education.

1. Impact of Pre-Kindergarten Programs on Children's Development

What do we know about the short-term and long-term impact of pre-kindergarten child development programs? This is a fundamental question for all child welfare, including its educational component. Many researchers have noted that numerous children, especially from low-income families, enter kindergarten already behind their age peers because of a lack of stimulating environments and experiences, and Cameron et al. (2020) recently made the case for universal early childhood education for young children in care. Good pre-K programs help children prepare for kindergarten and for their later schooling. In a timely review of the scientific literature, a pre-kindergarten task force of child development scholars from Duke University and the Brookings Institution (Phillips et al., 2017) produced a "consensus statement" on the impact of publicly funded pre-K programs on children's learning immediately following completion of pre-K and later in primary school. In their report, *Puzzling it Out: The Current State of Scientific Knowledge on Pre-Kindergarten Effects,* Phillips et al. (2017) formulated several major conclusions. First, research on pre-K children frequently finds that economically disadvantaged children show greater improvement in learning at the end of the pre-K year than do more economically advantaged children. These strong gains in learning are due to the disadvantaged children experiencing opportunities to acquire or enhance skills, knowledge, and attitudes linked with good school performance. Second, the trajectories taken by children's early learning depend on their experiences before and during pre-K but also in the early grades of primary school. Teachers' use of individualization and differentiation in classroom content and strategies seem especially important for longer-term learning in ensuring that children do not lose classroom time on material they have already mastered or that is too difficult for them. Third, much more evaluation, with high-quality research designs, is required to identify the cognitive skills, academic achievement, school retention, and social-emotional outcomes that pre-K programs actually influence, over the shorter and longer terms. Fourth, there is consistent evidence that children who attend public pre-K programs are more ready for school at the end of the pre-K year than children who do not attend. The evidence is robust that pre-K attenders benefit most frequently in literacy and numeracy, but evidence of their growth in social-emotional development and self-regulation is less abundant and suggests more modest progress. Fifth, evidence available on the longer-term effects of pre-K programs when introduced on a large scale is currently too limited to permit general conclusions. Existing evidence often points to measurable gains in learning during primary school, but sometimes there is no effect or even, for some programs, negative longer-term effects. Sixth, in future, progress is needed in designing, implementing, and evaluating pre-K programs, to enable children to make and retain even greater learning gains. Research partnerships between academics and field settings are one of the best ways of identifying pre-K and primary-school factors that contribute to positive long-term outcomes, especially when teaching interventions are implemented on a large scale. Increasingly, educational policy-makers are insisting on rigorous outcome measures and evidence of program effectiveness.

2. Early Childhood Education in Ontario

In a comprehensive report, *Affordable for All: Making Licensed Child Care Affordable in Ontario,* Cleveland (2018) addressed the question of what is the best way of improving the affordability and availability of licensed child care for infants, toddlers, and preschoolers in Ontario. His main recommendation was that the Government of Ontario should immediately implement free child care for children of pre-K or "preschool" age, 30 months to kindergarten age. Then, over a period of years, increased affordability should be phased in for infants and toddlers. In Ontario, in 2017, there were approximately 161,000 licensed centre spaces for infants, toddlers and preschoolers, that is, children aged 0–4, 106,000 (66%) of which were for pre-K children. Nearly 76% of Ontario's licensed child care centres were not-for-profits in 2017. Across Ontario, there were licensed spaces in centres and homes for infants, toddlers, and preschoolers to accommodate only about 23% of all children 0–4 years of age. (We have been unable to determine the proportion of the young children aged 0–4 who were served in these licensed spaces and were also children in out-of-home care. This is an important question because licensed centres and homes are typically of much higher quality than unlicensed child care, according to Cleveland [2018].)

Cleveland (2018) provided a summary of American and European studies of the effects of early childhood education on children that was in agreement with the consensus statement of Phillips et al. (2017) regarding the effects of public pre-K programs, while also including the effects on parents and on the cost-of-service provision to the Province of Ontario. Affordable child care would boost parents' employment and incomes and enhance women's participation in the labour force. Increased parental employment, in turn, would increase provincial tax revenues and reduce the net cost to Ontario of providing early childhood education and social assistance. For children, economically affordable early childhood education would promote children's intellectual, language, social, and emotional development and well-being, as well as improving their longer-term educational and employment prospects. Moreover, the quality of early childhood education and care has an important influence on the size of the effects on children's development.

3. The Motor, Social, and Cognitive Development of Young Children in Care, as Evaluated by the Ontario Looking After Children Project[1]

Young children learn about their environment through play and exploration, which stimulates growth in their sensory and perceptual systems and prepares the way for more complex cognitive functions, including language and self-regulation (Houwen et al., 2016; Osorio-Valencia et al., 2017). Children residing in out-of-home care, however, have often been exposed to maltreatment or neglect and experience delays in motor development (e.g., impairments to balance, speed, or spatial-perceptual skills) or deficits in attention, language, or executive functioning. These deficits, in turn, may be associated with lower measured IQ and academic underachievement (Osorio-Valencia et al., 2017; Houwen et al., 2016).

Early motor, social, and cognitive development plays an important role in young children's later academic success. In the general population, optimal motor developmental milestones in healthy infants are associated with later non-verbal, language, cognitive, and behavioural outcomes (Ghassabian et al., 2016). Attention, fine motor skills,

---

1.   We wish to thank Adrianna Côté, who carried out research based on OnLAC Project data related to young children during her BSc studies in psychology at the University of Ottawa, and Dr. Connie Cheung, who commented on an unpublished manuscript that was also based on OnLAC data related to young children in care. We have drawn upon their contributions in this section of Chapter 4.

and general knowledge are stronger predictors of reading, math, and science scores in primary school up to grade 5 than math and reading scores in kindergarten (Grissmer et al., 2010), and greater fine motor development is positively related to higher literacy and math skills in children (Pati et al., 2011). Moreover, the consequences of early life trauma from childhood abuse, neglect, and other adversities on the developing brain are well documented (Dube & McGiboney, 2018). Maltreatment early in life may compromise a child's language development and ability to regulate emotions, which in turn can jeopardize academic outcomes (Panlilio, Harden, & Harring, 2018). Conversely, academic success is a protective factor that contributes to positive physical, mental, emotional, and social well-being in children (Dube & McGiboney, 2018), which then promotes further learning and academic success (Panlilio et al., 2018).

Among children in care, research has often documented a relationship between poor educational outcomes and maltreatment experienced early in life (Tessier, O'Higgins, & Flynn, 2018; O'Higgins, Sebba, & Garner, 2017). Given that motor skills are considered a marker of school readiness (Cameron et al., 2012), we examined the relationship between activities by caregivers that promoted literacy and motor, social, and cognitive development among young children in care. We were able to control for a number of demographic, risk, and protective factors that past research suggests as potential confounds between literacy promotion and development: child sex, age, developmental delay, developmental disability, emotional and behavioural development, full-term birth, and general health. On the basis of previous research, we formulated two working hypotheses. First, we expected that early exposure to neglect or abuse would be associated in our sample of 520 young children in out-of-home care from the OnLAC Project with lower scores on our measure of overall development, the Motor and Social Development (MSD) Scale, than in children of the same age in the general population. Second, we anticipated that, net of the demographic, risk, and protective factors for which we were able to control, the more frequently the children's caregivers engaged with them in literacy-promoting activities, the higher would be the children's score on the MSD scale.

4. Participants

The sample was drawn from the OnLAC Project database, which at the time of data collection employed the 2010 version of the Assessment and Action Record (AAR-C2-2010; Flynn, Vincent, & Miller, 2011). The participants consisted of 520 young children, 56% boys (n = 289) and 44% girls (n = 231), who ranged in age from 12 to 47 months (M = 29.0, SD = 10.3); 70% had been full term at birth, 37% had a developmental delay, and 11% had a developmental disability. Twenty-nine percent were Indigenous and 10% were Black. The majority (87.5%) resided in foster homes, with the other 12.5% in kinship care homes. The primary language spoken in the foster or kinship homes was English, for 95.8% of the children.

5. Outcome Instrument

The MSD scale (U.S. National Longitudinal Survey of Youth, 1979) was embedded within the 2010 version of the AAR (AAR-C2-2010; Flynn, Vincent, & Miller, 2011). We used it as our measure of the level of the young child's motor, social, and cognitive development, relative to that of the general population of the same age (in months). Several national longitudinal studies in the general population in the United States, Canada, and the United Kingdom have employed the MSD scale (Grissmer et al., 2010). These studies indicate that family income has a positive effect on children's cognitive, motor, and social development (Aughinbaugh & Gittleman, 2003) and that mothers' level of formal education is associated with more favourable child birth weight, motor and social development, and early home learning environments (Carneiro, Meghir, & Parey, 2013).

The caregivers' literacy-promoting activities and the various demographic, risk, and protective factors for which we were able to control were part of the AAR instrument. Literacy promotion for children 1–2 years of age was assessed with a 10-item scale (sample items: "How often do you or your spouse or partner get a chance to do the following: Teach the child new words?" or "Read stories or show pictures or wordless baby books to the child?") Literacy promotion for children 3 years of age and over was evaluated with a 15-item scale (sample items: "How often do you or your spouse or partner get a chance to do the following: 'Teach the child to name printed letters and/or numbers?' or 'Encourage the child to use numbers in day-to-day activities, for example, counting the cookies on a plate?'") Prior to merging these two scales into a single measure that would cover the entire age range of the sample, we converted each scale to a T-score (M = 50, SD = 10). To derive the overall Cronbach's alpha of .59 for the merged literacy-promoting scale, we weighted Cronbach's alpha for the 10-item scale (.54) and for the 15-item scale (.68) by the number of children in each age group.

To test our first working hypothesis, we calculated the mean standard score of the sample on the MSD scale and compared it with the population mean (M = 100, SD = 15). To test the second hypothesis, we regressed the child's MSD score on the demographic variables of child sex and age, the risk variables of child developmental delay and developmental disability, and the four protective factors of child full-term birth status, general health, emotional and behavioural development [log10], and frequency of caregiver literacy-promotion activities.

6. Results

In our test of hypothesis 1, the mean standard score of the sample on the MSD scale was 88.67 (Mdn = 89.0; SD = 15.71), which was 0.76 SDs below the population mean of 100, a large effect size ($p < .001$). Thus, our first working hypothesis was supported. We had indeed found a lower average level of motor, social, and cognitive development in our sample of young children in care, compared with children of the same age in the general population.

Table 4.1 presents the results of our test of hypothesis 2. In our hierarchical regression model, we entered only those risk and protective variables that had been found to have a statistically significant zero-order correlation ($p < .01$) with the children's MSD score. At step 1, the control variables of sex and age accounted for a statistically significant increment in the variance accounted for in the MSD score (ΔR^2 = .03, $p < .001$), even though in the final model neither of the individual beta coefficients (i.e., partial standardized regression coefficients) was significant. At step 2, the two risk variables accounted for a large increment in the MSD variance (ΔR^2 = .22, $p < .001$), with both beta coefficients statistically significant in the final model. At step 3, the four protective variables explained an additional increment in the MSD variance (ΔR^2 = .07, $p < .001$), with all four beta coefficients significant in the final model. The model accounted for 32% of the total variance in the MSD score, and the largest beta coefficients were those for the presence of a developmental delay (β = -.30), the frequency of caregivers' literacy-promoting activities (β = .22), and the presence of a developmental disability (β = -.15).

7. Implications of the Results

It needs to be pointed out that the present regression model should be seen more as establishing a baseline for future research than as a formal hypothesis test. The reason is that we included in the regression model only those control, risk, and protective variables that we had already found to be significantly correlated with the child's MSD score.

The findings are cause for both concern as well as for cautious optimism. Alarming is the fact that despite an average age of only 29 months (range = 12–47 months), the young children in care were, on average, already three quarters of a standard deviation below children in the general population on motor, social, and cognitive development. As already noted, this is a large average effect size. It suggests that the children in the OnLAC sample would probably have benefited from high-quality pre-K programming, an intervention strategy advocated in the preceding section of this chapter.

Table 4.1. Beta coefficients from multiple regression of child's score on the Motor and Social Development scale on demographic, risk, and protective variables

Demographic Factors	Beta
Sex (1 = F, 0 = M)	.04
Age (in months)	-.03
Risk Factors	
Developmental disability (I = Yes, 0 = No)	-.15**
Developmental delay (1 = Yes, 0 = No)	-.30**
Protective Factors	
Full term at birth (1 = Yes, 0 = No)	.08*
Good general health (1 = Yes, 0 = No)	.08*
Emotional and behavioural development (log 10)	.09*
Frequency of literacy promotion by caregiver (T-score)	.22**

Notes. Sample composed of 520 children in care from OnLAC data set, aged 12–47 months (M = 29 months). Beta coefficients are standardized partial regression coefficients. R^2 = .32, $p < .001$.
*$p < .05$, **$p < .001$.
Source: Ontario Looking After Children Project data 2010–2015.

On the other hand, it was encouraging that the frequency of the caregivers' literacy-promoting activities in their day-to-day interactions with the children had a positive and statistically significant association with the latter's motor, social, and cognitive development. Caregivers, together with early childhood education, should thus be seen as important resources for promoting literacy and later academic achievement among young children in care, as Jackson and Hollingworth (2018) and Cameron et al. (2020) have argued.

Besides caregiver literacy-promotion activities, several other protective factors had statistically significant (albeit modest) associations with the child's motor, social, and cognitive development. It was not surprising that full-term status at birth had a net positive association with development, such that the child's full-term birth status, together with his or her possible prenatal exposure to drugs, alcohol, or other harmful substances or experiences, need to be routinely taken into account when plans of care are being formulated for young children in care.

The child's emotional and behavioural development is an important facet of overall development, and programs teaching social-emotional competence have been found to improve young children's prosocial behaviour (Schell et al., 2015). Finally, caregivers' activities in favour of literacy were positively linked to the young children's overall development. It is highly likely that virtually any young child in care would benefit from participating with a caregiver in activities such as reading a book together before bed, learning new words when out on errands, or singing action songs together. The fact that our relatively large Ontario sample of 520 young children in care scored on average three quarters of a standard deviation below children of the same age in the general population is an urgent summons to use all the educational science at our disposal to help children in care reach their full potential.

8. Developmental and Social-Emotional Screening and Monitoring of Young Children in Care with the Ages and Stages Questionnaires, as Evaluated by the Ontario Looking After Children Project

The gap of 0.75 standard deviations between the average level of development of young children in care in Ontario and their age peers in the general population, presented in the immediately preceding section, raises immediately the question of what, if anything, do we intend to do about it. Below, we discuss the findings from several of the randomized trials of tutoring with children in care that we have conducted in Ontario, along with much other systematic evidence, that tutoring should play a central role in efforts to close the educational achievement gap between children in care and those in the general population. Before we do so, however, we will present some further findings from the OnLAC Project on the overall and social-emotional development of young children in care in Ontario and on factors related to their progress. These findings derive from the use of the well-known screening and monitoring tools, the Ages and Stages Questionnaires, which we have embedded in the current version of the AAR (i.e., AAR-C2-2016). These tools consist of the Ages and Stages Questionnaires, Third Edition (ASQ-3), a general instrument for assessing overall early child development, and the Ages and Stages Questionnaire: Social-Emotional (ASQ:SE), for assessing social-emotional development. (Both instruments have been incorporated into the AAR-C2-2016 and are described in the *User's Manual for the AAR-C2-2016*; Miller, Vincent, & Flynn, 2017.)

9. Ages and Stages Questionnaires, Third Edition (ASQ-3)

According to the *ASQ-3 User's Guide* (Squires et al., 2009), the ASQ-3 is a caregiver-completed screening and monitoring tool that requires 10–20 minutes to complete on an individual child. Intended for children aged 1–66 months, it consists of questionnaires for 21 different age intervals, each questionnaire 30 items in length. In the OnLAC Project context, the ASQ-3 covers a slightly shorter age range (6–66 months) because the OnLAC Project serves virtually no children younger than 6 months, and thus includes 19 rather than 21 questionnaires. It comprises 5 developmental measures at each of the 19 age intervals:

- Communication skills: babbling, vocalizing, listening, and understanding;
- Gross motor skills: arm, body, and leg movements;
- Fine motor skills: hand and fingers movements;
- Problem-solving skills: learning and playing with toys; and
- Personal-social skills: solitary play and play with toys and other children.

With the ASQ-3, *a higher score signifies a higher level of skill or development on the part of the child.* An advantage of the ASQ-3 is that it makes use of learning activities (Twombly & Fink, 2013) that can help the child improve his or her current level of overall development.

10. Ages and Stages Questionnaire: Social-Emotional (ASQ:SE)

According to the *ASQ:SE User's Guide* (Squires, Bricker, & Trombly, 2003), the ASQ:SE, like the ASQ-3, is also a caregiver-completed screening and monitoring tool. It is intended for use with infants and children aged 3–65 months and consists of questionnaires for 6, 12, 18, 24, 30, 36, 48, and 60 months, which vary in length between 19 and 33 items (for technical details, see Miller et al., 2017). The instrument addresses seven social-emotional behavioural areas:

- Self-regulation ability: ability to calm, settle down, or adjust to stimulation;
- Compliance ability: ability to conform to direction by others and to rules;
- Communication ability: ability to respond to verbal or non-verbal signals;
- Adaptive functioning ability: ability to cope with physiological needs;
- Autonomy ability: ability to self-initiate or respond without guidance;
- Affect ability: ability to demonstrate own feelings and empathy for others; and
- Interaction with people ability: ability to initiate or respond to social responses.

With the ASQ:SE, *a higher score signifies a higher level of social-emotional difficulty on the part of the child.* There are empirically derived cut-off scores for each questionnaire. As with the ASQ-3, the ASQ:SE also makes use of learning activities (Twombly, Munson, & Pribble, 2018) to enable the child to improve his or her current level of social-emotional development. It is noteworthy that in their systematic review of social-emotional screening instruments for young children in child welfare, McCrae and Brown (2018) recommended the ASQ:SE because of its good internal consistency (alpha coefficient = .82) and good evidence of validity. Comparable evidence also exists for the internal consistency and validity of the ASQ-3.

10.1. Illustrative Uses of the ASQ and ASQ:SE in Child Welfare Contexts

In the last decade, the ASQ and ASQ:SE have found increasing use in practice and research by child welfare agencies or child development organizations directly relevant to child welfare practice or policy. What follows are a few examples from Canada and elsewhere.

In Quebec, Dionne et al. (2014) examined the use of the second edition of the ASQ with 282 young children (130 girls, 152 boys), aged 9–66 months and served by the Child and Family Centre, Mohawk Territory, Quebec. Teachers and parents of the children completed the tool. The parents and teachers agreed in 85% of the cases about referring the child for additional evaluation, and the use of the ASQ was judged culturally appropriate for use in the Indigenous community. Moreover, the internal consistency of the ASQ on the Indigenous sample was generally acceptable, with the authors suggesting further improvements and adaptations of the tool with Mohawk children.

McKelvey et al. (2017) used the ASQ-3 with a large sample of 2,004 young children, aged 32 months on average (range = 13–76 months). The children came from families in Arkansas who were almost all at or below 133% of the federal U.S. poverty line. The families were enrolled in one of three evidence-based home visiting programs, including Healthy Families America, a program for at-risk parents to prevent child abuse or neglect. Children identified as at risk on the ASQ-3 in one or more areas of child development (communication, problem-solving, gross motor development, fine motor development, or personal-social development) were also found more likely to have experienced four or more adverse childhood experiences.

Mastorakos and Scott (2019), in Ontario, studied a sample of 55 preschool children, aged 18 to 70 months (M = 41.7 months, SD = 13.0), to discover whether those who had been exposed to domestic violence (n = 23) exhibited hypervigilance and anxiety when exposed to angry or sad faces versus happy or neutral faces, compared with the non-exposed young children (n = 32). The researchers also investigated whether such vigilance was related to children's social-emotional development, as measured with the ASQ:SE-2. They found that 46% of the children previously exposed to domestic violence scored in the moderate to high-risk range for social-emotional problems, compared with only 13% of the non-exposed children. Also, the presence of greater social-emotional problems was related to an attentional bias away from sad and neutral faces but not from happy or angry faces. Mastorakos and Scott (2019) suggested that attention training might help exposed children to reduce hypervigilance and anxiety in the presence of negative stimuli and increase their attention to positive stimuli and their well-being.

McCrae, Cahalane, and Fusco (2011) derived directions for developmental screening in child welfare based on the use of both the ASQ and the ASQ:SE with a sample of 570 young children, aged 0–3. Both instruments are used in Pennsylvania to screen all children aged 0–3 who have been exposed to substantiated maltreatment. McCrae et al. (2011) found, on the ASQ, that 22% of the children scored in the problem range on at least one of the five developmental areas that had been assessed (14% were in the problem range on communication skills, 8% on fine motor skills, 8% on problem-solving skills, 7% on personal-social skills, and 6% on gross motor skills). On the ASQ:SE, 18% scored in the problem range on social-emotional concerns. Finally, when both overall and social-emotional development were taken together (i.e., when the assessment was based on both the ASQ and ASQ:SE), 31% of the children warranted a referral to early intervention services. Moreover, the rate of developmental and social-emotional concerns was higher when the screening was carried out by early-intervention personnel rather than by child welfare staff, 49% versus 27%. This suggested a need for further education and training of child welfare personnel in child development and the attainment of developmental milestones.

10.2. Results of Screening and Monitoring of Young Children in Care with the ASQ-3 and ASQ:SE, as Evaluated by the Ontario Looking After Children Project

Tables 4.2 and 4.3, respectively, show the screening and monitoring results obtained in the OnLAC Project with young children in care, aged 0–5, with the ASQ-3 (N = 834) and ASQ:SE (N = 910). (See the *User's Manual for the AAR-C2-2016* [Miller, Vincent, & Flynn, 2017] for instructions on scoring the ASQ-3 and the ASQ:SE from data obtained with the AAR-C2-2016 instrument.)

The results for the ASQ-3 (see Table 4.2) suggest that the development of a good number of very young children in care in Ontario is proceeding reasonably well, as on all five dimensions of development, about 60%–75% of the children score *above* the cut-off. However, according to Squires et al. (2009), such children should be *followed up* and *screened* at regular intervals (e.g., at 9, 18, 24, and/or 30 months). At the same time, in our sample, roughly 10%–15% of the young children in care scored *near* the cut-off, indicating a need for *monitoring* and perhaps *screening again* in a short time. Also, *referral* to a community program, such as Head Start, for developmental activities may be judged appropriate for children near the cut-off. Finally, depending

Table 4.2. Percentage of young children in the Ontario Looking After Children Project sample (*N* = 834), aged 0–5, scoring above, near, or below the ASQ-3 cut-off in five areas of development

	0–11 Months (*n* = 124)	12–23 Months (*n* = 214)	24 Months (*n* = 172)	3–5 Years (*n* = 324)
Communication Area	(%)	(%)	(%)	(%)
Above cut-off	85	72	63	67
Near cut-off	7	15	12	13
Below cut-off	8	13	25	20
Gross Motor Area				
Above cut-off	59	63	74	74
Near cut-off	13	14	11	11
Below cut-off	28	24	15	15
Fine Motor Area				
Above cut-off	59	63	74	74
Near cut-off	13	14	11	11
Below cut-off	28	24	15	15
Problem-Solving Area				
Above cut-off	61	63	61	73
Near cut-off	18	13	17	13
Below cut-off	21	23	23	15
Personal-Social Area				
Above cut-off	69	68	67	72
Near cut-off	15	14	13	14
Below cut-off	15	18	19	14

Note. Squires et al. (2009) note that children scoring *above* the cut-off on the ASQ-3 are *not identified* but should be *followed up* and *screened* at regular intervals. Children *near* the cutoff should be *monitored*, perhaps screened again in a short time, and *referred* for early interrvention services (e.g., a Head Start program in the community). Children scoring *below* the cutoff are *identified* and should be *referred* for further assessment and early intervention services.
Source: Ontario Looking After Children Project data, 2016–2018.

Table 4.3. Percentage of young children in the Ontario Looking
After Children Project sample (*N* = 910), aged 0–5, scoring below
the ASQ:SE cut-off

Age Group	Percentage *below* ASQ:SE Cut-Off
6 Months	100%
12 Months	95%
18 Months	83%
24 Months	83%
30 Months	82%
36 Months	65%
48 Months	70%
60 Months	54%
0–11 Months (n = 142)	97%
12–23 Months (n = 250)	87%
24–35 Months (n = 184)	80%
3–5 Years (n = 334)	61%

Note. Children scoring *below* the cut-off on the ASQ:SE are *not* identified and thus are seen as *not*
needing a referral for further assessment or early intervention at this time.
Source: Ontario Looking After Children Project data, 2016–2018.

on the age of the children and the area of development, about 10%–
25% scored *below* the cut-off. Squires et al. (2009) would recommend
that such children be *referred* for further assessment of their needs and
for potential enrollment in early intervention services.

In the OnLAC Project, we have used multiple regression to relate
a number of risk and protective factors to the overall level of development (as measured by the ASQ-3) of young children in care, aged 0–5.
Overall child development has been found to be positively associated
with the *protective factors* of more frequent literacy-promoting activities by caregivers ($p < .001$), fewer child social-emotional difficulties
($p < .001$), child female sex ($p < .01$), fewer children living in the home
($p < .05$), child placement in a kinship care home ($p < .05$), and a more
positive view of self by the child ($p < .05$). The *risk factors* of a greater
number of child socio-emotional difficulties ($p < .001$) and a greater
number of children living in the home ($p < .001$) have been found to be
negatively related to the child's overall development.

Table 4.3 displays the percentage of young children in care aged
0–5 who, in the OnLAC Project, manifested positive socio-emotional
development. That is, they scored *below* the ASQ:SE cut-off, were
thus *not identified,* and therefore were seen as *not needing* a referral

for further assessment or early intervention at that time. Associated with positive social-emotional development have been the *protective factors* of more positive parenting ($p < .01$) and higher levels of several skills assessed by means of the ASQ-3: communication skills ($p < .01$), personal-social skills ($p < .01$), and problem-solving skills ($p < .05$). *Risk factors* negatively linked with social-emotional development include developmental delay ($p < .001$), more frequent changes in caregivers ($p < .001$), older child age ($p < .001$), and African or Caribbean ethnicity ($p < .05$). Finally, we have found that young children's overall development (as reflected in the ASQ-3 total score) and social-emotional development (as reflected in the total ASQ:SE score) are strongly correlated ($r = -.51$, $p < .001$). This is actually a *positive* correlation because a *higher* score on the ASQ-3 and a *lower* score on the ASQ:SE are both *positive* in meaning. Thus, interventions that improve children's overall development are also likely to improve social-emotional development, and vice versa.

11. Educational Outcomes of Young People of Primary, Secondary, and Post–Secondary School Age in Ontario, as Assessed with the Assessment and Action Record

We note here that the AAR has good theoretical and operational links with the outcome of educational success. When we created the AAR in 2000, after receiving the original Social Sciences and Humanities Research Council of Canada (SSHRC) grant, the National Longitudinal Survey of Children and Youth (NLSCY) served as our template. At the time, the NLSCY, created by Statistics Canada in collaboration with then Human Resources and Social Development Canada, provided the main social policy framework and longitudinal data set for empirical research on the development of children, adolescents, and young adults in Canada. Over the years, we have replaced a number of NLSCY measures in the AAR with standardized instruments that we have judged to be of superior psychometric quality or greater utility in the child welfare context, such as our OnLAC measure of developmental assets.

Also, in a direct test of the comprehensiveness and content validity of the AAR and its predictive validity vis-à-vis educational outcomes among young people in care, Tessier, O'Higgins, and Flynn (2018) analyzed a cross-sectional OnLAC sample of 3,659 youths in care, aged 11–17. They tested the ability of the AAR to operationalize

20 conceptual variables identified in a systematic review by O'Higgins, Sebba, and Gardner (2017) as the key factors associated with educational achievement among children in kinship or foster care. In their study, Tessier et al. (2018) were able to operationalize in their OnLAC sample 15 of the 20 identified conceptual variables, using a total of 19 indicators from the AAR (several conceptual variables were operationalized with multiple indicators). At the final step of a hierarchical regression model, 12 of the 19 variables from the AAR were significant predictors of individual educational success. In three-year longitudinal analyses, based on a sample of 962 youths in care, five of the individual predictors were significant in the final regression model. In both the cross-sectional and longitudinal models, internal developmental assets were an especially important predictor of educational success.

12. Educational Performance in Reading and Math of Young People in Care of Primary- or Secondary-School Age, as Evaluated by the Ontario Looking After Children Project

Having seen how children in care who are younger than school age are faring in terms of their development in Ontario, we will now look at indicators of the progress of young people in care who are in primary, secondary, or post-secondary education. We use recent OnLAC AAR data from 2019 to answer this question. We do so, however, in the disturbing knowledge that, even before COVID-19, of the approximately 400,000 5-year-old children across Canada who were enrolled in kindergarten in 2020, roughly 100,000 (25%) will probably not be able to read and write well enough to keep up in grade 4 and it is likely that they will never catch up (O'Sullivan, 2020).

Tables 4.4.1 and 4.4.2 present data from 2019 for Ontario's performance indicators (PI) for education in reading and math for Ontario societies. These PIs are derived from OnLAC data for young people in care who were enrolled in 2019 in primary or secondary school in Ontario. The education PIs consist of brief ratings made each year by the young person's child welfare worker. The worker rates the young person's performance's abilities in school, first in reading and then in math, compared with his or her chronological age group and the grade in school in which a student of his or her chronological age is expected to be enrolled. The young person's performance in reading or math is rated by the worker as follows:

- as *excellent* if the young person is in the school grade appropriate for their chronological age (e.g., grade 8) but is actually reading or doing math at a higher-grade level (e.g., grade 9 or 10);
- as *good* if the young person is in the grade level appropriate for their age (e.g., grade 8) and is also reading or doing math at that same grade level (e.g., grade 8);
- as *fair* if the young person is in the school grade appropriate for their chronological age but is actually reading or doing math at a lower level (e.g., grade 7 or 6); and
- as *poor* if the young person is in a school grade lower than the appropriate grade for their chronological age (e.g., in grade 7 rather than grade 8) and is also reading or doing math at a lower level (e.g., grade 7 or 6).

The two items (performance in reading and performance in math) were highly correlated among both young children in care, aged 6–9 ($r = .83$) and older young people, aged 10–17 ($r = .71$), indicating that in both age groups, the two items were tapping the same construct of educational performance. Regarding the concurrent validity of the reading and math items, among 6-to-9-year-old children in care, performance in reading (as rated by the child welfare worker) correlated highly ($r = .74$) with a rating by the child's caregiver on a single-item measure of how well the child was doing in reading and other language arts (Flynn & Miller, 2017). Similarly, the worker's rating of the child's math performance correlated highly ($r = .66$) with the caregiver's rating of how well the child was doing in math. Similarly, among 10-to-15-year-olds in care, performance in reading (as rated by the worker) correlated highly ($r = .64$) with a rating by the young person's caregiver on a single-item measure of how well the young person was doing in reading and other language arts. Also, the worker's rating of the young person's performance in math correlated highly ($r = .61$) with the caregiver's rating of how well the young person was doing in math.

12.1. Performance in Reading in Primary School

Table 4.4.1 displays the results for performance in reading for 1,401 children of primary-school age (6–13 years) on this educational PI in 2019. Overall, the girls' performance in reading was better than

Table 4.4.1. Educational performance in reading of young people in care of primary-school age (6–13 years) in Ontario, by sex

	Females		Males		Total	
A. Performance in Reading (N = 1,401):	n	%	n	%	n	%
Excellent (above expected grade level)	70	11.4	83	10.5	153	10.9
Good (at expected grade level)	269	43.8	248	31.5	517	36.9
Fair (Below grade level)	181	29.5	244	31.0	425	30.3
Poor (Much below expected grade level)	94	15.3	212	26.9	306	21.8
Total	614	100.0	787	100.0	1401	100.0

$\chi^2(3) = 35.97$, $p < .001$, Cramer's $V = .160$ (95% CI = .115, .217).

that of the boys ($p < .001$), with a higher proportion rated as "good" and fewer as "poor." This is consistent with results favouring female educational performance and attainment in other studies of young people in care and in the general population (Kirk et al., 2012). Still, 44.8% of the girls (compared with 57.9% of the boys) were rated as only "fair" or "poor" in reading, suggesting a need for considerable improvement in many of the girls (and boys) in care if they were to succeed in their future schooling, as reading is key to performance in math and science as well.

12.2. Performance in Math in Primary School

In Table 4.4.2, in which the performance in math in 2019 is shown for 1,403 young people in care from the OnLAC Project, the girls again outperformed the boys ($p < .001$), although by a lesser margin than in reading. However, among both the girls (52.2%) and the boys (56.2%), more than half were rated as only "fair" or "poor." These findings are consistent with the position articulated by Phillips et al. (2017) and Cameron et al. (2020) on the need to make early intervention programs such as pre-K available in Ontario and Canada, especially for children who show early signs of falling behind academically. These results are also congruent with the sizeable gap in the average motor, social, and cognitive development of young children that we noted earlier in this chapter.

Table 4.4.2. Educational performance in math of young people in care of primary-school age (6–13 years) in Ontario, by sex

B. Performance in Math (1,403):	Females		Males		Total	
	n	%	n	%	n	%
Excellent (above expected grade level)	34	5.5	60	7.6	94	6.7
Good (at expected grade level)	260	42.3	285	36.2	545	38.8
Fair (Below grade level)	225	36.6	249	31.6	474	33.8
Poor (Much below expected grade level)	96	15.6	194	24.6	290	20.7
Total	615	100.0	788	100.0	1403	100.0

$\chi^2(3)$ - 21.67, $p < .001$, Cramer's V = .124 (95% CI = .080, .181).
Source: Ontario Looking After Children Project data from 2019.

12.3. Performance in Reading in Secondary School

The results for young people in care of secondary-school age (14–17 years) in 2019 are shown in Tables 4.5.1 and 4.5.2. Table 4.5.1 shows that a higher proportion of the girls were rated as either "excellent" or "good" in reading (62.2%), compared with less than half (45.3%) of the boys ($p < .001$). Concomitantly, fewer girls were rated as only fair or poor.

12.4. Performance in Math in Secondary School

As shown in Table 4.5.2, the girls were again more likely to be rated as "excellent" or "good" (49.7% vs. 35.9% for the boys) and less likely to be rated as "poor." When we compare the strength of the association between sex and performance in reading and math among the children of primary-school age and in the young people of secondary-school age, we note that in both age groups, Cramer's V is larger in the older group, for both reading and math performance. As mentioned earlier, this result suggests that as the curriculum becomes more difficult and demanding, the child who is struggling in primary school will find secondary school even more challenging. From this reality flows the necessity of intervening as early as possible, with more systematic screening and monitoring with the ASQ-3, more regular referrals to community pre-K programs and other early intervention services, and greater use of evidence-based programs such as academic tutoring (covered below in this chapter).

Table 4.5.1. Educational performance in reading of young people in care of secondary-school age (14–17 years) in Ontario, by sex

	Females		Males		Total	
Performance in Reading (N = 1,414):	n	%	n	%	n	%
Excellent (above expected grade level)	126	19.4	70	9.2	196	13.9
Good (at expected grade level)	311	47.8	276	36.1	587	41.5
Fair (below grade level)	131	20.2	232	30.4	363	25.7
Poor (much below expected grade level)	82	12.6	186	24.3	268	19.0
Total	650	100.0	764	100.0	1414	100.0

$\chi^2(3) = 77.86$, $p < .001$, Cramer's $V = .235$ (95% CI = .188, .287).
Source: Ontario Looking After Children Project data from 2019.

Table 4.5.2. Educational performance in math of young people in care of secondary-school age (14–17 years) in Ontario, by sex

	Females		Males		Total	
Performance in Math (1,403):	n	%	n	%	n	%
Excellent (above expected grade level)	49	7.6	46	6.1	95	6.8
Good (at expected grade level)	271	42.1	226	29.8	497	35.4
Fair (below grade level)	198	30.7	273	36.0	471	31.9
Poor (much below expected grade level)	126	19.6	214	28.2	340	23.1
Total	644	100.0	759	100.0	1403	100.0

$\chi^2(3) = 29.66$, $p < .001$, Cramer's $V = .145$ (95% CI = .100, .202).
Source: Ontario Looking After Children Project data from 2019.

13. Educational Performance of Ontario Young People in Care Compared with That of Ontario Students as a Whole in Primary or Secondary School, 2016–2017

Thanks to an information-sharing agreement between the Ontario Association of Children's Aid Societies (OACAS) and the Ontario Ministry of Education, we are now able to compare the educational performance of young people in care in 2016–2017 with that of students as a whole at the same levels in Ontario. The data in Table 4.6 reveal the large dimensions of the task facing societies and schools as

Table 4.6. Comparison of educational achievement in reading, writing, and math of Ontario students in out-of-home care versus Ontario students as a whole in 2016-2017 school year

	Reading		Writing		Math	
Educational Achievement Criterion	In-care (%)	Ont (%)	In-care (%)	Ont (%)	In-care (%)	Ont (%)
EQAO grade 3 results: Percent at or above provincial standard (levels 3 and 4)	41.2	73.9	47.6	73.3	29.3	62.4
EQAO grade 6 results: Percent at or above provincial standard (levels 3 and 4)	44.1	81.2	44.1	79.1	14.3	49.5
EQAO grade 9 academic math results: Percent at or above provincial standards (levels 3 and 4)	—	±	—	—	58.2	83.3
EQAO grade 9 applied math results: Percent at or above provincial standards (levels 3 and 4)	—	—	—	—	36.9	44.0

Note. EQAO = Educational Quality and Accountability Office (of Ontario).
Source: Ontario Educational Quality and Accountability Office (EQAO).

they try to help young people in care to raise their educational performance to levels as comparable as possible with those of students in the province as a whole. In reading and writing, as assessed in grades 3 and 6 by the Ontario Educational Quality and Accountability Office (EQAO), the percentage of children in care who attained the provincial standard of levels 3 or 4 (out of four possible levels, 1–4) was between 54% and 65% of the percentage of children in the province as a whole. Moreover, in grade 6 math, the percentage of children in care attaining the provincial standard was only 29% of the percentage of children in the province as a whole who did so. The gap was smaller in grade 9 academic math (70%) or applied math (84%), but in the latter grade, in neither the in-care group nor in the province as a whole did a majority of students attain the expected standard. It is clear that without widespread use of evidence-based learning interventions like those described later in this chapter—and from an early age—it will be very difficult to improve upon the current situation.

High-quality tutoring, the best intervention we can offer struggling children next to good classroom teaching, is especially needed in both reading and math.

In Table 4.7, the data for the high school years paint a similar portrait. In the case of grade 10 results, students in care who were "first-time eligible" successfully completed the Ontario Secondary School Literacy Test (OSSLT) only 60% as often, on average, as did students in the province as a whole. Of those who were "previously eligible," only 65% as a lot completed the OSSLT. Regarding the accumulation of credits in high school, which is a criterion of educational attainment to which some society educational consultants attribute greater credibility than they do to meeting the EQAO provincial standard of levels 3 or 4, 65% as many young people in care as young people in the province as a whole had attained the provincial standard. In grade 10,

Table 4.7. Comparison of educational achievement in literacy and credit accumulation at similar grade levels of Ontario students in out-of-home care versus students in the province as a whole in the 2016-2017 school year

Educational Achievement Criterion	Ontario Students in Out-of-Home Care (%)	Ontario Students as a Whole (%)
OSSLT grade 10 results: Percent who successfully completed the OSSLT when "first-time eligible" (FTE)	48.5	80.6
OSSLT grade 10 results: Percent who successfully completed the OSSLT when "previously eligible" (PE)	32.0	49.1
Grade 9 credit accumulation: Percent at or above the provincial standard	57.0	87.1
Grade 10 credit accumulation: Percent at or above the provincial standard	38.9	79.2
Grade 11 credit accumulation: Percent at or above the provincial standard	38.3	82.0
Percent of students receiving special education programs and/or services	59.8	17.9
Percent of students who were suspended at least once	18.4	2.67
Percent of students who were expelled at least once	0.2	0.02

Source: Ontario Association of Children's Aid Societies and Ontario Ministry of Education.
OSSLT = Ontario Secondary School Literacy Test.

however, this had declined to 49% and, in grade 11, to 47%. Regarding special education, 3.34% as many young people in care had been enrolled in special education programs or services. Concerning suspensions, 6.89% as many young people in care had been suspended at least once, and 10 times as much had been expelled at least once.

14. Educational Outcomes of Young People in Care of Post-Secondary Age (18–21 Years) in Ontario, as Evaluated by the Ontario Looking After Children Project

In order to have as large a sample as possible of young people of post-secondary age, we created an unduplicated sample of all young adults in Continued Care and Support for Youth (CCSY) who had been 18–21 years of age when they had completed the AAR in either 2016, 2017, 2018, or 2019. (Young adults aged 18–21 were not considered to be technically "in care," such that the Ministry of Children, Communities and Social Services [MCCSS] had not mandated the use of the AAR with 18-to-21-year-olds, but only with young people aged 0–17.) Because it was not required by MCCSS, many societies did not use the AAR with 18-to-21-year-olds, despite its acknowledged utility with this age group. Of the 301 young adults aged 18–21 in this unduplicated sample, 151 were aged 18 (50.2%), 94 were 19 (31.2%), 54 were 20 (17.9%) and only 2 were 21 (0.7%).

The top panel (A) of Table 4.8 indicates that the young women were more likely to be enrolled in a post-secondary program than the young men. Relatively few members of our OnLAC sample of post–secondary school age (18–21) were currently in a university program (5.8%), versus almost three times as many enrolled in a community college or career college program (14.6%), with most of the latter (39 of 44) in community college. The combined percentage in post-secondary programs was still relatively small (19.3%). Most worrying was the fact that 44.2% and virtually as high a proportion of young women as young men, were seemingly not enrolled in school at all, and this at a period in their lives when building human and social capital was fundamental to their personal futures. The bottom panel (B) of Table 4.8 shows that of the 270 young adults in extended care and maintenance (ECM) of post-secondary age who reported the highest grade, diploma, or technical trade program that they had currently completed, only 3.3% had obtained a university degree, community college diploma, or post-secondary technical/trade credential. The

Table 4.8. Educational outcomes of OnLAC Project young people in care of post-secondary age (i.e., 18–21 years) in 2016–2019 (*N* = 301)

A. Type of Educational Program in Which Youth Was Currently Enrolled (*N* = 301).	Females		Males		Total	
	n	%	*n*	%	*n*	%
University undergrad program	9	5.8	5	3.4	14	4.7
Community college/Private career college	28	18.2	16	10.9	44	14.6
High school/Secondary school	27	17.5	45	30.6	72	23.9
Alternative or adult high school	24	15.6	14	9.5	38	12.6
Not currently in school	66	42.9	67	45,6	133	44.2
Total	**154**	**100.0**	**147**	**100.0**	**301**	**100.0**

$X2(4) = 11.40$, $p = .022$; Cramer's $V = .195$, $p = 022$ (95% CI = .115, .322).

B. Highest Degree, Diploma, or Grade Youth had Currently Completed (*N* = 270).	Females		Males		Total	
	n	%	*n*	%	*n*	%
University degree, community college diploma, or technical/ trade program above high school	5	3.5	4	3.1	9	3.3
High school diploma (grade 12) or equivalent	77	54.6	52	40.3	129	47.8
Grade 11	40	28.4	53	41.1	93	34.4
Grade 10	9	6.4	9	7.0	18	6.7
Grade 9 or less	10	7.1	11	8.5	21	7.8
Total	**141**	**100.0**	**129**	**100.0**	**270**	**100.0**

$X2(4) = 6.30$, $p = .178$; Cramer's $V = .153$, $p = .178$ (95%, CI = .090, .292).

Source: Ontario Looking After Children Project data.

difference between the young women and young men in this regard was not statistically significant. In this still relatively young sample, almost half (47.8%), not surprisingly, were completing the last year of high school (grade 12). However, about a third were still in grade 11 and one in seven (14.5%) was still in grades 10, 9, or lower.

Clearly, the overall progress of this age cohort needs to be improved. For this to occur, however, improved support and results will first be required at the pre-K and primary-school levels, where basic academic skills are formed. We turn now to describing evidence-based interventions that, if applied, will enable greater educational achievements to become a reality at all levels, over the shorter and longer terms.

15. Interventions to Improve Learning Outcomes in Young People in Care

One of the ambitions of the present book is to encourage direct service persons, supervisors, managers, caregivers, and policy-makers in child welfare to genuinely adopt evidence-based interventions and policies in serving young people who are in out-of-home care or still with their families of origin. Only care that is supported by strong evidence of effectiveness will be able progressively to close the large educational, mental health, and employment gaps that often separate the achievements of young people who have been maltreated or neglected from those of their more advantaged peers in the general population. Unevaluated approaches have not worked in the past, nor will they do so in future. The time has long since arrived for educational, social, and psychological science to occupy a central role in guiding the choice of programs and policies that we use in child welfare services in Ontario, Canada, or other countries. Fifteen years ago already, a Canadian study identified the most pressing research question that child welfare practitioners and managers had formulated for researchers in the field: *How well are current services working for clients, both in the short-term and across the lifespan?* (Vandermeulen, Wekerle, & Ylagan, 2005). In other words, practitioners and managers in child welfare want to provide *effective* services, and this desire is not new. Now is the time to honour this wish.

Fortunately, we now have numerous evidence-based interventions at our disposal to promote the learning and well-being of young people in child welfare, and we will describe many of them now. After covering a wide range of evidence-based interventions for younger and then older children and young people, we will outline an important new meta-analysis on educational tutoring, as well as our own randomized trials on tutoring with young people in care in Ontario. Based on a strong research consensus and as we have mentioned previously, high-quality tutoring is the single most effective intervention that we have to improve the reading and math skills of young people in care. However, it needs to be employed in schools and child welfare organizations much more frequently than it has in the past. Persuaded that many practitioners and policy-makers in child welfare do not use evidence-based interventions because they do not know about them, we now provide overviews of four highly accessible online sources of validated interventions capable of improving learning and well-being outcomes for children and youths in care. Our descriptions here of evidence-based interventions that can be used in child welfare introduce the topic but certainly do not pretend to exhaust it.

16. What Works Clearinghouse (WWC)

The What Works Clearinghouse (WWC) is part of the U.S. Institute of Educational Sciences (http://ies.ed.gov/ncee/wwc/findwhatworks. aspx). It provides much information on a wide range of topics relevant to interventions with young children, such as early childhood education. For each intervention, the WWC provides an *improvement index* (i.e., the average gain in terms of percentiles) that previous research suggests may be expected for students receiving the intervention), a rating of *effectiveness* in producing desired outcomes, and the amount of *evidence* available (small vs. medium to large). These are all things that a high-expectancy, outcomes-focused practitioner, manager, or policy-maker will be looking for.

For example, the WWC's (2009) practice guide, *Organizing Instruction and Study to Improve Student Learning,* provides a number of practical suggestions, each rated according to the strength of the evidence in its favour. A few examples of the suggestions associated with this particular practice guide, together with the rated strength of the evidence in favour of each suggestion, with further detailed information also provided should the reader wish to consult it, are as follows:

- *Space learning over time.* Arrange to review key elements of course content after delay of several weeks to several months after initial presentation (moderate evidence).
- *Interleave worked example solutions with problem-solving exercises.* Have students alternate between reading already worked solutions and trying to solve problems on their own (moderate evidence).
- *Use quizzing to promote learning.* Use quizzes to re-expose students to key content (strong evidence).

17. The Educational Endowment Foundation Toolkits

The Educational Endowment Foundation (EEF) in the United Kingdom is an independent charity whose goal is to pursue greater social equality and mobility by enabling young people from a range of socioeconomic backgrounds to pursue post-secondary education and realize their full potential. The EEF has produced two useful and accessible summaries of educational research, the Early Years Toolkit and the Teaching and Learning Toolkit. Both toolkits are designed to help school and social agency personnel make well-informed decisions about how to improve learning outcomes, especially for disadvantaged young people. The toolkits present a large number of evidence-based approaches to improving teaching and learning, each summarized in terms of its average *impact*, its *cost*, and the strength of the *evidence* supporting it. The toolkits do not make definitive claims as to what will work to better outcomes in a given setting. Rather, they provide high-quality information about what is likely to be beneficial, based on existing evidence. Both toolkits are updated on a regular basis as new findings from high-quality research become available.

18. Early Years Toolkit from EEF in the United Kingdom (0–3 Years of Age)

The Early Years Toolkit provides information on twelve complementary approaches to improving the cognitive, social, emotional, and physical development and learning of young children aged 0–3 (https://educationendowmentfoundation.org.uk/evidence/early-years-toolkit). It is thus highly congruent with the focus on development and well-being of the present book. As noted earlier, for each of the twelve approaches, the Early Years Toolkit has rated its impact (i.e., the average months of learning that prior research indicates will be gained by a child in a year of exposure to the approach), cost, and the amount of evidence available. The toolkit also presents handy summaries of the available research and suggestions for teachers, tutors, and others who want to obtain maximum benefit from the toolkit.

We have listed the twelve approaches in the Early Years Toolkit in Table 4.9, and EEF has provided more information on the website. For example, *communication and language approaches* have been found to have a *high impact* (an average achievement gain of six months over a school year) and *very low cost*, based on *extensive evidence. Parental*

Table 4.9. Early Years Toolkit from UK's Educational Endowment Foundation (0-3 years)

Learning approaches	Impact and months gained on average in 1 year of exposure	Cost	Amount of Evidence
Communication and language approaches	High impact, +6 months	Very low cost	Based on extensive evidence
Early numeracy approaches	High impact, +6 months	Very low cost	Based on extensive evidence
Earlier starting age	High impact, +6 months	Very high cost	Based on moderate evidence
Play-based learning	Moderate impact, +5 months.	Very low cost	Based on very limited evidence
Self-regulation strategies	Moderate impact, +5 months	Very low cost	Based on limited evidence
Digital technology	Moderate impact, +4 months	Moderate cost	Based on limited evidence
Early literacy approaches	Moderate impact, +4 months	Very low cost	Based on moderate evidence
Parental engagement	Moderate impact, +4 months	Moderate cost	Based on Moderate evidence
Extra hours	Moderate impact, +3 months	Very high cost	Based on limited evidence
Physical development approaches	Moderate impact, +3 months	Very low cost	Based on moderate evidence
Social and emotional learning strategies	Moderate impact, +3 months	Moderate cost	Based on very limited evidence
Built environment	Very low or no impact, 0 months	Low cost	Based on very limited evidence

Note: Table 4.9 has been adapted from the EEF's Early Years Toolkit
(see https://educationendowmentfoundation.org.uk/evidence/early-years-toolkit).
Source: The United Kingdom's Educational Endowment Foundation.

engagement (i.e., encouraging parents to read and talk with their children at home or participate in activities in the early years setting), on the other hand, has a *moderate impact* (an average gain of five months), at *moderate cost,* based on *moderate evidence.* The EEF has taken pains to place research-based evidence at the ready disposal of service personnel who may not be used to employing such findings but who want to provide effective help. Also, as more evidence accumulates, the EEF will update the Early Years Toolkit.

19. Teaching and Learning Toolkit from EEF in the United Kingdom (5–16 years)

With funding from the Sutton Trust, the EEF (https://educationen-dowmentfoundation.org.uk/evidence-summaries/teaching-learning-toolkit/), and Durham University (all in the United Kingdom), the EEF has produced a technical manual that furnishes many details about how the Teaching and Learning Toolkit and the Early Years Toolkit were constructed and will be periodically revised (https://edu-cationendowmentfoundation.org.uk/public/files/Toolkit/Toolkit_Manual_2018.pdf). In Table 4.10, we have reproduced a somewhat shorter version of the Teaching and Learning Toolkit, one limited to the learning approaches in the EEF Toolkit that we saw as most rel-evant to the education of children and young people in care. Also, in relation to the impact of the learning approach of mentoring, our interpretation of the relevant research differs from that of the EEF, and it is our interpretation that we placed in Table 4.8. Our view of the impact of tutoring is more positive than that of the EEF and the researchers at Durham University, based on three high-quality meta-analyses and one literature review of research on mentoring (Dubois et al., 2002; Dubois et al., 2011; Rhodes & Dubois 2008).

The EEF toolkits provide many useful tips for implementing the various learning approaches covered. For example, in relation to "one-to-one tutoring" (for which they use the British term "tuition"), the Teaching and Learning Toolkit suggests that potential adopters assess the following issues prior to implementation. First, one-to-one tutoring is very effective but may be relatively expensive. So, small-group tutoring should be considered, and the outcomes need to be evaluated. Second, adding tutoring to and linking it with school work is likely to enhance its impact. Third, it is important to train and pro-vide support to tutors. Fourth, choose a tutoring program that has already been shown to be effective.

20. What Works for Children and Young People with Literacy Difficulties? The Effectiveness of Intervention Schemes

Brooks (2016) reviewed studies in the United Kingdom on the effec-tiveness of 81 interventions for struggling readers and writers. He sought to answer two questions (Brooks, 2016, p. 11): "What interven-tion schemes are there which have been used in the UK in an attempt

Table 4.10. Teaching and learning toolkit from UK's Educational Endowment Foundation

Learning approaches	Impact and months gained on average in 1 year of exposure	Cost	Amount of evidence
Arts participation	Low impact +2 months	Low cost	Based on moderate evidence
Behaviour interventions	Moderate impact +3 months	Moderate cost	Based on extensive evidence
Collaborative learning	Moderate impact +5 months	Very low cost	Based on extensive evidence
Digital technology	Moderate impact +4 months	Moderate cost	Based on extensive evidence
Early years interventions	Moderate impact +5 months	Very high cost	Based on extensive evidence
Extending school time	Low impact +2 months	Moderate cost	Based on moderate evidence
Feedback	High impact +8 months	Very low cost	Based on moderate evidence
Homework (primary school)	Low impact +2 months	Very low cost	Based on limited evidence
Homework (secondary school)	Moderate impact +5 months	Very low cost	Based on limited evidence
Individualized instruction	Moderate impact +3 months	Very low cost	Based on moderate evidence
Learning styles	Low impact +2 months	Very low cost	Based on limited evidence
Mastery learning	Moderate impact +5 months	Very low cost	Based on moderate evidence
Mentoring	Modest impact +2 months	Moderate cost	Based on extensive evidence
Meta-cognition and self-regulation	High impact +7 months	Very low cost	Based on extensive evidence
One-to-one tutoring	Moderate impact +5 months	Moderate cost	Based on extensive evidence
Small-group tutoring	Moderate impact +5 months	Moderate cost	Based on extensive evidence
Oral language interventions	Moderate impact +5 months	Very low cost	Based on extensive evidence
Parental engagement	Moderate impact +3 months	Moderate cost	Based on moderate evidence

Learning approaches	Impact and months gained on average in 1 year of exposure	Cost	Amount of evidence
Peer tutoring	Moderate impact +5 months	Very low cost	Based on extensive evidence
Phonics	Moderate impact +4 months	Very low cost	Based on very extensive evidence
Reading compre-hension strategies	High impact +6 months	Very low cost	Based on extensive evidence
Social and emotional learning	Moderate impact +4 months	Moderate cost	Based on extensive evidence
Sports participation	Low impact +2 months	Moderate cost	Based on limited evidence
Summer schools	Low impact 2 months	Moderate cost	Based on extensive evidence

Note: Table 4.10 has been adapted from EEF's Teaching and Learning Toolkit. We view mentoring, one-to-one tutoring, and small-group tutoring more positively than does EEF's Teaching and Learning Toolkit because we appear to have drawn upon a broader and partly more recent body of research (namely, three meta-analyses and one literature review). For details, see sections 22–26 of this chapter.
Source: The United Kingdom's Educational Endowment Foundation.

to boost the reading, spelling or overall writing attainment of lower-achieving pupils between the ages of 5 and 18, and have been quantitatively evaluated here?" And, "What are those schemes like, and how effective are they?"

In this, the fifth edition, Brooks reiterated several realistic and optimistic conclusions that he had formulated in earlier editions (Brooks, 2016, pp. 15–16). First, "ordinary teaching" (that is, no treatment) does not enable children with literacy difficulties to catch up. Thus, although good classroom teaching is crucial, research indicates that children who have fallen behind need more help than the classroom normally can give, and this aid needs coordination and training. Second, large-scale schemes are costly but worthwhile, such that long-term impact and future savings need to be taken into consideration, especially with the neediest students. Third, it is possible to have a real impact, with at least twice the standard rate of progress. If the intervention meets the child's needs, high expectations are merited and rapid improvement may be anticipated.

21. Best Evidence Encyclopedia

Produced by Robert Slavin and his colleagues at the Center for Research and Reform in Education at Johns Hopkins University, the Best Evidence Encyclopedia (BEE; http://www.bestevidence.org) has extensive reviews of programs in early childhood education (to improve literacy in preschool children); mathematics (elementary, middle, and high school); reading (for beginning, elementary, and struggling readers); and science (elementary and secondary). Comprehensive reviews of programs and their effectiveness are available within these categories. For example, Slavin et al. (2009; 2011) provided a comprehensive review of high-quality studies of the achievement-related outcomes of a range of approaches to helping struggling readers: one-to-one tutoring, small-group tutorials, classroom instructional processes (e.g., cooperative learning), and computer-assisted instruction. They suggested that one-to-one tutoring is very effective in improving reading and that small-group tutoring, although effective, is not as effective as one-to-one tutoring. Cooperative learning can also be an effective approach for struggling readers.

22. Tutoring: An Evidence-Based, Effective Intervention for Struggling Students

Robert Slavin is a strong proponent of tutoring, based on the extensive evidence available. He has often stated in his peer-reviewed publications and blog that "There is nothing nearly as effective as one-to-one or one-to-small group tutoring" (Slavin, 2020). He has also asserted that in situations such as the current COVID-19 crisis, "Nothing else can be put in place as quickly [as tutoring] with as high a likelihood of working." Indeed, the success and feasibility of tutoring explain why England and the Netherlands have implemented national tutoring programs to mitigate the negative effects of school closures brought about by COVID-19. In this section of the chapter, we will make the case for tutoring, both in the general population and among young people in care. We believe there is now sufficient evidence to justify much more frequent and widespread use of academic tutoring of reading and math with young people struggling with basic academic skills. Society child welfare workers, supervisors, educational consultants, and caregivers—not to mention young people in care themselves—need to harness the great potential of tutoring to improve their charges' performance in reading and math, the basis of their future educational achievement, which itself is a major source of self-confidence and well-being. Serious training and ongoing support of tutors need to be core components of educational planning in schools and child welfare agencies, whether the tutors be paraprofessionals (e.g., teaching assistants), volunteers, or caregivers.

In making our argument, we summarize the findings of a recent meta-analysis of exclusively experimental (i.e., randomized) studies of tutoring. This study covers the period 1980–2020 and is the first systematic review and comprehensive meta-analysis of experimental research on pre-K to grade 12 tutoring ever completed. It qualifies as one of the most compelling pieces of evidence—among the many available—of the effectiveness of tutoring. It also buttresses the case in favour of tutoring that researchers such as Slavin et al. (2009), Forsman and Vinnerljung (2012), the EEF, and others have been making for a decade or more. We begin with a summary of the main results and implications of the new tutoring meta-analysis and framework, and then provide a succinct overview of the findings from our own and others' research in Ontario on the effectiveness of tutoring with young people in care. Our objective is to encourage societies and the schools with which they interact to adopt the most effective, evidence-based educational interventions that are currently available. It is these that are likely to make a noticeable difference in the educational success of the children and young people in their care.

23. A Meta-Analysis of Randomized Evaluations of Tutoring Studies and a Systematic Framework for Pre-Kindergarten-to-Grade-12 Tutoring of Children and Youth

Nickow, Oreopoulos, and Quan (2020, p. 1) define *tutoring* as "one-on-one or small-group instructional programming by teachers, paraprofessionals, volunteers, or parents," qualifying it as "one of the most versatile and potentially transformative educational tools in use today." For them, tutoring is a form of educational technology whose goal is to increase the efficiency of learning and which is intended to supplement, not replace, classroom-based education. In their meta-analysis, they develop a framework for tutoring that examines different types of programs, both to examine overall effects but also to determine how these effects covary with program characteristics. In so doing, they provide the first meta-analysis of experimental (i.e., randomized) findings and an integrated framework for tutoring as a domain of theory and practice, enabling comparisons among different tutoring models, from pre-K through secondary school.

Nickow et al. (2020) addressed two research questions: (1) What are the impacts of pre-K-to-grade-12 tutoring on learning outcomes? And, (2) How do the effects of tutoring vary by characteristics of the interventions? In answering the first research question, they found that tutoring had an important positive impact on learning, namely, an overall pooled effect size of +0.37 standard deviations (*SD*). There was a wide range of outcomes, from -0.80 to +1.57 *SD*. Also, they speculated that the possible mechanisms through which tutoring achieves its impacts for students who have fallen behind include more instruction time, customization of learning (i.e., teaching at the right level for the student), encouragement of greater engagement, rapid feedback, and greater connectedness via the tutor–student relationship.

Regarding the second research question, Nickow et al. (2020, p. 28) found that "tutoring interventions exert substantial effects on learning across a wide range of program characteristics." Certain program characteristics, however, were associated with larger impacts on learning. First, on average, effects were similar in size for *literacy* (0.35 *SD*) versus *math* (0.38 *SD*). However, while effect sizes for literacy tutoring tended to decline with grade level, math tutoring tended to show the opposite tendency, with impacts increasing from pre-K and kindergarten to grade 1 and to grades 2 through 5.

Second, Nickow et al. (2020) calculated the average impact of different types of tutors. The first type was *certified classroom teachers,* in a program like Reading Recovery. The second type was *paraprofessionals,* such as school staff or undergraduate or graduate students in education, in a program such as Number Rockets, which is a first-grade math program. The third type was *non-professionals,* such as community members or retired adults who volunteer as reading tutors in Experience Corps with children in early elementary grades. The final type were *parents,* who tutor their own children at home, using an intervention such as paired reading. On average, the effects of tutoring were larger for teachers (0.50 *SD*) and paraprofessionals (.40 *SD*) than for non-professionals (0.21 *SD*) or parents (0.23 *SD*). However, Nickow et al. noted that even effects of 0.20 to 0.25 *SD* may be considered substantial if their cost is low, as is the case for parent tutoring interventions. Moreover, Nickow et al. noted an example of a paired reading program delivered by parents in Hong Kong that had an impact of $SD = 0.37$, at the mean of the study as a whole.

Third, regarding *delivery mode*, Nickow et al. (2020) found on standardized test scores that a one-to-one tutor-to-student ratio (0.38 SD) had roughly the same average impact as a one-to-two ratio (0.29 SD) or one-to-three or more (0.36 SD), and the latter seemed to be especially effective in grades 2–5. Fourth, on another aspect of delivery mode, namely, *timing during the day*, average effects were considerably stronger when tutoring took place during school hours (0.82 SD) than after school (0.19 SD).

Fifth, in terms of *dosage*, average effects were stronger with more tutoring sessions per week: 0.41 SD with four to five days per week, versus 0.34 SD with three days per week, versus 0.24 SD with one to two days per week. However, in grades 2–5, effects were stronger for three days per week than for four to five days per week, and only one session per week did not appear to generate large effect sizes. Sixth, average effects were larger with interventions of *less than 20 weeks*, versus *those longer than 20 weeks*, although this may be because tutoring by teachers tends to be shorter than by non-professionals. Finally, effects were larger, on average, with tutoring in the *earlier grades*: 0.45 SD in pre-K versus 0.42 SD in grade 1, 0.29 SD in grades 2–5, and 0.16 SD in grades 6–11.

In addition, Nickow et al. (2020) also focused on the outcomes of 12 relatively *large-scale evaluations*, chosen from among the 96 in their sample. Echoing Brooks' (2016) positive perspective on the merit of large-scale programs, noted earlier, Nickow et al. (2020, pp. 42–43) concluded that "large-scale impact evaluations show substantial effects of generally comparable magnitude to efficacy trials and other smaller-scale studies. Taken collectively, the [large-scale] studies […] indicate that tutoring programs can exert strong impacts for a wide range of samples and over diverse intervention characteristics." These large-sample trials also showed that tutoring by teachers, paraprofessionals, and non-professionals could all generate large effect sizes (there were no large-scale parent tutoring programs in their study sample).

Nickow et al. (2020) compared their results, obtained with tutoring, with alternative pre-K-to-grade-12 interventions. They noted that a meta-analysis by Dietrichson et al. (2017) had produced an overall average effect size of 0.36 SD, virtually identical to their overall estimate of 0.37 SD. Moreover, Dietrichson et al. had found that tutoring generated a stronger effect, on average, than feedback and progress monitoring (0.32 SD), small-group instruction of six or more students (0.24 SD), and cooperative learning (0.22 SD). Similarly, Pellegrini et al. (2018) reviewed eight types of elementary-level math programs, which had been evaluated in a total of 78 studies, and concluded that tutoring interventions had easily the largest average effect sizes (specifically, 0.26 SD for one-on-one tutoring and 0.32 SD for small-group tutoring). Most of the other categories had much smaller average effects (less than 0.10 SD). Finally, Inns et al. (2019) found average effect sizes of roughly comparable size for one-to-one tutoring (0.31 SD) and small-group tutoring (0.20 SD) in elementary school, leading them also to recommend tutoring.

Nickow et al. (2020) completed their landmark meta-analysis of randomized evaluations with several practical suggestions for the further development and implementation of tutoring as an educational intervention. First, they felt that paraprofessional tutoring, in particular, offered particularly great potential and should receive priority for expansion, given the possibility of major effects at relatively low cost, even for one-to-one or high-dosage tutoring. Second, they suggested that tutoring could undergo considerable growth at the secondary level, with possible extension to subjects such as science or social studies. Third, they cautioned that the smaller effects they found in after-school and parent tutoring programs indicate that it may be difficult to make sure that tutoring actually occurs in such contexts and that delivering tutoring in sufficiently high doses is an important program consideration. Fourth, they pointed to the need for free, public tutoring programs, to ensure that tutoring does not become available only to children of the affluent. Fifth, they concluded their important paper with an endorsement of tutoring that is worth quoting in its entirety for the field of child welfare, where improving educational outcomes is a long-standing, urgent priority:

> Tutoring programs rank among the most flexible and potentially transformative learning program types available at the PreK-12 levels. While this proposition has been clear for some time, the present review has, for the first time, synthesized and quantitatively analyzed experimental evidence on all programs for which such evidence is available that would be widely identified as tutoring. With effect sizes averaging at over a third of a standard deviation and impacts consistently significant across a

wide range of program and study characteristics, our review's meta-analytic findings demonstrate not only the power of tutoring but its versatility. As customized learning grows in prominence across today's educational systems, there is little doubt that tutoring programs will constitute a key workhorse policy model. (Nickow et al., 2020, pp. 57–58)

24. Four Randomized Controlled Trials in Ontario of Tutoring Young People in Care

Nickow et al. (2020) remarked that a relatively distinct literature on the tutoring of young people in care had already begun to emerge, citing as proof and including in their meta-analysis three randomized trials of tutoring with children in care that had already been completed in Ontario. Two of these studies were collaborations between Ontario societies and OnLAC Project researchers at the University of Ottawa (Marquis, 2013; Hickey & Flynn, 2019), and the third was a collaboration between two Ontario societies and researchers at Lakehead University in Thunder Bay (Harper & Schmidt, 2016). A fourth randomized tutoring trial with young people in care had been carried out in Ontario by Hickey and Flynn (2020) but was not included in the meta-analysis by Nickow et al. (2020) because its design did not meet their inclusion criteria. (Although randomized, it had compared two active tutoring treatments rather than comparing an active tutoring treatment with a passive control group.) Given the focus of the present volume on the findings of the OnLAC Project, and the direct relevance of tutoring to the task of improving the educational outcomes of young people in care in Ontario and elsewhere, we summarize here the main goals, features, and results of these four Ontario randomized tutoring trials.

The meta-analysis by Nickow et al. (2020) included 96 individual studies and 732 learning outcomes or effects. In each study, the researchers reduced multiple correlated effects to a single pooled estimate. Each pooled estimate was calculated as a standardized mean-difference effect size (SD), as the difference between the treatment and control group means, translated into units of the pooled standard deviation (SD) and expressed as Hedge's g (very similar in magnitude to Cohen's d but corrected for bias in smaller samples). For the three Ontario tutoring trials with young people in care included in the meta-analysis of Nickow et al. (2020), the pooled effect sizes were quite similar. For Marquis (2013), which used caregivers as tutors, the pooled effect size (g) was 0.26; for Harper and Schmidt (2016), which had non-professionals (university students) as tutors, the pooled effect size was 0.28; and for Hickey and Flynn (2019), with paraprofessional (trained persons) as tutors, the pooled effect size was 0.21.

24.1. Marquis (2013): One-to-One Tutoring of Children in Care

The first randomized trial of tutoring in Ontario that was included in the meta-analysis by Nickow et al. (2020) was Robyn Marquis' (2013) doctoral thesis in clinical psychology at the University of Ottawa, with Robert Flynn as her thesis advisor. Marquis (2013) extended the research questions, analyses, and findings derived from the data set generated by an earlier randomized tutoring trial with young people in care (Flynn et al., 2012), and Marquis and Flynn (2019) later added other analyses and results, based on the same data set.

The basic goal of Marquis (2013), and of the original trial by Flynn et al. (2012), was to test the hypothesis that one-to-one tutoring by caregivers could improve the basic skills in reading and mathematics of young people in care, which are often weak. Of the research sample of 64 children in care (after attrition), aged 6–13, 30 had been randomly assigned to direct-instruction tutoring, based on Maloney's (1998) *Teach Your Children Well* program and workbooks, and 34 to a wait-list control group. All 64 had undergone pre-test and post-test assessments with the age-standardized Wide Range Achievement Test (WRAT4; Wilkinson & Robertson, 2009) and other measures. The young people in the tutoring group received an intervention designed to provide three hours a week of individual tutoring from their caregivers, for up to 30 weeks. The tutoring intervention included two hours of one-to-one direct instruction in reading, 30 minutes of reading aloud by the young person in care to the tutor or another adult, and 30 minutes of self-paced instruction in math for the young person, under the supervision of the caregiver.

The tutoring program produced statistically significant gains, on average, on the WRAT4 sub-tests of Sentence Comprehension (Hedges' g = 0.38, $p < .05$) and Math Computation (g = 0.46, $p < .01$), but not on Word Reading or Spelling. The tutoring program was well received by the children and caregivers. As one of the first successful randomized trials with children in care in the international child welfare literature, the study showed that tutoring in literacy and numeracy could be an effective and operationally feasible intervention for children in care (for details, see Marquis, 2013; Flynn et al., 2012; Marquis & Flynn, 2019).

24.2. Harper and Schmidt (2016): Small-Group Tutoring of Indigenous Children in Care

The second randomized trial of tutoring involving young people in care in Ontario was carried out as Julie Harper's doctoral thesis in clinical psychology at Lakehead University, from which Harper and Schmidt (2016) published their paper. Two local societies (one of which was Indigenous) collaborated on the project, of which Fred Schmidt was the thesis co-advisor and Robert Flynn an external member of the thesis committee. The aim of Harper's analysis was to investigate the effectiveness of tutoring, especially with Indigenous young people in care. Of the research sample of 91 young people, of whom 78% were Indigenous, 45 were randomly assigned to the tutoring condition (after attrition) and 46 to a wait-list control condition. Both conditions lasted for up to 30 weeks. Harper and Schmidt (2016) also employed Maloney's (1998) Teach Your Children Well tutoring method, with volunteer university students (rather than caregivers) as tutors. The children were tutored in small groups of three to six, formed according to skill level, and were assessed at the pre-test and post-test with the WRAT4 and other measures.

Harper and Schmidt (2016) found that the tutoring intervention produced statistically significant effects on several WRAT4 sub-tests: Word Reading ($g = 0.40$, $p < .001$), Spelling ($g = .25$, $p = .02$), and Math Computation ($g = 0.34$, $p = .04$), but not on Sentence Comprehension (see Harper & Schmidt, 2016, for details). They concluded that their findings showed that the tutoring of children in care of mainly Indigenous cultural background, delivered in a small-group format, was effective in improving both literacy and numeracy skills, thus extending the results of the previous Ontario randomized trial reported on by Flynn et al. (2012) and Marquis (2013).

24.3. Hickey and Flynn (2019): One-on-One Tutoring of Children in Care

The third randomized trial of tutoring with young people in care in Ontario was conducted from the University of Ottawa, in conjunction with the OnLAC Project. It was part of Andrea Hickey's doctoral thesis in clinical psychology, of which Robert Flynn was the thesis advisor. The research evaluated the effectiveness of TutorBright, a new tutoring program for improving young people's basic skills in reading and math that, like Maloney (1998) had, was also based on direct-instruction methods. A local society was interested in implementing the program with young people in care who were struggling in reading or math, but first it wanted evidence that TutorBright was indeed effective.

The research sample consisted (after attrition) of 70 children in care in Ontario, aged 5–16 and enrolled mainly in primary grades 1–8, with a few in secondary grades 9–11. Of the sample, 34 young people were randomly assigned to the tutoring intervention and 36 to a wait-list control condition. All the children in care had also been pre-tested and post-tested with the age-standardized Woodcock-Johnson III Tests of Achievement (Woodcock, McGrew, & Mather, 2001) and other measures. The TutorBright approach uses one-on-one, in-home tutoring, trained tutors, detailed instructors' manuals, student workbooks, and customized homework help. In the tutoring condition, the tutors met individually with the young people in care in their respective foster homes for 2 one-hour sessions per week, for up to 50 hours of tutoring. On average, the young people received 47 tutoring sessions and 48.66 hours of tutoring.

The TutorBright intervention produced statistically significant gains on the Woodcock-Johnson III sub-tests of Reading Fluency ($g = 0.16$, $p < .05$), Passage Comprehension ($g = 0.34$, $p < .05$), Broad Reading ($g = 0.14$, $p < .06$), and Math Calculation ($g = 0.39$, $p < .05$). However, there were no significant gains on Letter-Word Identification, Spelling, Math Fluency, or Broad Math (for details, see Hickey & Flynn, 2019).

24.4. Hickey and Flynn (2020): Shorter Versus Longer Versions of One-to-One Tutoring of Children in Care

The fourth randomized trial of tutoring involving young people in care in Ontario was conducted at the University of Ottawa, also as part of Andrea Hickey's doctoral thesis in clinical psychology, with Robert Flynn as the thesis advisor. The study was carried out in collaboration with two local societies, in conjunction with the OnLAC Project. The trial used Maloney's (1998) *Teach Your Children Well* (TYCW) method and addressed the practical question of whether a shorter, 15-week version of TYCW would be as effective as the longer, standard version of 25 weeks that Marquis (2013), Flynn et al. (2012), and Harper and Schmidt (2016) had evaluated. If so, the shorter version of TYCW could be implemented more easily and less expensively by local societies, perhaps twice a school year rather than only once. (As mentioned previously, because this randomized trial had compared two active treatments, rather than comparing an active treatment with a wait-list control condition, it did not satisfy the inclusion criteria of Wissow et al. [2020] and was not included in their meta-analysis.)

The 36 young people in care in the 15-week tutoring group and the 36 in the 25-week tutoring group (after attrition) were assessed at a pre-test and post-test with the Woodcock-Johnson III (WJIII) achievements tests (Woodcock et al., 2001). At the post-test, there were initially no statistically significant mean differences between the shorter and longer versions of TYCW tutoring on any of the Woodcock-Johnson III sub-tests, and it was only after the removal of a statistical outlier that a significant difference ($p < .05$) emerged on one WJIII sub-test, Math Fluency. Given the relative lack of differences in effects of the two interventions, Hickey and Flynn (2020) pooled the two groups to form a single tutoring group ($N = 72$) and tested for differences between the merged group's pre-test and post-test means. On all the WJIII sub-tests except Spelling, there were significant differences in the pre-test and post-test means, almost all at the $p < .001$ level (for details, see Hickey & Flynn, 2020). Overall, the findings suggested that societies or schools interested in implementing TYCW tutoring would do well to choose the 15-week rather than the 25-week version. However, careful consultation of the meta-analysis by Nickow et al. (2020) would also be highly recommended, as the authors provide good descriptions and suggestions regarding a broad range of tutoring models that could potentially prove very helpful to young people in care who are struggling in reading or math.

A promising start has thus been made on the development of tutoring as a practical, evidence-based intervention with children in care in Ontario. What is needed now is more frequent collaboration in applied research and program development among academic researchers, child welfare agencies, schools, and government funders. A sustained collaborative effort, coupled with better training and compensation of tutors and the adoption of the most promising tutoring models described by Nickow et al. (2020) and in the present chapter could quickly make tutoring a major vehicle for improving the educational success of struggling young people in care, at both the primary and secondary levels. Moreover, without such an effort, the long-standing educational problems of a substantial proportion of young people in care may prove virtually intractable.

25. More Proven Programs in Tutoring

We have provided what we hope is convincing and rapidly evolving evidence that tutoring is an effective intervention with young people in both the general and in-care populations, if tutors are well trained and the program is adequately supported and funded. For child welfare organizations or schools, however, the important question remains of which tutoring programs appear to be effective and thus worth implementing and evaluating. Besides the programs we have mentioned in this chapter, Robert Slavin, until his death the director of the Center for Research and Reform in Education at Johns Hopkins University, listed in his blog of November 12, 2020, what he calls "proven programs" in reading or math tutoring. These are programs that have been used successfully with young people in the general school population, but many could no doubt be adapted for use with young people in care who need individual or small-group tutoring.

Table 4.11 lists 20 tutoring programs in reading or math from Slavin's blog of November 12, 2020, that have effect sizes of +0.20 or larger and are also delivered by trained teaching assistants or paid volunteers. Such projects are likely to be less expensive and more feasible for child welfare organizations or schools than programs delivered by certified teachers. (See Slavin's blog of November 12, 2020, for his full list of proven programs.)

26. ProvenTutoring.org

Robert Slavin remarked that few of the 120,000 primary and secondary schools in the United States regularly used any of the 120+ proven reading or math programs that showed significant positive effects and met the standards of effectiveness for the Every Student Succeeds Act (ESSA). He noted that this lack of adoption in education contrasted strongly with medicine, where treatments shown to be effective in rigorous studies were usually widely adopted by medical practitioners (partly under pain of lawsuits if they did not, we may add). Similar

Table 4.11. More proven tutoring programs in reading and math

Tutoring Program	Reading or Math	Tutors	Group Size	Effect Size
Sound Partners	Reading	TAs or paid volunteers	One-to-one	0.58
SPARK	Reading	TAs or Paid Volunteers	One-to-one	0.51
SMART	Reading	TAs or Paid Volunteers	One-to-one	0.48
Reading Rescue	Reading	TAs or Paid Volunteers	One-to-one	0.87
Tutoring with the Lightning Squad	Reading	TAs or Paid Volunteers	One-to-one	0.43
Quick Reads	Reading	TAs or Paid Volunteers	Small groups	0.21
Pirate Math (Fuchs)	Math	Teaching Assistants	One-to-one	0.37
Galaxy Math (Fuchs)	Math	Teaching Assistants	One-to-one	0.24
Fractions (Fuchs)	Math	Teaching Assistants	Small groups	0.51
ROOTS	Math	Teaching Assistants	Small groups	0.32
Focus Math	Math	Teaching Assistants	Small groups	0.24

Note. Adapted from Robert Slavin's blog, November 12, 2020, Johns Hopkins University, Center for Research and Reform in Education (https://robertslavinsblog.wordpress.com/2020//11/12/a-called-shot-for-educational-research-and-impact/). Only those tutoring programs delivered by TAs (teaching assistants) or paid volunteers and with an effect size of 0.20 or larger are listed here, as these are likely to be most feasible for implementation in child welfare organizations or many schools. See Slavin's blog for programs delivered by certified teachers or with effect sizes smaller than 0.20.

Source: Adapted from Robert Slavin's blog, November 12, 2020, Johns Hopkins University, Center for Research and Reform in Education.

processes of evidence-to-practice adoption are also commonplace in fields such as agriculture or technology.

In order to create a similar climate of adoption of evidence-based programs in education, Slavin and his colleagues founded in 2021 a coalition called ProvenTuroring.org. It consists of 14 programs in field use that have been proven to be effective with college-educated teaching assistants as tutors. The goal is to expand to a total of 100,000 tutors, serving some 4,000,000 children in the United States. We believe that the Ontario Association of Children's Aid Societies, local societies, and the Ministries of Education and of Children, Community, and Social Services (MCCSS) should follow this development closely. Ideally, Ontario would bring a small team from ProvenTutoring.org into the province to provide training, as has begun to happen in the United States, and the movement for rigorous tutoring would grow from there, with further training and adoption. This will no doubt prove to be far more effective than launching tutoring in Ontario with unevaluated programs or unprepared tutors, which is likely to yield disappointing results. In the meantime, the group of randomized trials of tutoring that have had their roots in the OnLAC Project constitutes a promising start on tutoring effectiveness research and practice in Ontario, Canada, and internationally (Flynn et al., 2012; Marquis, 2013; Marquis & Flynn, 2019; Harper & Schmidt, 2016; Hickey & Flynn, 2019; 2020).

27. Concluding Comment: Implementing Quality Standard 10 on Educational Achievement in Ontario's New Framework for Licensed Residential Services in Ontario

In September 2019, MCCSS issued the initial draft of *Developing a Quality Standards Framework for Licensed Residential Services in Ontario.* The objective of this new framework within child welfare is to improve the quality and outcomes of the residential services that young people experience in the province and align these services better with the heightened goals of the new child welfare legislation introduced in Ontario in 2017. It is a fitting conclusion to the present chapter on education to comment on how the OnLAC Project is able by its very nature to contribute much to the attainment of these improvements.

The OnLAC Project already furnishes rich information about individual young people in care that can illuminate their service needs and the quality of their present residential services. This is thanks to the comprehensive nature of the conversational interview conducted each year with the AAR, in which the young person in care (if aged 10 or over), caregiver, and worker participate. The new Quality Standards Framework sees the following information as central, and all of it is already gathered by the annual AAR interview:

- The young person's outcomes during the past year and likely service needs over the year to come, permitting informed placement decisions.

- The young person's physical, emotional, and mental health and well-being.
- The young person's experience and voice over the past year on many closely related topics, such as schooling, dress, room and setting, relationships with family, caregivers, and staff, hobbies, sports and recreation, and support for career choices.
- The young person's individual and cultural identity.
- The young person's educational achievement.
- The young person's experience of careful preparation and support in transition to independence and adulthood.

The OnLAC research team obviously supports education as a strong and essential plank within the new policy on licensed residential services, given education's critical role in shaping young peoples' futures, but we also support the other planks as well. Overall, we believe the AAR already sheds much light on the most important aspects of a young person's residential situation. During the next revision of the AAR, we stand ready to revise the instrument so that it becomes even more aligned, both conceptually and empirically, with the new residential services framework.

References

Aughinbaugh, A., & Gittleman, M. (2003). Does money matter? A comparison of the effect of income on child development in the United States and Great Britain. *The Journal of Human Resources*, 38, 416–440.

Brooks, G. (2016). *What works for children and young people with literacy difficulties? The effectiveness of intervention schemes* (5th ed.). Dyslexia-SpLD Trust.

Cameron, C. E., Brock, L. L., Murrah, W. M., Bell, L. H., Worzalla, S. L., Grissmer, D., & Morrison, F. J. (2012). Fine motor skills and executive function both contribute to kindergarten achievement. *Child Development*, 83, 1229–1244.

Cameron, C., Höjer, I., Nordenfors, M., & Flynn, R. (2020). Security-first thinking and educational practices for young children in foster care in Sweden and England: A think piece. *Children and Youth Services Review*, 119, Article 105,523. https://doi.org/10.1016/j.childyouth.2020.105523

Carneiro, P., Meghir, C., & Parey, M. (2013). Maternal education, home environments, and the development of children and adolescents. *Journal of the European Economic Association*, 11, 123–160.

Cleveland, G. (2018). *Affordable for all: Making licensed child care affordable in Ontario.* (Executive Summary). University of Toronto Scarborough.

Dionne, C., McKinnon, S., Squires, J., & Clifford, J. (2014). Developmental screening in a Canadian First Nation (Mohawk): Psychometric properties and adaptations of Ages and Stages Questionnaires (2nd ed.). *BMC Pediatrics*, 14(23), 1–8.

Dietrichson, J., Bog, M., Filges, T., & Klint Jorgensen, A. M. (2017). Academic interventions for elementary and middle school students with low socioeconomic status: A systematic review and meta-analysis. *Review of Educational Research*, 87(2), 243–282.

Dube, S. R., & McGiboney, G. W. (2018). Education and learning in the context of childhood abuse, neglect and related stressor: The nexus of health and education. *Child Abuse and Neglect* 75, 1–5.

Dubois, D. L., Holloway, B. E., Valentine, J. C., & Cooper, H. (2002). Effectiveness of mentoring programs for youth: A meta-analytic review. *American Journal of Community Psychology*, 30, 157–197.

DuBois, D. L., Portillol, N., Rhodes, J. E., Silverthorn, N., & Valentine, J. C. (2011). How effective are mentoring programs for youth? A systematic assessment of the evidence. *Psychological Science in the Public Interest*, 12(2), 57–91.

Flynn, R. J., Marquis, R. A., Paquet, M-P., Peeke, L. M., & Aubry, T. D. (2012). Effects of individual direct-instruction tutoring on foster children's academic skills: A randomized trial. *Children and Youth Services Review*, 34, 1183–1189.

Flynn, R. J., & Miller, M. (2017). *Review of the reliability and validity of current and potential performance indicators derived from OnLAC for Ontario's children's aid societies.* Centre for Research on Educational and Community Services, University of Ottawa.

Flynn, R. J., Vincent, C., & Miller, M. (2011). *User's mI for the AAR-C2-2010.* Centre for Research on Educational and Community Services, University of Ottawa.

Forsman, H., & Vinnerljung, B. (2012). Interventions aiming to improve school achievements of children in out-of-home care: A scoping review. *Children and Youth Services Review*, 34(6), 1084–1091.

Ghassabian, A., Sundaram, R., Bell, E., Bello, S. C., Kus, C., &Yeung, E. (2016). Gross motor milestones and subsequent development. *Pediatrics*, 138, Article e20154372.

Grissmer, D., Grimm, K. J., Aiyer, S. M., Murrah, W. M., & Steele, J. S. (2010). Fine motor skills and early comprehension of the world: Two new school readiness indicators. *Developmental Psychology*, 46, 1008–1017.

Harper, J., & Schmidt, F. (2016). Effectivevess of a group-based academic tutoring program for children in foster care: A randomized controlled trial. *Children and Youth Services Review*, 67, 238–246.

Hickey, A. J., & Flynn, R. J. (2019). Effects of the TutorBright tutoring programme on the reading and mathematics skills of children in foster care: A randomised controlled trial. *Oxford Review of Education, 45*(4), 519–537.

Hickey, A. J., & Flynn, R. J. (2020). A randomized evaluation of 15 versus 25 weeks of individual tutoring for children in care. *Children and Youth Services Review* 109, Article 104,697, 1–11. https://doi.org/10.1016/j.childyouth. 2019.104697

Houwen, S., Visser, L., van der Putten, A., & Vlaskamp, C. (2016). The inter-relationships between motor, cognitive, and language development in children with and without intellectual and developmental disabilities. *Research in Developmental Disabilities, 53–54,* 19–31.

Inns, A. J., Lake, C., Pellegrini, M., & Slavin, R. E. (2019). A quantitative synthesis of research on programs for struggling readers in elementary schools. *Best Evidence Encyclopedia.* Center for Research and Reform in Education, Johns Hopkins University.

Jackson, S., & Hollingworth, R. (2018). Children in care in early childhood. In L. Miller, C. Cameron, C. Dalli, & N. Barbour (Eds.), *The SAGE handbook of early childhood policy (pp.* 354–367). Sage.

Kirk, C. M., Lewis, R. K., Brown, K., Nilsen, C., & Colvin, D. Q. (2012). The gender gap in educational expectations among youth in the foster care system. *Children and Youth Services Review 34,* 1683–1688. https://doi. org/10.1016/j.childyouth.2012.04.026

Maloney, M. (1998). *Teach Your Children Well: A solution to some of North America's educational problems.* QLC Educational Services.

Marquis, R. (2013). *The gender effects of a foster parent-delivered tutoring program on foster children's academic skills and mental health: A randomized field trial* [Unpublished PhD dissertation in clinical psychology]. University of Ottawa.

Marquis, R. A., & Flynn, R. J. (2019). Gender effects of tutoring on reading and math skills in a randomized controlled trial with foster children of primary-school age. In P. McNamara, C. Montserrat, & S. Wise (Eds.), *Education in out-of-home care: International perspectives on policy, practice and research* (pp. 119–134). Springer.

Mastorakos, T., & Scott, K. L. (2019). Attention biases and social-emotional development in preschool aged children who have been exposed to domestic violence. *Child Abuse and Neglect, 89,* 78–86.

McCrae, J. S., & Brown, S. M. (2018). Systematic review of social-emotional screening instruments for young children in child welfare. *Research on Social Work Practice, 28*(7), 767–788.

McCrae, J. S., Cahalane, H., & Fusco, R. A. (2011). Directions for developmental screening in child welfare based on the Ages and Stages Questionnaires. *Children and Youth Services Review, 33,* 1412–1418.

McKelvey, L. M., Conners Edge, N. A., Fitzgerald, S., Kraleti, S., & Whiteside-Mansell, L. (2017). Adverse childhood experiences: Screening and health in children from birth to age 5. *Families, Systems, and Health*, 35(4), 420–429.

Mensah, F. K., & Hobcraft, J. (2008). Childhood deprivation, health and development: associations with adult health in the 1958 and 1970 British prospective birth cohort studies. *Journal of Epidemiology and Community Health*, 62, 599–606.

Miller, M., Vincent, C., & Flynn, R. (2017). *User's ml for the AAR-C2-2016*. Centre for Research on Educational and Community Services, University of Ottawa. https://ruor.uottawa.ca/handle/10393/37843

Ministry of Children, Communities, and Social Services of Ontario. (2019, September) *Developing a quality standards framework for licensed residential services in Ontario: Discussion guide.*

Ministry of Education of Ontario. (2019). *Provincial society student profile report, 2016–2017.*

National Longitudinal Survey of Youth. (1979). *Motor and social development (MSD)*. U.S. Bureau of Labor Statistics.

Nickow, A. J., Oreopoulos, P., & Quan, V. (2020). *The impressive effects of tutoring on preK-12 learning: A systematic review and meta-analysis of the experimental evidence* [EdWorking PAperp 20-267]. Retrieved from Annenberg Institute at Brown University. https:33doi.org/10.263003/ehoc-pc52

O'Higgins, A., Sebba, J., & Gardner, F. (2017). What are the factors associated with educational achievement for children in kinship or foster care: A systematic review. *Children and Youth Services Review*, 79, 198–220.

Osorio-Valencia, E., Torres-Sánchez, L., López-Carrillo, L., Rothenberg, S. J., & Schnaas, L. (2018). Early motor development and cognitive abilities among Mexican preschoolers. *Child Neuropsychology*, 24(8), 1015–1025. https://doi.org/10.1080/09297049.2017.1354979

O'Sullivan, J. (2020, September 12). Literacy deficiency. *The Globe and Mail*, p. 8.

Panlilio, C. C., Harden, B. J., & Harring, J. (2018). School readiness of maltreated preschoolers and later school achievement: The role of emotion regulation, language, and context. *Child Abuse and Neglect*, 75, 82–91.

Pati, S., Hashim, K., Brown, B., Fiks, A. G., & Forrest, C. B. (2011). Early identification of young children at risk for poor academic achievement: Preliminary development of a parent-report prediction tool. *BMC Health Services Research*, 11, 197.

Pellegrini, M., Lake, C., Inns, A., & Slavin, R. E. (2018). Effective programs in elementary mathematics: A best-evidence synthesis. *Best Evidence Encyclopedia*. Center for Education and Reform, Johns Hopkins University.

Phillips, D. A., Lipsey, M. W., Dodge, K. A., Haskins, R., Bassok, D., Burchinal, M. R., Duncan, G. J., Dynarski, M., Magnuson, K. A., & Weiland, C. (2017). *Puzzling it out: The current state of scientific knowledge on pre-kindergarten effects*, 19–30. Brookings Institution and Duke Center for Child and Family Policy.

Rhodes, J. E., & Dubois, D. L. (2008). Mentoring relationships and programs for youth. *Current Directions in Psychological Science, 17*(4), 254–258.

Schell, A., Albers, L., von Kries, R., Hillenbrand, C., & Hennemann, T. (2015). Preventing behavioral disorders via supporting social and emotional competence at preschool age. *Deutsches Arzteblatt International,* 112, 647–654.

Slavin, R. (2020, November 12). A "called shot" for educational research and impact. [Blog post] Centre for Research and Reform in Education, Johns Hopkins University. https://robertslavinsblog.wordpress.com/2020/11/12/a-called-shot-for-educational-research-and-impact/

Slavin, R. E., Lake, C., Davis, S., & Madden, N. A. (2011). Effective programs for struggling readers: A best-evidence synthesis. *Educational Research Review, 6*(1), 1–26. http://dx.doi.org/10.1016/j.edurev.2010.07.002

Squires, J., Bricker, D., & Twombly, E. (2003). *The ASQ:SE user's guide for the Ages and Stages Questionnaires: Social-Emotional.* Paul H. Brookes.

Squires, J., Twombly, E., Bricker, D., & Potter, L. (2009). *ASQ-3 user's guide: Ages and Stages Questionnaire, Third Edition.* Paul H. Brookes.

Tessier, N. G., O'Higgins, A., & Flynn, R. J. (2018). Neglect, educational success, and young people in out-of-home care: Cross-sectional and longitudinal analyses. *Child Abuse and Neglect, 75,* 115–129.

Twombly, E., & Fink, G. (2013). *ASQ-3: Learning activities.* Paul H., Brookes.

Twombly, E., Munson, L. J., & Pribble, L. M. (2018). *ASQ:SE-2: Learning activities and more.* Paul H. Brookes.

U. S. Institute of Education Sciences. (2009). *Organizing instruction and study to improve student learning.* What Works Clearinghouse practice guide.

Vandermeulen, G., Wekerle, C., & Ylagan, C. (2005). Introduction to the special edition on child welfare-research collaborations: Teamwork, research excellence, and credible, relevant results for practice. *OACAS Journal,* 49(1), 1–3.

Wilkinson, G. S., & Robertson, G. J. (2006). *Wide-Range Achievement Test, Fourth Edition.* Psychological Assessment Resources.

Woodcock, R., McGrew, K., & Mather, N. (2001). *Woodcock-Johnson III Tests of Achievement manual.* Houghton-Mifflin.

Chapter 5

An Educational Snapshot of a Young Person in Care, Using Assessment and Action Record Information

Elisa Romano, Lauren Stenason, Erik Michael, and Meagan Miller

I n this chapter, we present a concrete example or "snapshot" of how information from the Assessment and Action Record (AAR) can be used to plan for needed services to support the educational well-being and functioning of young people in care. We first begin with a brief consideration of the applied ways in which the AAR can be used, as well as barriers to its use in practice. We then present the Educational Snapshot and illustrate its applied use by way of a case example.

1. How Is the AAR Used?

As the primary assessment tool of the Ontario Looking After Children (OnLAC) Project, the AAR is used to monitor outcomes for young people who have been in out-of-home care for at least one year. The AAR is completed on an annual basis through a "conversational interview" or discussion that includes the child welfare worker, resource caregiver, and young person (if aged 10 or older; Flynn et al., 2004). The AAR contains a wealth of developmentally sensitive information for young people in care across various domains of functioning. It can provide a comprehensive picture of a young person's current strengths and areas of need through its reliance on input from multiple informants and across several levels of influence (e.g., within young people themselves, in a young person's relationships, and in a young person's connections within the community).

These various features of the AAR undoubtedly hold much relevance for the child welfare sector. *Child welfare workers* and *caregivers* can make use of AAR information for a particular young person to help guide service planning and delivery and monitor outcomes in a way that is tailored to the young person's specific circumstances. Using AAR information in this manner would be consistent with one of the tool's primary goals, which is to help improve developmental outcomes and permanency planning for young people in care (Flynn et al., 2004). At the *organizational level*, AAR information may be used in aggregate form by service and executive directors to identify society-level trends in the well-being and functioning of the young people whom they serve. Such material is significant for purposes of informing resource allocation and planning, as well as increasing organizational accountability through outcome monitoring and program evaluation (Stenason, Romano, & Cheung, 2020). At the *provincial level*, the Ontario Association of Children's Aid Societies (OACAS) and the Ontario Ministry of Children, Community and Social Services (MCCSS) may use AAR information to inform current or prospective policy decisions.

2. Obstacles to Using the AAR in Practice

Although the annual completion of the AAR is mandated across Ontario child welfare, there remains a great deal of variability in the applied use of the data, especially at the individual worker, caregiver, and society levels (Romano et al., 2020). To improve the regular use of AAR information within child welfare practice, we worked alongside three large, urban-based Ontario societies to complete a pilot project aimed at enhancing understanding of the ways in which AAR data could be used to inform service planning and delivery in conjunction with other sources of information about young people—all within a conceptual and evidence-informed framework. We focused on educational functioning as it was identified by our partners as being a key concern for young people in care. We developed and offered AAR-based training to various child welfare stakeholders that included executive and service directors, workers and supervisors, and resource caregivers (i.e., foster, adoptive, and kin) in order to better ensure positive and sustained outcomes. Additional information on training content, delivery, and evaluation may be found in Romano et al. (2020) and Stenason et al. (2020). In brief, the majority of the feedback on the AAR-based trainings was positive, but there remained barriers to AAR use that included the following: receiving individual AAR data for young people in a timely manner so that the information could be considered when plans of care were being developed; understanding AAR data in the current format; and interpreting the meaning of AAR data due to limited knowledge by stakeholders of statistical concepts such as means and percentiles.

3. What Is the Education Snapshot?

In response to the feedback we received, both formally through our pilot project and anecdotally during ongoing discussions with our partner societies, we developed the Education Snapshot, with an initial focus on young people 10–15 years of age. We were committed to developing a profile around educational functioning that would:

1. Summarize, in an easily understandable and brief format, data from variables in the AAR that have been found through research to impact educational functioning;
2. Situate variables within a conceptual framework that recognized the various systems in which young people in care are embedded (i.e., ecological model);
3. Balance young people's needs and strengths;
4. Include multiple perspectives from young people, resource caregivers, and child welfare workers; and
5. Be fairly easy to develop and provide to child welfare workers in a way that lines up with the timing for their plans of care.

In terms of our conceptualization, we relied on the ecological framework (Bronfenbrenner, 1979) to examine how the different systems in which young people are embedded, as well as the relationships between these various systems, can impact educational functioning. We focused on three systems or levels of influence: (1) the young person's characteristics and well-being; (2) the caregiving environment; and (3) the school setting. As such, we incorporated information from the AAR that fits within these three systems and that influences educational outcomes.

The Appendix to Chapter 5 (Appendix F—see Appendix) presents the Education Snapshot, which consists of three main sections.

The *first section* (four pages) includes a cover page with information about the young person and the society, a table of contents, an introduction, and a scoring page. The introduction outlines the organization of the AAR data in terms of the ecological framework and orients the user to consider the information within an evidence-informed practice framework—alongside other sources of information about the young person and through an equity, diversity, and inclusion perspective. The scoring page provides guidance regarding data interpretation and the ways in which information may be used (e.g., more in-depth understanding of the young person's educational needs). The *second section* (four pages) presents AAR data for a particular young person. In line with the ecological framework, there is information about youth-, family-, and school-level variables that can impact educational functioning. We also include material based on the full AAR developmental assets measure that includes a mix of youth-, family-, and school-level variables. The *third section* (seven pages) consists of a worker worksheet, glossary of terms, supervisor checklist, reference table, and acknowledgements. The goal of the worksheet is to give workers the opportunity to interact with and critically consider the AAR data through a set of questions. The worksheet also asks workers to consider how they might share the Education Snapshot results with the young person and their resource caregivers, as well as how they will consider the results in supervision. Finally, the checklist is geared towards child welfare supervisors as a way to better ensure that the findings from the Education Snapshot are being considered in supervision to inform service planning and delivery and outcome monitoring.

4. Case Example

Dylan[1] is a 14-year-old male who was born in eastern Ontario. His mother is Jamaican-Canadian, born in Toronto, and his father is of European descent, originally from Montréal. Having had their own experiences of childhood trauma, Dylan's parents struggled with mental health and substance use throughout Dylan's childhood. During the periods of Dylan's childhood when his parents were actively using substances, he was often left alone overnight with limited food. He was exposed to his parents' substance use and

---

1.   The case example and data presented here are fictional and used to illustrate the use of the Education Snapshot in practice.

to parties they had at the family's apartment. Dylan remembers waking up one night to his parents being unconscious on the kitchen floor. One night when Dylan was 8 years old, police found him walking alone along a busy road. Dylan's parents were not home at the time and had not been present for several days. Following this incident, Dylan was placed in temporary kinship care with his maternal grandparents in Toronto for three months. During this time, Dylan's parents participated in inpatient mental health and substance use treatment and eventually regained custody of their son.

Although Dylan's parents maintained their sobriety, they experienced much stress because of financial struggles. Dylan's parents began getting into frequent arguments and subsequently separated when he was 12 years old. Dylan lived with his mother, who worked three jobs so he was often left alone in the home. While Dylan's father continued to struggle with substance use they did not have frequent contact, Dylan still reported feeling close to his father. When his father was around, they got along well and loved watching soccer together.

When Dylan was 13 years old and had just started grade 8, he began working in the evening as a dishwasher at a local restaurant as he was trying to financially support himself and his mother. Dylan was a strong student who was popular at school and enjoyed playing on the school soccer team, but his teacher was concerned about his increasing absences and noticed that, when he was in school, he appeared tired. He began to withdraw from peers and often complained of hunger. Dylan was reluctant to disclose more information to his teacher, and his teacher and the school were unable to reach either of Dylan's parents. Dylan's teacher subsequently called the local children's aid society to report her concerns. Upon investigation, Dylan's mother was found to be recovering from a substance use binge. The home was in a state of chaos, and the water had been shut off.

Shortly after his elementary school graduation, Dylan was placed in a foster home with a White married couple called Susan and Bob. Dylan's maternal grandparents reported being too old and having too many health problems to properly care for Dylan. Currently, Dylan is in his first year of high school, and he has been living with his caregivers for 1.5 years. He has weekly visits with his mother. There are no additional young people living in the home. Susan and Bob describe Dylan as withdrawn and say he hardly speaks to them. When asked what he feels and needs, he shrugs his shoulders and says, "I don't know." Dylan rejects his caregivers' efforts to talk with him about his biological family and spends most of his time alone in his room. Recently, Dylan has begun yelling and arguing with his caregivers, and he has been experiencing mood swings and irritability. Dylan's teacher reports similar concerns in that he appears more withdrawn and more reactive than usual. Recently, Dylan was involved in a physical altercation at school with a peer, and both boys were suspended for several days. School staff, Susan, and Bob desperately want to help him but are unsure about how best to support him.

Dylan, his female caregiver, and his child welfare worker (Isabelle) recently sat down together to complete the AAR over two meetings, each lasting about one hour. Isabelle has just received the Education Snapshot and is in the process of completing the worksheet in order to better understand Dylan's educational strengths and needs, plan for supervision, and begin preparing for her feedback meeting with Dylan and his caregivers.

5. Worksheet

Below, we present the worksheet questions and the worker's answers to illustrate some of the ways to critically consider the AAR data presented in the Education Snapshot. The wording is in the first person from the perspective of a worker who is completing the form.

There are many factors related to a young person's identity that impact their lived experience and our conceptualization of their strengths and needs. Some factors related to a young person's identity include religion or spiritual affiliation, language, racial and ethnic identity, cultural background, biological sex (e.g., male, female, intersex), sexual orientation (e.g., heterosexual, gay, lesbian, bisexual, queer, two-spirit), gender identity (e.g., male, female, transgender, non-binary, gender non-conforming), gender expression, and socioeconomic status. What are some ways in which factors related to the young person's identity impact their lived experience? How might these factors tie into the young person's strengths and needs, as identified in this AAR Snapshot?

Dylan is a young person of bi-racial background, which we know will impact his lived experience. Could we consider how racism might present itself in the systems with which Dylan interacts? For example, Dylan might be experiencing racist remarks and micro-aggressions within the school environment, which may explain his concerns around bullying/cyberbullying and possibly the physical altercation that resulted in his suspension. Could the bullying/cyberbullying also (or instead) be related to students knowing his family background and that he is in care? He does say he feels safe most of the time at school, as well as travelling to and from school, so I need to better understand safety concerns (if any) at school. I will need to look into aspects of both physical and psychological safety (e.g., asking Dylan what helps him to feel safe and supported at home and at school).

Dylan's racial background is different from that of his caregivers. What is being done to ensure Dylan feels connected to his community? Are his low scores around placement satisfaction and relationship with primary caregiver (identified by him as Susan) partly due to them needing to better understand his experience as a Black male youth? What can Susan and Bob do to facilitate and maintain Dylan's connection to his community?

Dylan is involved in activities (e.g., the school soccer team). Is this sufficient in helping him feel connected to others and to his culture, or would Dylan benefit from participating in additional activities? How can his visits with his mother help? Dylan does not have much contact with his maternal grandparents because they live out of town. Would he like to re-establish regular contact (e.g., phone calls) to help with his sense of belonging and connection to his culture and extended family? Dylan also identified his birth father as a confidant. What can be done to continue building in consistent contact? What role can I play in helping to connect Dylan's birth father to substance use supports so that he can play a more consistent and positive role in Dylan's life?

Review the responses in the previous sections of the Snapshot:

How many green? 6

How many yellow? 3

How many red? 3

Based on these results, what are some areas of strength for this young person? How can these strengths continue to be reinforced?

Strengths fall in the youth and school domains.

Susan (female caregiver) is reporting few behavioural challenges and high prosocial behaviours. Maybe I can continue to reinforce this by involving Dylan in activities that build on his prosocial skills. Talk to him about what he enjoys doing and any activities that he wants to pursue. Is he enjoying his current activities (e.g., being on the soccer team)? Also, talk to him about what is helping with his behaviour.

While Dylan's performance in reading and math was reported as "Good," there are some concerns with his educational success, and he was recently suspended from school. What could be some possible explanations for this discrepancy? What can be done to keep Dylan engaged in his studies and ensure he has stability at school? While Dylan has not missed much school, his suspension is a major concern, and I need to collaborate with the school, Susan, and Bob to determine what is going on at school or at home that is causing Dylan to feel disconnected and/or unsafe and, in turn, more reactive. Could Dylan be experiencing trauma reminders that result in him withdrawing or becoming more reactive? Is he having difficulty coping with his transition into care? How can we all collaborate to ensure Dylan experiences success and engagement both at home and at school?

Dylan is not reporting any substance use. I need to continue to monitor and provide Dylan with accurate information on substance use, especially given his biological parents' struggles in this area.

Dylan has not experienced much adversity this past year, and he says he has people in whom he can confide. I am listed as one of those people so maybe I can spend a bit more time with him.

He lists his grandparents and his birth father but does not see them too often. Perhaps the contact can be increased and become more regular.

Dylan has a number of internal assets. Look through them and consider how they can continue to be promoted in his day-to-day life. For example, he is interested in school, has a good sense of self, and has interpersonal skills. He also holds important values around honesty, social justice, and personal responsibility. I can speak to him about the reasons I scored him as having these internal assets and see if he agrees and then think about ways to keep building these assets (e.g., mentorship to children, child welfare youth advocacy group).

What are some areas that may require additional supports and what resources are available to address these concerns?

There are some concerns. At school, Dylan says he is experiencing bullying, yet also reports feeling safe. Try to get a better understanding so we can come up with a solution (if needed).

For academics, I reported that he was doing well in reading and math, but my scores and those of Susan and Dylan suggest that school work needs to be monitored. Check how my perspective/understanding is similar or different from theirs. Follow up with his homeroom teacher also to get their perspective.

Dylan is reporting mental health difficulties. I need to gather more information—maybe look at the items that make up the Positive Mental Health (i.e., well-being) scale to see exactly what he is reporting. Check with Dylan to better understand his concerns and see what options may be available (e.g., mental health services) and his openness to exploring this option.

Dylan is having problems at home. Speak with him about his relation-ship with Susan and Bob. Does he feel comfortable to share some of his concerns with them? Dylan does not list them as confidants. How can I help? Speak with the caregivers to get their perspective, especially because there seems to be more conflict between them and Dylan recently. What might be going on? Consider an intervention to address these relationship difficulties. Do Susan and Bob need more support and guidance in supporting Dylan's needs?

There are a number of external assets that are missing or that I am uncertain about. There is a greater need to work on Dylan's external sup-ports (relative to his internal assets, although these are still important). He seems to need more positive adult relationships. How can I facilitate creating new relationships for him and how can I strengthen the positive relationships Dylan already has in his life?

How does this information fit with other information you have about this young person (e.g., observations of and interactions with the young person and other important individuals in the young per-son's life)?

How is this information inconsistent with other information you have about this young person? What might explain the differences?

For fit, the information around Dylan's educational functioning seems con-sistent overall when his perspective and that of Susan and his homeroom teacher are considered. This is also what I have understood in interacting with Dylan. However, I should double-check on the academics and any bul-lying/cyberbullying that Dylan might be experiencing. This is especially important given his recent suspension.

What doesn't fit? I need more information about his home environ-ment because Dylan's report seems different than Susan's. When I visit the home, Dylan seems comfortable with Susan and Bob and has told me wants to continue living with them. I need to think about how to strengthen this relationship. Perhaps the caregivers need some supports to focus more atten-tion on the relationship and not primarily on Dylan's behaviour? Maybe the caregivers need strategies that are trauma-informed so they can meet Dylan's needs? It could also be that the increasing conflict with Susan and Bob is not directly related to them but to something else that might be going on with Dylan — school? Visits with mother? Greater desired contact with grandpar-ents and/or father? How can we promote increased autonomy given Dylan's age, while still ensuring he feels supported?

What are some points that are important to discuss in supervision?

Continued supports at school for academics. Assess safety concerns.

Increased involvement in activities/groups to promote Dylan's sense of well-being, with attention to his preferences and to issues around his racialized background. Greater contact with maternal grandparents and birth father?

Assessment of his placement and relationship with his caregivers, with the goal of perhaps introducing more resources to improve their trauma-informed parenting skills.

After better understanding of his mental health concerns, perhaps consider psychological services.

For any interventions (school, mental health), how to ensure they are evidence-informed?

Discuss the best way to present the Education Snapshot to Dylan and his caregivers.

Increased involvement in activities/groups to promote Dylan's sense of well-being, with attention to his preferences and to issues related to his racialized background. Greater contact with maternal grandparents and birth father?

Assessment of his placement and relationship with his caregivers, with the goal of perhaps introducing more resources to improve their trauma-informed parenting skills.

After better understanding of his mental health concerns, perhaps consider psychological services.

For any interventions (school, mental health), how to ensure they are evidence-informed?

Discuss the best way to present the Education Snapshot to Dylan and his caregivers.

How do you plan to share the information presented in this *Education Snapshot* with the young person and caregivers?

Discuss with supervisor but it may be best to start with individual meetings with Dylan and then with his caregivers, especially given Dylan's concerns about his home and his relationship with his caregivers. This information will help me better understand these AAR results.

When I speak with everyone and share the Snapshot, present the framework (individual-, family-, and school-level variables as well as assets). Start with highlighting strengths and then work together to find ways to continue strengthening these areas. Do not use the word "problems" but rather areas of need. Generate solutions together and make sure everyone's perspective is heard. Focus on evidence-based solutions (consult with supervisor and resources).

6. Conclusion

In developing the Education Snapshot, our goal was to illustrate the various ways in which child welfare workers and supervisors can use some of the AAR data to more fully understand the educational strengths and needs of a young person. We believe that the organization of data within a conceptual framework that considers youth-, family-, and school-level variables brings greater clarity around the influences on a young person's educational outcomes. As a result, it is expected that service planning around a young person's educational needs will be enhanced. We have also put much consideration into developing an Education Snapshot that represents the perspectives of all informants and that is organized in an easy-to-use manner to better ensure its applied and sustained use over time. Finally, the inclusion of a worksheet is intended to facilitate a worker's examination of the AAR data by providing a set of questions to consider, and the inclusion of a supervisor checklist is intended to ensure that AAR data are considered as part of supervisory practice and to highlight the important roles of both workers and supervisors in using AAR data for service planning, delivery, and outcome monitoring. As the Education Snapshot is integrated into practice, further information and/or training to support its use will be available to child welfare practitioners as needed.

References

Bronfenbrenner, U. (1979). *The ecology of human development*. Harvard University Press.

Flynn, R. J., Ghazal, H., Legault, L., Vandermeulen, G., & Petrick, S. (2004). Use of population measures and norms to identify resilient outcomes in young people in care: An exploratory study. *Child and Family Social Work*, 9(1), 65–79. https://doi.org/10.1111/j.1365-2206.2004.00322.x

Romano, E., Stenason, L., Weegar, K., & Cheung, C. (2020). Improving child welfare's use of data for service planning: Practitioner perspectives on a training curriculum. *Children and Youth Services Review*, 110, Article 104783. https://doi.org/10.1016/j.childyouth.2020.104783

Stenason, L., Romano, E., & Cheung, C. (2020). Using research within child welfare: Reactions to a training initiative. *Journal of Evidence-Based Social Work*, 18(2), 214–234. https://doi.org/10.1080/26408066.2020.1820413

Chapter 6

Cultural and Personal Identity

There is no single definition of "identity." The development of identity is complex, multidimensional, and fluid (McMurray et al., 2011). Positive identity development embodies a sense of belonging through safe and secure relationships, having opportunities to test identities through age-related and social activities, and having experiences that promote self-efficacy and confidence to construct a sense of agency (Munford & Sanders, 2015). Unger (2015) notes that a strong personal identity, personal control and efficacy, a sense of belonging, cultural adherence, and supportive relationships all serve as important protective factors that contribute to resilience. This chapter examines the culture and identity development of Indigenous Peoples, people of colour (Black, Asian, Latin, and Arab-Canadian), and Franco-Ontarian children and young people in child welfare. These racial or ethnic groups face greater obstacles to identity development within Canadian society, including the child welfare system. With the right support, children and young people in care can form a rich sense of self and connection to their culture.

1. Indigenous Youth and Child Welfare

The Indigenous population in Canada is greatly overrepresented within the child welfare system. According to the Canadian Child Welfare Research Portal, the number of children in the general population in out-of-home care in 2013 was 62,400. For every 1,000 children in Canada, 8.6 children were in out-of-home care in 2013. Over the last ten years, the number of children in out-of-home care has fluctuated roughly between 62,000 and 64,000 (Jones, Sinha, & Trocmé, 2015). According to the 2016 census of the population, 4.9% of the total population of Canada is Indigenous (Statistics Canada, 2017). Across Canada, 7.7% of children aged 0–14 are Indigenous but make up 52.2% of children in care. In Ontario, 4.1% of the population is Indigenous and under the age of 15; however, 30% of children in care are Indigenous (Ontario Human Rights Commission, 2018). In 2019, 3,924 Assessment and Action Records (AAR) were completed and submitted to the Ontario Looking After Children (OnLAC) Project; of those, the racial identity of young people aged 0 to 18 was 57.8% White/European descent, Indigenous 20.3%, Black (African/Afro-Caribbean) 13.4%, and other racial identities 8.5%.

The overrepresentation of Indigenous children and youth in child welfare is a complex issue that extends back to a long historical pattern of the removal of Indigenous children from the care of their families. When the French and British began arriving in North America in the sixteenth century, Indigenous Peoples helped them navigate land and rivers for safe travel, were active agents in commercial trade, and became military allies. British and French traders fought for control over trade, and often this resulted in battles where Indigenous communities made alliances. This era was one of military and economic collaboration. However, after the War of 1812, the need for alliances diminished and the number of settlers rose. With this came an increase in settlers and desire for land to farm and build industry. Indigenous communities on desirable land were now seen as an impediment. The European view that Indigenous communities were autonomous changed, and the push to assimilate Indigenous Peoples into Euro-Canadian culture grew enormously. Indigenous Peoples were organized into reserves and, in many cases, were relocated to designated areas where they were given plots of land to cultivate and would be indoctrinated and assimilated into Euro-Canadian culture (Miller, 1996).

One major aspect of this assimilation project was residential schooling, where children were removed (in many cases forcibly) from their families and communities and sent to boarding schools with the objective to "civilize" and assimilate them into mainstream Euro-Canadian culture. The government created standards for instruction in the schools, but churches acted on behalf of the government in the daily operation, education, Christianization, and "civilization" of the children. Government believed education would rid Indigenous children of ignorance and superstition, and they would be turned into "useful members of society and contributors to, instead of merely consumers of, the wealth of the country" (Miller, 1996, p. 264). It is important to note that some Indigenous communities saw value in the prospect of formal schooling for their children, recognizing that they had to adjust to the changing socioeconomic environment. However, when it became apparent the system was maltreating the children, Indigenous Peoples began to refuse to send their children to the schools and to pressure the government to change how the schools were operated (Miller, 1996). Many children were forcibly removed from their homes after attendance at the schools was mandated by law. Forcible removal from their families was a traumatic experience, as the children experienced relational disruptions.

There were 139 residential schools operating between 1883 and 1996, although most schools had closed by 1979, and only 12 remained until the final school closed in 1996. Over 150,000 children were forced to attend residential schools, with many experiencing physical, emotional, and sexual abuse or dying each year from tuberculosis and malnutrition. It is estimated that the number of deaths was over 6,000, making the odds of death while in residential schooling 1 in 25 (Schwartz, 2015). The recent discovery of mass graves of over 1,000 children on the grounds of Kamloops Indian Residential School in British Columbia and Cowesses Indian Residential School in Saskatchewan and the likely discovery of many more in the future has brought this issue very much to the fore. The earlier estimates of deaths and missing children are now being revised as perhaps closer to 10,000, and local Indigenous leaders are asking for an inquiry and for the church and government to release all administrative records related to the schools (Austen & Bilefsky, 2021).

The government began to phase out residential schooling after the Second World War ended. It was at this time that the federal government took over the administration of the schools, with the intent of moving towards ending the system entirely. In 1947, the Canadian Welfare Council and the Canadian Association of Social Workers recommended changes to the Indian Act to allow provinces and territories to provide on-reserve health, welfare, and education services to Indigenous people. In reality, however, these changes put more power into the hands of the provincial governments, which made agreements with child welfare services, including decisions about child welfare that continued to be made from a Euro-Canadian perspective.

The Sixties Scoop (beginning in the 1960s but lasting almost three decades to the late 1980s) saw a large number of Indigenous children apprehended very rapidly. It is estimated that roughly 20,000 children were taken during this period, often without parental or band consent (McKenzie et al., 2016). Large numbers of children were apprehended because of cultural practice, as Indigenous communities were seen as not in sync with Euro-Canadian culture. In the 1960s, the child welfare system did not require child welfare workers to have any specific training to care for Indigenous children or communities. Child welfare workers removed children from reserves based on the smallest pretext, thinking they were removing the children from a life of poverty, unsanitary conditions, or malnutrition (Mackenzie, 2016). Children were placed into foster or adoptive homes. In some cases, children were sold to the United States to adoptive parents for labour (Mackenzie, 2016). Seventy percent of children apprehended during the Sixties Scoop were placed in non-Aboriginal adoptive or foster homes, and in some cases, they were denied their heritage. In, fact, some adoptive and foster parents told the children they were French or Italian instead of Indigenous. Because birth records were sealed and could only be opened if both the child and parent consented, children who suspected they might be Indigenous were unable to confirm this (Indigenous Foundations, 2009).

The impact of residential schooling on Indigenous individuals, families, and communities has been intergenerational. Parental loss, institutional care, forced acculturation, acculturation stress, and discrimination and racism affected almost all students in residential schools. These factors are associated with impacts later in childhood, adolescence, and adulthood, including mental disorders, traumatic reactions, poor educational attainment, and marginalization (Barnes & Josefowitz, 2019). Residential schooling was destructive for families and communities, resulting in models of parenting based on many negative experiences. The latter included punitive institutional settings; emotional responses lacking the warmth and intimacy of childhood; the repetition of physical and sexual abuse; the loss of knowledge, language, and traditions; the devaluing of Indigenous identity; and the essentializing of Indigenous identity as intrinsic and unchanging (Kirmayer, Simpson, & Cargo, 2003). The result was the "loss of individual and collective self-esteem, individual and collective disempowerment, and, in some instances, the destruction of communities" (Kirmayer et al., 2003, p. 518). It is important to discuss intergenerational damage from residential schooling because many former students of residential schools have retained these negative behaviours. Also, research has shown that Indigenous Peoples experience poor health outcomes as compared to their non-Indigenous peers, and this is related to the impact of colonial disruption (Czyewski, 2001, p. 8). As also noted in Chapter 7 of the present volume, research in childhood maltreatment has found a link that suggests changes in brain functioning can be passed from one generation to another (Ehlert, 2013). Increasing evidence points to a strong interrelationship between epigenetic processes (changes in gene expression, as opposed to modification of the genetic code), genetic temperament, and the body's stress-related hormonal and immune systems (Ehlert, 2013).

According to Cindy Blackstock (2007), Indigenous children are twice as likely to be reported for neglect. Neglect includes poverty, poor housing, and substance misuse, but parents have little ability to control two of these three factors in the short-term. As Blackstock (2007) notes, children were not removed because they were at greater risk with their families, but because these families were at greater risk of social exclusion, poverty, and poor housing. According to Fallon et al. (2013), what are needed are community-based responses that are coupled with provincial/territorial and federal support in order to address the widespread social, economic, and cultural risk factors in Indigenous communities. The 2013 *Ontario Incidence Study of Reported Child Abuse and Neglect* showed that Indigenous children are 130% more likely to be investigated than White children. Allegations of abuse or neglect that involve Indigenous families are 15% more likely to be substantiated, and Indigenous children are 168% more likely to be placed in out-of-home care, compared to White children (Fallon et al., 2016).

Despite a shift in policy and practice that acknowledges the over-representation of Indigenous young people in out-of-home care, little progress has been made to address it. Quinn et al. (2022) found in both the 2013 and 2018 *Ontario Incidence Study of Reported Child Abuse and Neglect* that First Nations youth were two times more likely than White youth to be placed in out-of-home care. The authors suggest a systemic overhaul that is community-based and focused on a model of prevention, rather than investigation.

The overrepresentation of Indigenous children and young people in care must be contextualized, as it is rooted in social and economic systems. According to Trocmé et al. (2010, p. 2083), "current conditions have been shaped by colonial, Canadian, and provincial/territorial policies and practices that dispossessed people from traditional lands, disrupted functioning economic systems, suppressed First Nations cultures and languages, and separated generations of children from their parents." Findings from the CIS-2008 found case characteristics such as maltreatment type, child functioning, and harm levels do not account for the significant overrepresentation of Indigenous children in child welfare. Instead, poverty, poor housing, and substance misuse are the main causes for Indigenous children and young people coming into care.

The authors of the recent *First Nations/Canadian Incidence Study of Reported Child Abuse and Neglect* (Fallon et al., 2021), used the title of their report to denounce the continued overrepresentation of First Nations children in Canadian child welfare. The report is the fourth national study of reported and investigated child maltreatment in Canada and a major resource for better understanding of the long-standing issue of overrepresentation. It is a major resource for knowledge about Indigenous and non-Indigenous young people in child welfare in Canada and covers the following major topics:

- *The Indigenous identity of the child:* Nineteen percent of the nearly 300,000 child maltreatment investigations carried out in Canada in 2019 involved Indigenous children (close to 46,000). Child maltreatment investigations of First Nations children, aged 0–15, were 3.6 times more likely than those involving non-Indigenous children.
- *Child functioning:* At least one concern regarding child functioning was noted in 37% of child maltreatment investigations involving First Nations children, compared with 32% in investigations involving non-Indigenous children.
- *Primary-caregiver risk factors:* At least one primary-caregiver risk factor was noted in 74% of investigations involving First Nations children, versus 57% of inquiries involving non-Indigenous children. Caregivers of First Nations children were more likely to have complex needs, fewer social supports, and mental health or substance issues than caregivers of non-Indigenous children.

- *Housing conditions:* Families in investigations involving First Nations children were more likely to face major structural challenges, including poverty and unsafe or overcrowded housing, thus limiting their capacity to provide for their children.
- *Primary type of maltreatment:* Investigations of neglect were the key driver of the overrepresentation of First Nations children in the child welfare system, with the rate of substantiated investigations focused on neglect 8.5 times higher for First Nations compared with non-Indigenous children.

In an OnLAC study of resilient outcomes among First Nations young people, Filbert and Flynn (2010) found that young people with higher levels of cultural assets (opportunities to participate in First Nations culture) had lower levels of behavioural difficulties. Additionally, First Nations youth who had greater numbers of developmental assets showed greater resilience in terms of prosocial behaviour, academic performance, general self-esteem and fewer behavioural difficulties. For First Nations youth, strengths and culture-based approaches are important because they allow young people to reclaim and reaffirm culture and counter the negative history of colonialism. The social and historical context of First Nations youth places them at higher risk for mental health problems, whereas according to Snowshoe et al. (2015), focusing on cultural connectedness helps one to think from a resiliency and strength-based approach, rather than from a deficit-based approach.

Children in care, unlike their peers in the general population, must manage challenges arising from their adverse experiences and child welfare status. Being in care can compromise knowledge of personal history and engender a sense of loss and not belonging (Winter & Cohen, 2005). According to Saewyc et al. (2013), cultural connection is associated with higher rates of self-esteem, school and family connectedness, and less drinking and destructive behaviour.

The preservation of family relationships, where possible, and access to child welfare records are important to establishing and maintaining family backgrounds, as well as cultural and personal identity development (McMurray et al., 2011; Murray & Goddard, 2014). An Australian study found that good record keeping and having a "portable personal record" were especially important for children whose significant relationships had been most disrupted (Kertsez et al., 2012,

p. 51). Documentation of life stories can be an invaluable resource to explore and construct identities, understand childhood experiences, and resolve identity issues (Kertsez et al., 2012; Murray & Goddard, 2014), since the in-care population can experience gaps in "biological memory," especially from multiple placements (Watson, Latter, & Bellew, 2015, p. 90).

Many Indigenous children apprehended during the Sixties Scoop and whose heritage was kept secret did not experience issues of psychological and emotional stress due to identity suppression until later in life, when they finally learned about their birth family or heritage. Raven Sinclair (2007, p. 66) argues that these experiences create "tremendous obstacles to the development of a strong and healthy sense of identity for the transracial adoptee." In child welfare, lifebooks are an important tool to help children in out-of-home care or who have been adopted to record memories and track life events as they move to different placements. Lifebooks help children keep a connection between their past and present experiences, as well as integrate them in a constructive way. The OnLAC Year 13 AAR report showed that caregivers reported that 94% of children aged 0–4 (n = 1020) had an up-to-date album and 95% of children aged 5–11 (n = 1654) had a personal album. For ages 12–17, the percentage declined to 87% (n = 3627), and by age 18 and older (n = 126), the percentage of young adults who had a personal album had declined to 73%. In OnLAC year 2017, 89% of caregivers reported children and young people aged 0 to 17 had a lifebook, versus 83.9% of young adults 18 and over. The percentage of lifebook use fluctuates slightly throughout the years, but it is consistently reported that the older the young people in care, the less likely they are to have an up-to-date lifebook. The reasons for this could be related to the fact that older youths have other ways to track their personal experiences, especially through social media such as Facebook or Instagram, which can act as a sort of virtual lifebook for posting pictures and capturing memories.

2. Educational Success and Culture

Indigenous young people have a secondary-school graduation rate of 36%, versus 72% for the non-Indigenous population (Assembly of First Nations, 2012). Success in the education system is negatively correlated with poverty rates, and 50% of First Nations children live in poverty (Assembly of First Nations, 2012). Education is important, not only for employment and income levels, but, according to Kirmayer et al. (2007), it is also a protective factor for positive mental health. Young people with higher levels of positive mental health also have positive attitudes towards school, good peer relations, and a positive cultural identity (Kirmayer et al., 2007; Forsman et al., 2016).

Over 50,000 Indigenous students attend public elementary and secondary schools in Ontario, and 70% live in urban areas. Studies of educational success find that many Indigenous students struggle in school because their cultural and linguistic traditions are not represented (Cherubini et al., 2010). There is a discrepancy between traditional Indigenous and Eurocentric models of learning. For example, Eurocentric teaching styles are frequently task-oriented, linear in process, and passive, whereas Indigenous teaching styles are often holistic, cooperative, and active.

Advocating for an emphasis on Indigenous history and culture in the education system has risen in the last 15 years, and in 2009 the Ontario Ministry of Education created the Equity and Inclusive Education Strategy. The objective was to build an inclusive education system that removed discriminatory biases and barriers to student success and well-being that relate to ethnicity, race, faith, family structure, socioeconomic status, sexual orientation, ability, and mental health. Culturally relevant education is a form of education that is culturally sensitive, inclusive, and appropriate to those cultures that exist within the school population. The issue of culturally relevant education needs attention, especially as the number of Indigenous students in public schools increases. As Cherubini et al. (2010, p. 342) remarked, "public education in Ontario is experiencing an unprecedented and steady growth in the number of Aboriginal children in classrooms, and yet the predominantly non-Aboriginal teachers are ill prepared to provide the learning environments necessary to promote self-determination." Culturally relevant education correlates with raising achievement levels, creating equitable environments for learning, and increasing motivation in students (Longboat, 2012).

Gordon and White's (2014) research on Indigenous educational completion in Canada tracked high school and post-secondary completion rates from 1996 to 2011. They found that since the 1996 census, there had been an increase in post-secondary graduation rates. Young people who could be classified as either non-status First Nations or Métis and living off-reserve were most likely to graduate from a post-secondary institution. Gordon and White emphasized that during the same period, non-Indigenous populations also made gains in higher educational attainment levels and graduation from post-secondary institutions. "The number of Indigenous degree holders is increasing both absolutely and proportionally, but the increase in non-Indigenous university completion is even greater. This gap is slowly widening; from 12 percentage points in 1996 to 16 percentage points in 2011" (Gordon & White, 2014, p. 18). As a result, even though more Indigenous people are graduating from post-secondary institutions, their rates of graduation are not at the same rate as non-Indigenous people, and as a result, there are still major socio-cultural and economic barriers for Indigenous people that need to be addressed to close this gap (Gordon & White, 2014).

Mashford-Pringle's (2012) study of the Aboriginal Head Start Urban and Northern Communities (AHSUBC) program in Ontario is an off-reserve learning program that focuses on children aged 3 to 5 and their families, helping Indigenous families navigate two cultures. The program helps the children learn about their bicultural life from parents and extended family in order to help navigate society outside their homes. The program found that participation in the program improved health status, commitment to culture and linguistic revitalization, and improved healthy living practices with families and communities (Mashford-Pringle, 2012). Participants in AHSUBC gained knowledge in interacting with children, and their understanding of biculturalism rose.

Greenberg and colleagues (2016) created an exploratory model of educational outcomes that incorporated risk and protective factors for First Nations youth in out-of-home care in Ontario. The cross-sectional OnLAC sample was composed of First Nations young people, aged 12 to 17, who had participated in the completion of an AAR between 2010 and 2014. The results of their preliminary findings indicated that soft drug use, learning-related difficulties, increased cultural assets (a counter-intuitive result about which we comment later in the chapter), and total behavioural difficulties were risk factors for positive educational outcomes. Predictive protective factors for positive educational outcomes were developmental assets and positive life experiences. Overall, developmental assets were the most influential factor. The more developmental assets the youth had, the more positive the educational outcomes. Also, the more self-identified positive life experiences the young people had had, the higher they scored on positive educational outcomes.

3. Suicidality Prevention and Culture

Suicide and self-inflicted injuries are the leading cause of death of First Nations youth and adults to age 44 (Health Canada, 2003). Indigenous people are five to six times more likely to commit suicide than non-Indigenous populations. According to Statistics Canada, female First Nations youth are more likely to have thought about attempting suicide than First Nations males (33% compared to 29%) and are more likely to have attempted suicide (19% compared to 13% of males) (Health Canada, 2003). Twenty-one percent of First Nations females aged 15 to 17 have reported attempting suicide, three times the rate of males in the same age group (Health Canada, 2003).

Chandler and Lalonde (1998) found that cultural autonomy is a protective factor in regard to suicidality/self-harm. Their 1998 study of First Nations suicide levels in British Columbia began by questioning why the overall suicide rate for First Nations is three to five times higher than the country average. By looking more closely at individual First Nations communities, they uncovered a trend that showed that the rates of suicidality and self-harm varied depending on the number of protective factors a community had and the practices employed to preserve culture. Suicide rates are not evenly distributed across Indigenous communities, and over half of the communities Chandler and Lalonde studied in British Columbia did not have any known suicides, while others had rates 500 to 800 times the national average. Chandler and Lalonde found that those communities that had preserved and promoted cultural heritage had lower rates of suicide. Control over traditional lands, self-government, education, health care, police, fire, and traditional practices all served as protective factors that were linked to decreased rates of youth suicide. The association between community effort and outcomes revealed that success with lowered levels of suicidality was not random, and Chandler and Lalonde (1998, p. 68) argued that "the success that these communities have achieved has clear implications for policy-makers and service providers."

Lalonde's (2006) research on identity formation and resilience in Indigenous communities has implications for Indigenous communities' levels of suicidality. Lalonde began with the question of resilience, which is not something inherent within children (or people in general) but rather a part of a process of the interaction between the child, family, neighbourhood, and social and cultural environment. Individuals able to express how their sense of self endured over time—changing, yet also permanent, either through an *essentialist* strategy (physical features remain, such as eye colour) or *narrative* strategy (a story that connects parts of one's changing life)—experienced lower levels of suicidality. Almost 600 children and youth were interviewed. Those who were not able to use either an essentialist or narrative strategy to express how their person stayed the same yet also endured over time were all persons who, at the time of their interview, had been in a psychiatric setting and actively suicidal (Lalonde, 2006).

Lalonde (2006) found that the wide variation of suicidality levels in different communities was related to their capacity to adapt to the high risks associated with being an Indigenous community. This, in turn, was related to the process of individual identity formation and the capacity for self-continuity, as well as the promotion of culture by the community as a whole. The promotion of culture was also vital to the ability of individuals to form identity. Lalonde (2006) concluded that community rates of suicide risk were different because different communities were more successful in their resistance to the history of acculturation and the threat to cultural existence. That is, communities that made efforts to regain legal title to traditional lands, establish self-government, control education, health care, fire, and police services, or erected facilities within the community that were devoted to traditional culture, events, and practices were equipped to protect their culture, and this was a protective factor for the entire community.

Aside from the work of Chandler and Lalonde, there is little research that examines the high suicide rates of Indigenous people in depth by community. Most research on this topic examines Indigenous experiences across entire provinces and territories, or even the entire country. What makes the work of Chandler and Lalonde important and unique is their examination of individual communities, rather than province- or country-wide studies. Most work on suicidality does uncover the relation of suicidality to socioeconomic factors in communities (including poverty, unemployment, overcrowded housing, access to affordable nutritious food, and clean water), but does not examine the difference in rates of suicide in communities, which varies greatly from zero to five or six hundred times the national average. The Health Canada report, *Acting on What We Know: Preventing Youth Suicide in First Nations* (2003) found that there were specific risk factors for First Nations in relation to suicide and self-harm. These risk factors were economic marginalization, rapid culture change and culture discontinuity, forced assimilation, forced relocations, residential school experiences, and clustering effects due to close ties and identity among youth in small communities (Health Canada, 2003). The report found three major protective factors, including perceived parent/child connectedness, emotional well-being (especially for girls and women), and success at school. In regard to the prevention of suicide in First Nations communities, the report advocated a strong emphasis on youth identity, resilience, and culture, as these act as protective factors vis-à-vis suicidality (Health Canada, 2003).

Greenberg et al. (2016) examined risk and protective factors for suicidality and self-harm in First Nations youth in care. The model included dichotomous variables based on reported experiences by the young people of suicidality/self-harm within the previous 12 months. The respondents answered "yes" or "no" to whether they had attempted to harm themselves, had seriously contemplated suicide, or had attempted suicide. Greenberg et al. (2016) found that the risk factors most highly correlated with suicidality and self-harm among First Nations young people in their sample were sex, age, stress symptoms, and soft drug use. Females were 124% more likely to experience suicidality/self-harm than males. The younger the youth's age, the more likely they were to experience suicidality/self-harm. With each additional year in age, the odds of suicidality/self-harm decreased by 20%. The odds of suicidality and self-harm were greater by 12% for respondents who used soft drugs. The odds of suicidality/self-harm were also 58% greater for every one unit increase in the youth's stress symptoms score.

In their results, Greenberg et al. (2016) found that positive mental health and family-based care were protective vis-à-vis suicidality and self-harm. The young people in the sample experienced a 2% decrease in suicidality/self-harm for every one-unit increase in positive mental health. There was a 41% decrease for suicidality/self-harm for those in family-based care versus group care. (On this latter placement-related finding, see also Chapter 7 in this volume.)

Greenberg et al. (2016) found that the higher the young person's cultural assets score, the lower their positive educational outcomes score. The authors argued that this counter-intuitive result could be due to the fact that the education system does not have in place enough culturally relevant education programs and training for teachers in Ontario. Not all students have equal access to programs to help with cultural connectedness, nor do all schools have programs to help students bridge gaps in culture and education. As a result, it is possible that students who believe that they have high levels of cultural assets would have a more difficult time in schools where the curriculum is Eurocentric rather than culturally appropriate, with their culture not widely represented. According to a report by the Assembly of First Nations, "For Indigenous students, the sense of belonging at school is often the single most important factor of educational success especially where generations before have been marginalized at school" (Longboat, 2012, p. 78). The presence of Indigenous staff contributes to a sense of belonging, but there is a shortage of Indigenous educators/staff in schools. Policy-makers need to mandate participation and leadership in the school system by Indigenous educators and knowledgeable non-Indigenous educators in order to help students learn about their history.

Bania's (2017) report, *Culture as Catalyst: Preventing the Criminalization of Indigenous Youth,* explored the importance of cultural connectedness and its importance to youth development for Indigenous children and young people. Bania's report stressed the significance of resilience and strength-based approaches that connect to Indigenous culture to help Indigenous young people flourish in schools. Studies in Canada have found that the more children and youth are connected to culture, the lower the risk factors for Indigenous people and their connection to violence (Bania 2017). Strengths in Motion is an example of a program that can inspire further dialogue, highlight practical strategies and find synergies between a strength-based approach to child well-being and the Indigenous idea of "living well" through community, family, and societal supports. This program focuses on children in child welfare and the importance of culturally appropriate, strength-based supports in school in order to help develop a positive view of self, leadership skills, problem-solving skills, social competence, sense of purpose, and hope for the future (Bania, 2017).

The impact of the Strengths in Motion program in a Thunder Bay school with a population that is 50% First Nations, compared with a school with no program, found that students in Strengths in Motion were more focused on helping others, had increased school engagement and involvement, and felt better about themselves, their competencies, and classroom environments. Students also made better choices and their academic achievement was higher than First Nations students without the program (Bania, 2017). There is a need for culturally specific programs, as they help children, young people, and their families negotiate the Eurocentric system and provide a place where students can see themselves reflected in the curriculum.

In light of the fact that Indigenous youth in the general population are at a much greater general risk in their daily lives, it is important to discuss the risk and protective factors for positive educational outcomes and suicidality/self-harm for First Nations young people in out-of-home care. The new Child, Youth, and Families Act has included major changes to child protection laws, including a focus on culturally relevant services, particularly for Indigenous and African-Canadians. The Call to Action mandate of the Ontario Association of Children's Aid Societies (OACAS) has committed societies to working with community partners to create a child welfare system that achieves the best outcomes for all children, youth, and families. Included in their plan to make this a reality is a focus on culturally responsive services and a commitment to acknowledging the role of child welfare in the oppression of Indigenous children, youth, and families and taking steps towards reconciliation. To do this, there are many examples of partnerships between community programs and schools that can be drawn upon for implementation in other communities. Child protection workers' training could also include learning about colonialism and the history of residential schools in Canada. Learning these things can help workers understand why certain regulations must be followed when working with Indigenous children and young people in the child welfare system. The Foster Family Coalition of the Northwest Territories has added such topics to their training of child welfare workers and foster families. This kind of training can help workers and caregiving families understand the backgrounds of children coming into care (Mosher, 2017).

The AAR includes questions about identity and identity-related experiences of young people, including a sense of belonging to the young person's culture (fostered through family and social relationships), and opportunities to learn about traditions, customs, ceremonies, or events related to the young person's ethnic or cultural background. Table 6.1 shows that across racial identities, young people aged 10–17 in the OnLAC Project feel they have a strong sense of belonging to their culture, either "a great deal" or to "some" degree.

Table 6.2 shows that the vast majority of young people aged 0 to 18+ responded that they have adequate opportunities to participate in traditions, customs, ceremonies, or events related to their ethnic or cultural background. We can see from the 2019 results that there was a discrepancy based on race for those who answered "yes" versus "no," but within each category, the lowest percentage of responses was 88%, which is still very high. This raises the question of why the rate of "yes" answers was lower than the 94% reported for young White/ European people.

By promoting protective factors, it might be possible to mitigate some of the risk factors and foster good outcomes for children and young people in care. In the case of child welfare, exploring the protective factors for positive educational outcomes for First Nations youth in out-of-home care could prove helpful to combat the lower educational attainment levels First Nations young people generally achieve in Canada. Protective factors from this discussion could also help to highlight ways to aid in lowering suicidality/self-harm rates in First Nations youth in out-of-home.

Table 6.1. Young person has a strong sense of belonging in the young person's culture, fostered through family and social relationships (young people aged 10–17)

	White/ European	Indigenous	Black	Other
A great deal	40.5	34.2	47.3	42.1
Some	51.0	57.7	49.8	48.6
Very little	8.5	8.1	2.9	9.3

Source: Ontario Looking After Children Project data from 2019.

Table 6.2. Adequate opportunities for the young person to participate in traditions, customs, ceremonies, or events related to the young person's ethnic or cultural background (young people aged 0–18+)

	White/ European	Indigenous	Black	Other
No	6.0	12.0	10.5	10.6
Yes	94.0	88.0	89.5	89.4

Source: Ontario Looking After Children Project data from 2019.

4. Racial or Ethnic Minorities in Child Welfare

While it is true that Indigenous children and youth are by far the most overrepresented minority group in the child welfare system in

Canada, there is also growing concern about the overrepresentation of people of colour, including those of Black (African and Caribbean descent), Latin, and Asian descent. The *Canadian Incidence Study of Reported Child Abuse and Neglect* (CIS-2003, Trocmé et al., 2005), which included 11,562 cases of children 15 years of age or younger, revealed that African and Latino young people (including residents and refugees) had the highest investigation rates for neglect (after Indigenous children), while Asian children had the highest level of investigation and substantiation for corporal punishment. Otherwise, Asian children were actually under-represented in other categories (Lavergne et al., 2008).

Lavergne et al. (2008) argued that child vulnerability factors and parental and housing risk factors alone were insufficient to explain the overrepresentation for people of colour, although these factors were important in Indigenous cases. Instead, Lavergne et al. stated that the results of these investigations could reflect racial bias in identifying and reporting maltreatment. Additionally, immigrant parents were thought to face additional challenges, including adapting their role as a parent in a context where values and child rearing models may be different (Lavergne et al., 2008).

While there has been an increase in the recognition that Indigenous families and families of colour must overcome more systemic problems, such as entering the job market, discrimination, poverty, single parenting, inadequate housing, and physical and mental health problems, these issues need to be addressed at a broader level. The Government of Ontario recently drafted a three-year Anti-Racism Strategic Plan, which included a commitment to break down barriers for racial equity. The mandate includes reviewing government policies, programs, and services to make way for racial or ethnic groups to have access to improved opportunities and outcomes. The plan targets racism in policy development and decision-making and evaluates programs and monitors decision-making from an anti-racism perspective (Government of Ontario, 2017). This mandate includes examining the current model of the Ministry of Children, Community and Social Services (MCCSS). Funding has been given to the Ontario Association of Children's Aid Societies (OACAS) for the One Vision One Voice Project, to help develop tools to meet the needs of African-Canadian families and young people in child welfare.

The One Vision, One Voice Project has developed a framework to improve outcomes for African-Canadian young people and families. The Children's Aid Society of Toronto reported in 2013 that 40.8% of children and youth in out-of-home care were Black. The latter are 40% more likely to be investigated compared to White children and 18% more likely to have their abuse substantiated (OACAS, 2016). In Ontario, only Indigenous children have greater disparities than African-Canadians. The OACAS report argued that this overrepresentation is related to levels of poverty, which in turn may lead to neglect and abuse. But the report also suggested that decision-making within child welfare agencies could also be a factor, indicating that systemic racism may result in children from racial or ethnic groups being more likely to be apprehended than those from White homes (OACAS, 2016).

As part of its Anti-Racism Strategic Plan, the Ontario government introduced the Ontario Black Youth Action Plan (OBYAP) to help young people access supports and opportunities closer to home, including mental health, mentors, skill development programs, and family support. There has also been an increase in Indigenous cultural competency training. The Government of Ontario has implemented mandatory Indigenous cultural competency and anti-racism training for all employees in Ontario public services. This training includes discussion of terminology, diversity, colonial history, and violence against Indigenous women. These kinds of training sessions are important to help create anti-oppression frameworks. Yee, Hackbusch, and Wong (2015) argue that an anti-oppression framework can be used as a tool in order to critique, understand, and improve the current practices of child welfare agencies. Understanding the colonial past and how it continues to operate currently can help child welfare develop new practices to address systemic racism by including multiple viewpoints in the administrative and policy decision-making processes (Yee et al., 2015).

Antwi-Boasiako et al. (2022) examined the overrepresentation of Black youth in the Ontario child welfare system. They found racist bias and a lack of cultural sensitivity among referral sources and child welfare workers, which was upheld by a dearth of diversity, training, culturally appropriate assessment tools, and recognition of and collaboration with Black families as stakeholders and experts. The authors emphasized the need for organizations to diversify the workforce, obtain cultural sensitivity training, and provide support for Black families (and other racial or ethnic cultures), in order to ensure young people can remain with their families of origin. As with the overrepresentation of Indigenous children in Ontario child welfare, a systemic shift is needed in order to address the inherent racism and bias present within.

Due to mounting public concern, the Ontario Human Rights Commission (OHRC) launched an investigation into Indigenous and racialized young people in the child welfare system. The OHRC requested information about the collection of identity-based data and the tracking by societies of families receiving services. The OHRC report in 2018, *Interrupted Childhoods: Over-Representation of Indigenous and Black Children in Ontario Child Welfare,* found that Black children (African-Canadian, African-Caribbean, continental African) were overrepresented in approximately 30% of societies in their sample (2018, p. 48). This overrepresentation occurred mostly in urban areas and the Greater Toronto Area. The report made 25 recommendations for societies, the Government of Ontario, and OACAS. The Ontario government needed a provincial strategy to identify and assess the social and economic conditions of families and to link them to disproportionality and disparity. The government should also require child welfare workers to be trained on how to collect human-rights-based data and on anti-racism. The report recommended that OACAS implement the Truth and Reconciliation Commission recommendations that are relevant to its *Call to Action* mandate and create an equity sector to monitor and collect data. Individual societies are required to comply with government regulations to acquire and report data in a standardized way.

Regarding further work in this area, research in Canada concerning Black young people in child welfare is quite limited, and OHRC has specifically demanded that identity-based data be collected by societies across Ontario in a systematic way that is also culturally sensitive and appropriate. While many societies have been concerned with racial disproportion and disparity, the implementation of a deliberate and holistic approach to data collection is needed. Agencies also need dedicated resources to conduct analysis of this data as well as staff that is trained in the collection of data, anti-racism approaches, and cultural sensitivity. The data standards for the collection of identity-based data will be used by societies as well as research initiatives such as the OnLAC Project. The new data standard, which is currently in use, was created to help provide information relevant to analyzing systemic racial discrimination and disparities. The measure itself is under review, and may not stay "as is" in the future.

However, its inclusion as a part of data collection now and in whatever form in the future measure will aid in the collection of data and add to the ethnicity-based data collected by societies for many years. Collecting identity-based data will allow agencies and researchers to look at numerical data in order to help with policies, practices, and decision-making processes within organizations to uncover systemic discrimination and better understand factors that contribute to systemic racial inequalities in access to services or differences in substantiated versus unsubstantiated child welfare cases.

5. Francophone Ontarians

According to the 2016 census, 20.4% of people in Canada reported speaking French as their first language (Statistics Canada, 2016), a decline from the 23% disclosed in the 2011 census. According to the 2011 data, the majority of those who spoke French at home and lived outside of Quebec resided in either New Brunswick or Ontario. In Ontario, 596,000 people spoke French at home and were by far the largest linguistic minority in the province (Statistics Canada, 2011b). In the OnLAC sample from 2017, 1.9% of the 4,771 children and young people aged 0 to 17 indicated they spoke French as a first language, with no other languages. In this group, 37% of the children and youth had completed an AAR in French; 3.4% of the 4,771 children and youth with completed AARs reported French as one of their primary languages.

Canada is constitutionally a bilingual country. In 1968, the Official Languages Act was passed, thereby giving French and English equal official status in Canada and preferred status relative to other languages. In response to this, the Province of Ontario opted to develop its own French Language Services Act (FLSA). The FLSA states services of the provincial government will be provided in French in geographically designated regions, but the FLSA does not give French official language status in Ontario. Societies across Ontario are funded provincially and governed by the Child and Family Services Act (CFSA). They are, however, private and independent organizations, and as such are not legally required to operate in both official languages. However, the CFSA does specify that service providers are to make services available to children and families in French "where appropriate." The 2009–2010 report to the Ontario government by the Ontario French Language Services Commissioner recommended that the Ministry of Children and Youth Services (the predecessor of MCCSS) ensure that societies "actively" offer French-language services and create a network of French-language service providers if they cannot offer services themselves (Lemay, 2012).

Services provided in one's first language are likely to be considerably more effective than if delivered in another language, as language and culture are intertwined. Young people in care who speak French as their first language live in various regions of Ontario. While clusters of Francophones in Eastern and Northeastern Ontario may make it more feasible to offer services in French on a regular basis, all children and young people should, as much as possible, have access to services in their first language, regardless of where they live.

Language is a key component of human service. Assessment and diagnosis are based on questions being asked and answers being given, and intervention mainly involves dialogue and discussion. Thus, linguistic competence is a key factor. The issue here is partly one of practicality and effectiveness, which applies to all languages. However, for Francophones, it is also a question of historic rights and the struggle against assimilation. The CFSA requires that services be provided in French to Francophones. Indeed, even those who are linguistically competent in English have a right in Ontario to be served in French.

6. Conclusion

When the Charter of Rights and Freedoms was created in 1982, Section 27 included what is regarded as a testament to multiculturalism in Canada because it required the entire Charter to be interpreted in a multicultural context. Section 27 reads: "This Charter shall be interpreted in a manner consistent with the preservation and enhancement of the multicultural heritage of Canadians." Less than 10 years later, in 1988, then prime minister Brian Mulroney enacted the Canadian Multiculturalism Act to affirm Section 27 of the Charter, thus ensuring that people of all origins receive equal treatment, be allowed to promote and preserve their cultures, and federal and provincial governments undertake projects and programs that contribute to the multicultural heritage of Canada. Multiculturalism in Canada is a part of public policy and programming, but it is about more than cultural policy, it is an issue of equity. Berry (2013) argues that Canadian policy revolving around multiculturalism has a focus on equity and inclusion, and this is a response to evidence that not all cultures within Canada's diverse society are treated equally. Public programming, therefore, has a focus on "equitable participation" in order to focus on issues of racism and alienation. Society building focuses on a common citizenship, including equity for all, and Canadian multiculturalism is not only about cultural diversity. There is also a civic component that directs lawmakers and policy-makers to focus on equity and the importance of an integrative model of multiculturalism (Berry, 2013).

Because multiculturalism in Canada is sanctioned by law, it could be a useful tool to help support the needs of children whose background is in a minority culture within the child welfare system. Young people in care are already at risk because of their in-care status, but if they are also people of colour, their risk is twofold. The challenge of integration rather than assimilation for all people of colour is one that needs to be considered in child welfare. By using the legality of multiculturalism to discuss the needs of children and youth in care, child welfare organizations could advocate that governments (provincial and federal, for Indigenous children) provide resources to ensure that young people remain connected to their cultures and not feel alienated. The development of identity is important, and connection to their cultural backgrounds helps to ensure continuity in their lives to build resilience. There is a great need for services that foster good outcomes for children and youth in care. The work that OACAS has been doing in mandating changes that focus on the need for culturally responsive services, and programs such as Strengths in Motion with its focus on the development of positive mental health and education, are important in improving positive outcomes for young people. The recent changes to the Child and Family Services Act have also included a new emphasis on making services available and culturally appropriate for young people, to ensure that they receive the best support possible. These kinds of changes are important because they focus on the needs of racial or ethnic cultures and enhance the development of personal identity, a sense of belonging, and cultural attachment, all of which are protective factors that contribute to successful educational attainment, positive mental health, and resilience. Combined with the recommendations from the Ontario Human Rights Commission, these developments put child welfare in a good position to address discrimination and disparities. The focus on collecting identity-based data to make more informed policy decisions is especially important, as it promises to build on the strengths of young people in care and help them achieve a successful future in the world at large.

Much of the research conducted using OnLAC data was done prior to the advent of the First Nations Data Governance Strategy (2020). Completion of the Assessment and Action Record is mandated by the Ontario Ministry of Children, Community and Social Services, but participation in the provincial OnLAC Project by way of data submission to the University of Ottawa remains voluntary. Should a society choose to participate in the provincial OnLAC Project, that society's confidential data remains its property, and is returned to the society at least annually or more frequently, upon request. The University of Ottawa OnLAC team is committed to the principles outlined in the First Nations Data Governance Strategy and to collaboration with societies and Indigenous community partners, and supports societies in their autonomy to choose to participate in the OnLAC Project and use the data collected how they see fit.

The University of Ottawa OnLAC team acknowledges, encourages, and supports an ongoing review of the AAR. In order to ensure that the tool remains relevant to the needs and life experiences of young people in care, revision is needed on a regular basis (at least every five years), but a review of the current AAR-C2-2016 has been on hold for several years now. Revisions are an intensive and important process to ensure that measures included in the tool are culturally sensitive and are able to examine outcomes in child welfare based on changing needs and policies. Revisions work should continue to include community partners, including members of Indigenous and Black communities as experts. At the time of publication, a new revisions committee has not been struck, but the University of Ottawa OnLAC team continues to engage with OACAS regarding the importance of this much-needed work.

References

Aboriginal Children in Care Working Group. (2015). *Aboriginal children in care: report to Canada's premiers*. The Canada's Premiers website: http://canadaspremiers.ca/phocadownload/publications/aboriginal_children_in_care_report_july2015.pdf

Antwi-Boasiako, K., Fallon, B., King, B., Trocmé, N., & Fluke, J. (2022). Understanding the overrepresentation of Black children in Ontario's child welfare system: Perspectives from child welfare workers and community service providers. *Child Abuse & Neglect*, 123, Article 105425. https://doi.org/10.1037/cap0000154

Assembly of First Nations. (2012). A portrait of First Nations education: Fact sheet. *Chiefs Assembly on Education.* http://www.afn.ca/uploads/files/events/fact_sheet-ccoe-3.pdf

Austen, I., & Bilefksy, D. (2021, June 24). Hundreds more unmarked graves found at former residential school in Canada. *The New York Times.* https://www.nytimes.com/2021/06/24/world/canada/indigenous-children-graves-saskatchewan-canada.html

Bania, M. (2017). *Culture as catalyst: Preventing the criminalization of indigenous youth.* Crime Prevention Ottawa. https://www.crimepreventionottawa.ca/wp-content/uploads/2019/02/Ottawa-Street-Violence-Gang-Strategy-2017-2020-final2.pdf

Barnes, R., & Josefowitz, N. (2019). Residential schools in Canada: Persistent impacts on Aboriginal students' psychological development and functioning. *Canadian Psychology*, 60(2), 65–76. https://doi.org/10.1037/cap0000154

Berry, J. W. (2013). Research on multiculturalism in Canada. *International Journal of Intercultural Relations*, 37(6), 663–675. https://doi.org/10.1016/j.ijintrel.2013.09.005

Blackstock, C. (2007). Residential schools: Did they really close or just morph into child welfare? *Indigenous Law Journal*, 6(1), 71–78.

Chandler, M. J., & Lalonde, C. (1998). Cultural continuity as a hedge against suicide in Canada's First Nations. *Transcultural Psychiatry*, 35(2), 191–219. https://doi.org/10.1177/136346159803500202

Cherubini, L., Hodson, J., Manley-Casimir, M., & Muir, C. (2010). Closing the gap at the peril of widening the void: Implications of the Ontario ministry of education's policy for aboriginal education. *Canadian Journal of Education*, 33(2), 329–355. https://www.jstor.org/stable/10.2307/canaje-ducrevucan.33.2.329

Czyewski, K. (2011). Colonialism as a broader social determinant of health. *The International Indigenous Policy Journal*, 12(1), 1–14. https://doi.org/10.18584/iipj.2011.2.1.5

Ehlert, U. (2013). Enduring psychological effects of childhood adversity. *Psychoneuroendocrinology*, 38(9), 1850–1857. https://doi.org/10.1016/j.psyneuen.2013.06.007

Fallon, B., Black, T., Van Wert, M., King, B., Filippelli, J., Lee, B., & Moody, B. (2016). *Child maltreatment-related service decisions by ethno-racial categories in Ontario in 2013 – August 2016.* Canadian Child Welfare Research Portal. http://cwrp.ca/sites/default/files/publications/en/176e_v_0.pdf

Fallon, B., Chabot, M., Fluke, J., Blackstock, C., MacLaurin, B., & Tonmyr, L. (2013). Placement decisions and disparities among aboriginal children: Further analysis of the Canadian Incidence Study of reported child abuse and neglect part A: comparisons of the 1998 and 2003

surveys. *Child Abuse & Neglect*, 37(1), 47–60. https://doi.org/10.1016/j.
chiabu.2012.10.001

Fallon, B., Lefebvre, R., Trocmé, N., Richard, K., Hélie, S., Montgomery, M.,
Bennett, M., Joh-Carnella, N., Saint-Girons, M., Filippelli, J., MacLaurin,
B., Black, T., Esposito, E., King, B., Collin-Vézina, D., Dallaire, D., Gray,
R., Levi, J., Orr, M., Petti, T., Thomas Prokop, S., & Soop, S. (2021).
*Denouncing the continued overrepresentation of First Nations children in
Canadian child welfare: Findings from the First Nations/Canadian Incidence
Study of Reported Child Abuse and Neglect-2019.* Assembly of First Nations.

Filbert, K. M., & Flynn, R. (2010). Developmental and cultural assets and resilient outcomes in First Nations young people in out-of-home: An initial
test of an explanatory model. *Children and Youth Services Review*, 32(4),
560–564. https://doi.org/10.1016/j.childyouth.2009.12.002

First Nations Information Governance Centre. (2020). *A First Nations data governance strategy.* Introducing a First Nations Data Governance Strategy.
https://fnigc.ca/wp-content/uploads/2020/09/FNIGC_FNDGS_report_
EN_FINAL.pdf

Forsman, H., Brännströma, L., Vinnerljung, B., & Hjern, A. (2016). Does poor
school performance cause later psychosocial problems among children
in foster care? Evidence from national longitudinal registry data. *Child
Abuse & Neglect*, 57, 61–71. https://doi.org/10.1016/j.chiabu.2016.06.006

Gordon, C. E., & White, J. P. (2014). Indigenous educational attainment in
Canada. *The International Indigenous Policy Journal*, 15(3), 6–34. https://
doi.org/10.18584/iipj.2014.5.3.6

Government of Ontario. (2017). *A better way forward: Ontario's 3-year anti-racism
strategic plan.* https://files.ontario.ca/ar-2001_ard_report_tagged_final-s.pdf

Greenberg, B., Miller, M., Michael, E., & Flynn, R. (2016, September). *Risk
and protective factors influencing educational success and suicidality for
First Nations youth-in-care in Ontario, Canada* [Conference presentation].
The XIV International Conference EUSARF 2016: Shaping the Future,
Oviedo, Spain.

Health Canada. (2003). *Acting on what we know: Preventing youth suicide in First
Nations.* http://www.hc-sc.gc.ca/fniah-spnia/pubs/promotion/_suicide/
prev_youth-jeunes/index-eng.php#s34

Indigenous Foundations. (2009). *Sixties Scoop.* First Nations and
Indigenous studies: The University of British Columbia. http://
indigenousfoundations.arts.ubc.ca/home/government-policy/sixties-
scoop.html

Jones, A., Vandna, S., & Trocmé, N. (2015). *Children and youth in out-of-home
care in the Canadian provinces.* Canadian Child Welfare Research Portal.
http://cwrp.ca/sites/default/files/publications/en/167e.pdf

Kertesz, M., Humphreys, C., & Carnovale, C. (2012). Reformulating current
record keeping practices in out-of-home care; recognising the centrality

of the archive. *Archives and Manuscripts*, 40(1), 42–53. https://doi.org/10.1080/01576895.2012.668846

Kirmayer, L., Brass, G. C., Holton, T., Paul, K., Simpson, C., & Tait, C. (2007). *Suicide among Aboriginal people in Canada*. The Aboriginal Healing Society. http://www.douglas.qc.ca/uploads/File/2007-AHF-suicide.pdf

Kirmayer, L., Simpson, C., & Cargo, M. (2003). Healing traditions: Culture, community, and mental health promotion with Canadian Aboriginal peoples. *Australasian Psychiatry*, 11(1), S: S15–S23. https://doi.org/10.1046/j.1038-5282.2003.02010.x

Lalonde, C. E. (2006). Identity formation and cultural resilience in Aboriginal communities. In R. J. Flynn, P. M. Dudding, and J. G. Barber (Eds.), *Promoting resilience in child welfare* (pp. 52–71). University of Ottawa Press.

Lavergne, C., Dufour, S., Trocmé, N., & Larrivée, M. (2008). Visible minority, Aboriginal, and Caucasian children investigated by Canadian protective services. *Child Welfare*, 87(2), 59–76.

Lemay, R. A. (2012). Supporting the provision of French language child welfare services in Ontario: Some of the implications of section 2 of the Child and Family Services Act and the French Language Services Act (FLS). Ontario Association of Children's Aid Societies.

Longboat, D. K. (2012). *Soul of sovereignty: The impact of culturally responsive education on the academic achievement of First Nations students*. Assembly of First Nations. http://www.afn.ca/uploads/files/education/soul-of-sovreignty.pdf

Mashford-Pringle, A. (2012). Early learning for Aboriginal children: Past, present and future and an exploration of the Aboriginal head start urban and northern communities program in Ontario. *First Peoples Child & Family Review*, 7(1), 8–28. https://doi.org/10.7202/1068870ar

McKenzie, H. A., Varcoe, C., Browne, A. J., & Day, L. (2016). Disrupting the continuities among residential schools, the Sixties Scoop, and child welfare: An analysis of colonial and neocolonial discourses. *The International Indigenous Policy Journal*, 7(2). http://ir.lib.uwo.ca/iipj/vol7/iss2/4

McMurray, I., Connolly, H., Preston-Shoot, M., & Wigley, V. (2011). Shards of the old looking glass: Restoring the significance of identity in promoting positive outcomes for looked after children. *Child and Family Social Work*, 16(2), 210–218. https://doi.org/10.1111/j.1365-2206.2010.00733.x

Miller, J. R. (1996). *Shingwauk's vision: A history of native residential schools*. University of Toronto Press.

Miller, M., & Flynn, R. (2014). *Looking After Children Ontario provincial report (year 13)*. Centre for Research on Educational and Community Services, University of Ottawa.

Mosher, A. (2017, March 3). Training for N.W.T. child protection workers now includes learning about colonization. *CBC News*. http://www.cbc.

ca/news/canada/north/nwt-foster-care-training-includes-colonization-learning-1.4006671

Munford, R., & Sanders, J. (2015). Negotiating and constructing identity: Social work with young people who experience adversity. *British Journal of Social Work, 45*(5), 1564–1580. https://doi.org/10.1093/bjsw/bcu059

Murray, S., & Goodard, J. (2014). Life after growing up in care: Informing policy and practice through research. *Australian Social Work, 67*(1), 102–117. https://doi.org/10.1080/0312407X.2013.868010

Ontario Association of Children's Aid Societies. (2016). *One vision, one voice: Changing the Ontario child welfare system to better serve African-Canadians.* http://www.oacas.org/wp-content/uploads/2016/09/One-Vision-One-Voice-Part-1_digital_english.pdf

Ontario Human Rights Commission. (2018). *Interrupted childhoods: Over-representation of Indigenous and Black children in Ontario child welfare.* http://www.ohrc.on.ca/en/interrupted-childhoods

Quinn, A., Fallon, B., Joh-Carnella, N., & Saint-Girons, M. (2022). The overrepresentation of First Nations children in the Ontario child welfare system: A call for systemic change. *Children and Youth Services Review, 139,* Article 106558. https://doi.org/10.1016/j.childyouth.2022.106558

Saewyc, E. M., Tsurudo, S., Homma, Y., Smith, A., & Brunanski, D. (2013). Population-based evidence for fostering cultural connectedness to reduce inequalities among Indigenous Canadian adolescents. *Platform Abstracts, 52*(2), Supplement 1, S4. https://doi.org/10.1016/j.jadohealth.2012.10.014

Schwartz, D. (2015, June 2). Truth and Reconciliation Commission: By the numbers. *CBC News.* http://www.cbc.ca/news/indigenous/truth-and-reconciliation-commission-by-the-numbers-1.3096185

Sinclair, R. (2007). Identity lost and found: Lessons from the Sixties Scoop. *First Peoples Child and Family Review, 3*(1), 65–82. https://doi.org/10.7202/1069527ar

Sinha, V., Ellenbogen, S., & Trocmé, N. (2013). Substantiating neglect of First Nations and non-Aboriginal children. *Child and Youth Services Review, 35*(12), 2080–2090. https://doi.org/10.1016/j.childyouth.2013.10.007

Snowshoe, A., Crooks, Claire V., Tremblay, P. F., & Craig, W. M. (2015). Development of a cultural connectedness scale for First Nations youth. *Psychological Assessment, 27*(1), 249–259. https://doi.org/10.1037/a0037867

Statistics Canada. (2016). *Census profile, 2016 census.* http://www.12.statcan.gc.ca/census-recensement/2016/dp-pd/prof/details/page.cfm?Lang=E&Geo1=PR&Code1=01&Geo2=&Code2=&Data=Count&SearchText=Canada&SearchType=Begins&SearchPR=01&B1=All&TABID=1

Statistics Canada. (2013). *National Household Survey: Aboriginal Peoples – Aboriginal Peoples in Canada: First Nations People, Métis and Inuit, National Household Survey year 2011.* (Issue number: 2011001). http://www.12.statcan.gc.ca/nhs-enm/2011/as-sa/99-011-x/99-011-x2011001-eng.cfm

Statistics Canada. (2011a). *Linguistic characteristics of Canadians.* http://www.12.statcan.gc.ca/census-recensement/2011/as-sa/98-314-x/98-314-x2011001-eng.cfm

Statistics Canada. (2011b). *French and the* francophonie *in Canada.* http://www.12.statcan.gc.ca/census-recensement/2011/as-sa/98-314-x/98-314-x2011003_1-eng.cfm

Trocmé, N., Fallon, B., MacLaurin, B., Sinha, V., Black, T., Fast, E., Felstiner, C., Hélie, S., Turcotte, D., Weightman, P., Douglas, J., & Holroyd, J. (2010). *Findings from the Canadian incidence study of reported child abuse and neglect – 2008: Major findings.* Ottawa: Public Health Agency of Canada.

Trocmé, N., Fallon, B., MacLaurin, B., Daciuk, J., Felstiner, C., Black, T., Tonmyr, L., Blackstock, C., Barter, K., Turcotte, D., & Cloutier, R., (2005). *Canadian incidence study of reported child abuse and neglect – 2003: Major findings.* Ottawa: Minister of Public Works and Government Services Canada.

Unger, M. (2015). Resilience and culture: The diversity of protective processes and positive adaption. In C. Theron, L. Liebenberg, and M. Ungar (EDs.), *Youth resilience and culture: Commonalities and complexities, cross-cultural advancements in positive psychology, Vol.* 11 (pp. 37–48). Springer, Dordrecht. https://doi.org/10.1007/978-94-017-9415-2_3

Watson, D. L., Latter, S., & Bellew, R. (2015). Adopted children and young people's views on their life storybooks: The role of narrative in the formation of identities. *Children and Youth Services Review,* 58, 90–98. https://doi.org/10.1016/j.childyouth.2015.09.010

Winter, K., & Cohen, O. (2005). Identity issues for looked after children with no knowledge of their origins: Implications for research and practice. *Adoption & Fostering,* 29(2), 44–52. https://doi.org/10.1177/030857590502900206

Yee, J. Y., Hackbusch, C., & Wong, H. (2015). An anti-oppression (AO) framework for child welfare in Ontario, Canada: Possibilities for systemic change. *British Journal of Social Work,* 45(2), 477–492. https://doi.org/10.1093/bjsw/bct141

Chapter 7

Family and Social Relationships and Social Presentation

It is well established that experiences of childhood maltreatment and removal from the family home can have a detrimental impact on a number of developmental domains, including social relationships, psychological well-being, behavioural functioning, and cognitive and language skills (Boivin & Hertzman, 2012; Oswald, Heil, & Goldbeck, 2010). Such difficulties may continue into later life, if left unaddressed (Cicchetti, 2013). However, previous research has demonstrated that the presence of positive and supportive relationships can work to buffer the negative effects of such experiences (Masten & Shaffer, 2006; Sheridan, Eagle, & Dowd, 2013; Singer, Berzin, & Hokanson, 2013; Storer et al., 2014; Winter, 2015). Masten (2006) indicates that among the factors contributing to adaptive outcomes among maltreated children are relationships and strong connections with one or more effective parents or caregivers. She also names fundamental adaptive systems that, if present, provide children with the tools needed to recover from a wide range of adversities over the course of development, including attachment relationships that provide emotional security and protection, effective self-control systems that provide for the self-regulation of arousal, emotion, and behaviour, and community safety and emergency service systems. While each of these represents an important domain to consider when assessing child well-being, the current chapter focuses on the relationships between children in out-of-home care and the various individuals with whom they directly interact (e.g., family, peers).

With regard to family relationships, previous findings indicate that the relationships children living in out-of-home care have with their families (foster or biological) can have a significant impact on their current functioning (Bell & Romano, 2015; Cheung et al., 2011; Farineau et al., 2013; Legault, Anawati, & Flynn, 2006; Luke & Coyne, 2008). This was highlighted in a Canadian study by Bell and Romano (2015) in which eleven child welfare workers were interviewed to gain their perspectives on the factors associated with resilient functioning among children and young people living in out-of-home care. The critical importance of a child's relationships and social support underpinned all other domains discussed. In particular, child welfare workers emphasized the impact of a positive relationship between the caregiver and child. Such a relationship was described as nurturing within the context of a predictable and stable home environment. Workers also highlighted that integration into the family home by the caregiver, such as including the child in family vacation plans, was a contributing factor to resilient functioning. The need for a positive and supportive caregiver–child relationship is a common finding among both qualitative and quantitative studies utilizing samples of children in out-of-home care, caregivers, and child welfare professionals (Cheung et al., 2011; Daniel, 2006; Drapeau et al., 2007; Fernandez, 2006; Johnson-Garner & Meyers, 2003; Legault et al., 2006; McMurray et al., 2008; Schofield & Beek, 2009; Shuker, Sebba, & Hojer, 2020; Storer et al., 2014; Thomas & Reifel, 2010).

Regarding the child's relationship with his or her biological family members, findings have been mixed. For instance, regular contact with biological parents has been linked with greater prosocial behaviour (Bell et al., 2013), and reduced feelings of abandonment, grief, and depression that are often experienced by children when placed in out-of-home care (Sanchirico & Jablonka, 2000). However, previous findings have also indicated that contact with biological parents can contribute to the development of loyalty conflicts, which have been characterized by psychological distress and behavioural problems that arise from children's conflicting feelings of loyalty, trust, and affection towards their biological parents and their caregivers (Poulin, 1986). This conflict becomes particularly salient when a biological parent is not supportive of the child's placement in a foster family home. Regarding other biological family members, Gilligan (2006) noted that a broad set of social relationships, including individuals who naturally belong to the child's network (e.g., siblings, aunts, grandparents), is key to ensuring the child has stability and continuity in his or her relationships and support in place when needed. These bonds are also important in providing the child with a sense of support.

Turning to peer relationships, these become of increasing importance as children enter school age and adolescence; however, maltreated children often struggle within their friendships. In their review of the literature, Romano et al. (2014) concluded that maltreated children have a tendency to perceive hostility, threat, danger, and/or aggression in their interactions with others. Maltreated children have learned that others cannot be trusted because they can be sources of danger and harm, and these perceptions often get carried forth into their peer interactions. Such interactions are characterized by behaviours (e.g., approach-avoidance, hostility/aggression, fewer prosocial behaviours) that lead to difficulties in developing and/or maintaining relationships (Romano et al., 2014; Shonk & Cicchetti, 2001). Despite these difficulties, for some maltreated children, peers provide a form of relationship consistency and contribute to adaptive outcomes, particularly when connections with family members are weakened (Hedin et al., 2011). For example, among a Ontario Looking After Children (OnLAC) sample of 220 young people aged 14–17 living in out-of-home care, Legault et al. (2006) found that a greater number of perceived high-quality friendships, among other variables (e.g., perception of relationship with female caregiver, self-esteem), predicted lower anxiety and lower physical aggression. Such findings were echoed in a study by Farineau et al. (2013), which utilized a U.S. sample of 188 young people aged 11–16 living in long-term care. The findings revealed that in addition to the adolescents' relationship with their current caregiver, a positive perception of peer relationships was significantly related to greater levels of reported self-esteem. Therefore, maintaining positive peer relationships, where possible, may be of critical importance for maltreated children and young people living in out-of-home care.

Outside of family members and peers, children in out-of-home care interact with other individuals who can have an impact on their current well-being. Such individuals might include teachers, coaches, child welfare workers, and other professionals within the child welfare agency. Collins, Spencer, and Ward (2010) investigated the role of social support among a sample of 96 young adults who had lived in out-of-home care in an American northeastern state until the age of 18 years. The young adults identified several sources of support, including professionals (i.e., outreach workers), family members, and mentors (i.e., extended family, child welfare professionals, community members, friends, or older siblings). The young adults specifically highlighted the role that mentors played in their lives in terms of the longevity and consistency of these relationships. These individuals had remained reliable sources of support, providing ongoing encouragement and assistance when needed over a period of several years. Furthermore, the presence of a mentor was significantly associated with completion of high school and fewer episodes of homelessness (Collins et al., 2010).

Furthermore, in their chapter on young people in care, Britner, Randall, and Ahrens (2014) reviewed current theories and research regarding the impact of mentors on children and young people in out-of-home care. Across the literature, both naturally occurring mentors (i.e., non-parent adults providing support to a child or young person) and formal mentors were found to have a positive impact on the outcomes assessed. For example, in one of the reviewed studies (Munson & McMillen, 2009), having a natural mentor was linked with lower stress and higher life satisfaction as well as fewer depression symptoms and a lower likelihood of being arrested at 19 years of age. It is important to note, however, that additional research demonstrating the effectiveness of natural and formal mentors is needed. Britner et al. (2014) cautioned that the majority of the reviewed research consisted of qualitative data from small samples or limited quantitative investigations, though the results are encouraging.

While few studies have investigated the relationship between child welfare workers and children, such studies have revealed important findings (Augsberger & Swenson, 2015; Bell & Romano, 2015; Finlay, 2003; McLeod, 2010; Singer et al., 2013). For instance, Finlay (2003) concluded that children value their relationship with their worker, but they often report that workers are unavailable, change frequently, and do not listen to their concerns. It has also been reported that workers' administrative roles and heavy caseloads often compromise their ability to form relationships with the children in their care (Department for Education and Skills, 2007). Similarly, Bell and Romano (2015) found that most workers felt additional time to spend with the children on their caseload would be beneficial. However, despite these limitations, workers spoke of their efforts to foster supportive and long-lasting relationships with the children in their care. Bell (2002) refers to the worker–child relationship as a "secondary attachment." While child welfare workers are not a parent substitute, they nevertheless reflect some aspects of a parental role in their responsibilities for the children in their care. This finding is reflected in Table 7.1, which presents child and young person self-reports regarding their confidants. With the exception of their female caregiver, young people most often identified their child welfare worker as a confidant.

Finally, a young person's ability to develop and maintain relationships is in part impacted by his or her social presentation and understanding. Learning how to present well and relate appropriately to others has been recognized as an important aspect of human development. Burger (2015) notes that early childhood experiences and relationships play a significant role in the acquisition of social skills and this can, in turn, influence future learning and development. As noted earlier, experiences of maltreatment can lead to greater perceived hostility, threat, danger, and/or aggression in interactions with others, placing children at an increased risk of impaired social-emotional development (Romano et al., 2014). Such findings were corroborated in a systematic review and meta-analysis by Luke and Banerjee (2013) on the impact of parental physical abuse or neglect on children's social understanding (i.e., ability to understand feelings, beliefs, and desires, and their role in social behaviour). The authors reviewed 51 studies in which comparisons between maltreated and non-maltreated children had been conducted on the outcomes of emotion recognition, understanding, and knowledge. The meta-analysis included 19 studies, 16 of which revealed that maltreated children performed more poorly on emotion skills (recognition, understanding, and knowledge) in comparison with non-maltreated children. Furthermore, the systematic review demonstrated links between maltreatment and perspective taking, false belief comprehension, and hostile attribution bias. However, the authors caution that maltreated children should not be viewed as a homogeneous group. The assessment of a maltreated child's social understanding should encompass his or her strengths, difficulties, and any unique social experiences (Luke & Banerjee, 2013).

1. Findings from the Ontario Looking After Children Project

As part of the Assessment and Action Record (AAR-C2-2010; Flynn et al., 2011), young people 10–17 years of age living in out-of-home care provided a self-report regarding whom they could confide in, in response to this question: "Other than your close friends, do you have anyone else in particular you can talk to about yourself or your problems?" Using the OnLAC Project data from 2015–2016, responses to this question were examined for 10-to-12-year-olds, 13-to-15-year-olds, and 16-to-17-year-olds separately by sex (Table 7.1). In addition, the confidants reported by Indigenous (First Nations, Métis, or Inuit) children and young people were reported independently. The findings are encouraging in that many children and young people were able to identify individuals in whom they could confide. Both boys and girls most often indicated their female caregiver, although the number declined with age. This may be partially explained by the finding that older youth more often experienced less familial homes (i.e., independent living or group homes), compared with younger children, and thus had many fewer opportunities to develop stable relationships with caregivers. Other significant individuals identified included the child welfare worker, male caregiver (particularly among boys), teacher (particularly among younger children), birth mother, grandparents, and foster and biological siblings. Also of note is the young person's boyfriend or girlfriend, particularly among girls 16–17 years of age. These findings remained consistent across several years of OnLAC Project data collection (Miller & Flynn, 2011; 2011a; 2012; 2013). With regard to Indigenous young people, approximately one in ten identified either an Elder, cultural teacher, or Indigenous community member as their confidant.

As part of the AAR, young people 10–17 years of age also respond to questions regarding the quality of their caregiver relationships. On an annual basis, they answer the following four questions: How well do you feel they understand you? How much fairness do you receive from them? How much affection do you receive from them? Overall, how would you describe your relationship with them? Responses to the questions are summed for a total score ranging from 0 to 8, with higher scores indicating higher quality of the caregiver–child relationship, in the eyes of the young person in care.

Previous research (Flynn, Robitaille, & Ghazal, 2006) found that the caregiver–child relationship is a significant predictor of placement satisfaction. Using the OnLAC Project data from 2018–2019, average scores on the quality of the caregiver–child relationship by placement type (Figure 7.1) were examined. The findings revealed that children within kinship and foster family homes rated their caregiver

Table 7.1. Confidants as reported by the young person (N = 3,527)

Confidant	10–12 years N = 759		13–15 years N = 1,349		16–17 years N = 1,419	
	Boys n = 438	Girls n = 321	Boys n = 754	Girls n = 595	Boys n = 746	Girls n = 673
Female caregiver	68.5%	73.8%	60.2%	62.0%	42.4%	49.3%
Child welfare worker	59.6%	62.0%	53.4%	50.8%	50.9%	52.2%
Male caregiver	52.7%	46.7%	45.9%	30.1%	32.6%	22.0%
Teacher	44.7%	46.1%	31.8%	30.3%	22.5%	29.7%
Birth mother	32.4%	41.1%	34.1%	32.6%	32.3%	29.0%
Grandparents	31.7%	33.3%	28.0%	24.2%	24.8%	24.7%
Foster sibling(s)	28.5%	35.5%	22.1%	29.7%	17.8%	22.0%
Other (e.g., family doctor)	27.4%	27.7%	25.6%	28.1%	23.2%	25.6%
Brother	27.2%	24.0%	28.5%	24.2%	27.5%	20.4%
Sister	23.3%	37.4%	27.5%	32.8%	25.5%	31.8%
Other relative	17.8%	21.5%	21.0%	22.0%	18.6%	20.2%
Birth father	17.1%	14.0%	18.7%	15.0%	17.2%	13.5%
Friend of the family or a friend's parent	16.9%	26.8%	19.6%	25.5%	19.4%	28.4%
Coach or leader	8.9%	8.4%	10.3%	8.9%	9.8%	6.7%
Birth parent's partner	4.6%	5.0%	4.6%	5.4%	6.7%	4.8%
Sitter or baby sitter	5.7%	8.1%	1.3%	2.5%	0.7%	0.9%
Boyfriend/ girlfriend	2.7%	4.7%	8.9%	19.2%	16.6%	30.5%
	Indigenous 10–12 years N = 173		Indigenous 13–15 years N = 280		Indigenous 16–17 years N = 215	
	Boys n = 98	Girls n = 75	Boys n = 145	Girls n = 135	Boys n = 117	Girls n = 98
Elder	7.1%	5.3%	9.7%	4.4%	5.1%	11.2%
Cultural teacher	8.2%	8.0%	6.9%	3.7%	6.8%	6.1%
Indigenous community member	11.2%	8.0%	4.8%	7.4%	4.3%	10.2%
Healer	1.0%	1.3%	3.4%	0.7%	1.7%	4.1%

Source: Ontario Looking After Children Project data.

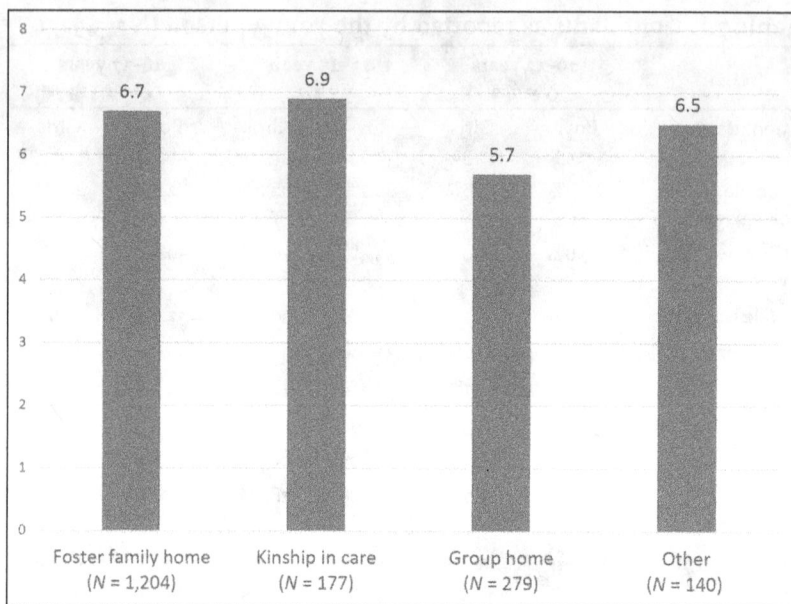

Figure 7.1. Placement type and average scores on quality of the caregiver–young person relationship for 10-to-17-year-olds.

Source: Ontario Looking After Children Project data.

relationship as higher in quality in comparison with children in group homes or other placement types (e.g., mental health facility). This is not surprising, given previous research that has emphasized the importance of having at least one stable positive and supportive caregiver, which is of a higher likelihood within kinship and foster family homes.

Placement satisfaction (as rated by the young person in care) was also examined by placement type (Figure 7.2). Note that the placement satisfaction scale ranges from 0 to 12, with higher scores indicating greater satisfaction. Similar to the quality of the caregiver–child relationship, children within kinship and foster family homes reported greater placement satisfaction than those placed in group homes or other placement types (e.g., mental health facility).

To add to these findings, OnLAC Project data from 2012–2013, based on a sample of 4,034 10-to-17-year-old young people in care ($M = 14.33$, $SD = 2.17$), was used to investigate the relationship between placement satisfaction and quality of the caregiver–child relationship. Over half of the young people (56.0%) were boys, and the majority

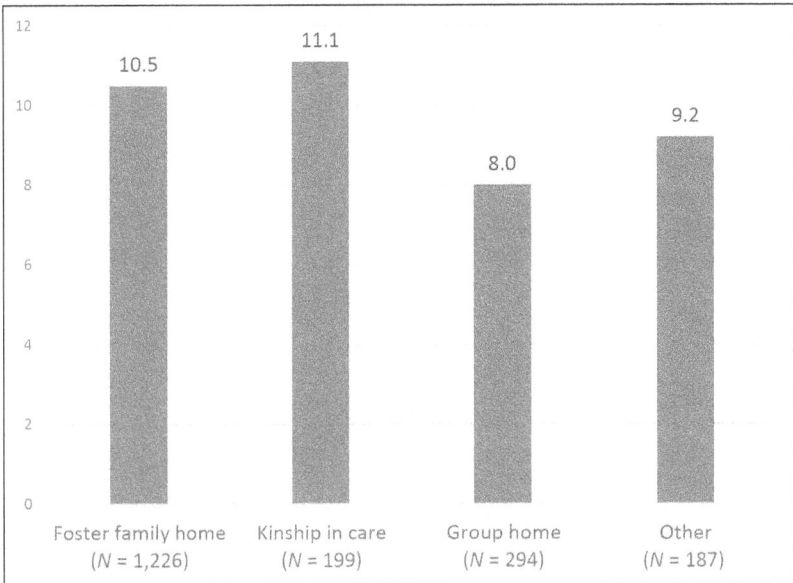

Figure 7.2. Placement type and average scores on placement satisfaction for 10-to-17-year-olds.

Source: Ontario Looking After Children Project data.

were living in foster homes (67.6%), with 18.1% in group homes and 9.7% in kinship homes. The reasons for admission to care were often multiple: neglect (59.0%), emotional harm (38.1%), physical harm (27.5%), domestic violence (21.3%), problematic behaviour (20.5%), abandonment/separation (20.3%), and sexual harm (7.2%).

Prior to conducting a hierarchical regression analysis, inter-correlations among the variables of interest were explored (Table 7.2). All the variables were significantly correlated with placement satisfaction. Older girls had lower levels of placement satisfaction, as did young people with a greater number of family-related adversities in the past year. Those reporting higher-quality relationships with their caregivers and friends reported higher placement satisfaction. Young people in kinship homes reported greater placement satisfaction, while those in group homes were less satisfied.

In our hierarchical regression results (Table 7.3), the young person's age, sex, and past-year family-related adversities were entered into the model at the first step. As a set, these variables accounted for 4% of the variance in the placement satisfaction score. At step 2, placement type was entered into the model and accounted for an additional

Table 7.2. Means (or percentages), standard deviation, and inter-correlations for all variables ($N = 4,034$)

	1	2	3	4	5	6	7	8
1. Placement satisfaction	—							
2. Sex (0 = male, 1 = female)	-.04*	—						
3. Age (years)	-.15**	.02	—					
4. Family-related adversities	-.11**	.08**	-.01	—				
5. Kinship placement	.10**	.03*	-.08**	-.02	—			
6. Group home placement	-.44**	-.10**	.16**	.01	-.16**	—		
7. Quality of caregiver–child relationship	.59**	-.05**	-.17**	-.08**	.05**	-.19**	—	
8. Relationship with friends	.18**	-.04**	-.04*	-.06**	.10**	-.13**	.16**	—
Mean (or percentage)	10.1	56%	14.3	0.7	10.1%	19.3%	6.5	3.2
SD	2.8	-	2.2	1.2	-	-	1.9	1.0

$*p < .05$, $**p < .01$, $***p < .001$
Source: Ontario Looking After Children Project data.

18% of the variance. At step 3, the addition of quality of the caregiver–young person relationship and friendships accounted for a further 25.3% of the variance in placement satisfaction.

At step 3, significant predictors of placement satisfaction included sex, past-year family-related adversities, placement in a group home setting, quality of the caregiver–young person relationship, and relationships with friends. Girls and young people with a greater number of past-year family-related adversities reported lower placement satisfaction, together with those living in group homes versus foster homes. The quality of the caregiver–young person relationship, as perceived by the young person, was the predictor of placement satisfaction that had the largest beta coefficient. Finally, the young person's perceived friendships also predicted greater placement satisfaction.

Table 7.3. Summary of hierarchical regression analysis for variables predicting placement satisfaction (N = 4,034)

Variable	β
Step 1	
Sex (0 = male, 1 = female)	-.03
Age (years)	-.15*
Family-related adversities	-.10*
Step 2	
Sex (0 = male, 1 = female)	-.07*
Age (years)	-.08*
Family-related adversities	-.09*
Kinship placement	.02
Group home placement	-.43*
Step 3	
Sex (0 = male, 1 = female)	-.04*
Age (years)	-.01
Family-related adversities	-.05*
Kinship placement	.01
Group home placement	-.34*
Quality of caregiver–child relationship	.51*
Relationship with friends	.05*

Note. R^2 = .04 for Step 1; ΔR^2 = .18 for Step 2; ΔR^2 = .25 for Step 3.
*$p < .001$.
Source: Ontario Looking After Children Project data.

2. Conclusion

The findings from the current chapter provide correlational evidence of the impact of a positive relationship between the caregiver and young person. When asked who they felt they could talk to about themselves and their problems, the majority of the young people in our sample identified their female caregivers. Furthermore, our hierarchical regression analysis showed that the quality of the caregiver–young person relationship (as seen by the young person) was the single best predictor of greater placement satisfaction, with controls for several other variables (i.e., the young person's sex and age, past-year family-related adversities, placement type, and relationships with friends). This is consistent with previous findings, which have pointed to the importance of a high-quality caregiver–young person relationship for young peoples' outcomes (e.g., Cheung et al., 2011; Legault et al., 2006; Thomas & Reifel, 2010). Furthermore, our findings echoed those of Flynn et al. (2006), who found a higher-quality relationship between the young person and female caregiver to be a robust predictor of placement satisfaction. When such a close relationship is characterized by understanding, fairness, and affection, a young person's positive adaptation and well-being is considerably more likely.

Our findings may also be read through the lens of the Developmental Relationships Framework, which was recently established by the Search Institute through intensive research, data analysis, and input from scholars and practitioners (Roehlkepartain et al., 2017). The framework builds upon the Search Institute's previous research on developmental assets and internal and external resources that contribute to the ability to thrive (see Chapter 2, this volume). A report by Roehlkepartain et al. (2017) defined developmental relationships as a mix of five elements—express care, challenge growth, provide support, share power, and expand possibilities—which can be expressed through 20 actions, such as be dependable, set boundaries, or collaborate. According to the authors, developmental relationships exist when they assist children or young people to discover who they are, develop abilities to shape their own lives, or learn how to engage with and contribute to the world around them. The application of this framework in child welfare in future research would permit a better understanding of how caregivers engage in developmental relationships with young people in their care. This is of particular interest in light of findings that developmental relationships can have an influence on multiple domains of a young person's functioning (e.g., educational attainment, psychological and emotional well-being) and prepare the way for successful transitions into young adulthood (Scales et al., 2016).

The developmental relationships framework could also be useful for assessing and supporting other relationships in a young person's life. In particular, our findings indicate that child welfare workers and teachers are key individuals with whom young people in care feel they can talk to about themselves and their problems. For Indigenous children and young people, such individuals include Elders, cultural teachers, and Indigenous community members. Roehlkepartain et al. (2017) suggest that different types of relationships can be developmental, and they list mentors and other non-family adults, parents, friends, teachers, and program leaders as potential candidates for participating in such relationships with young people. This highlights the necessity of paying attention to all the individuals with whom a young person interacts, across various contexts, and to support these relationships, where possible. Given the encouraging literature regarding the positive impact of natural and formal mentors for children and young people in out-of-home care (Britner et al., 2014), we should no doubt encourage the formation of developmental relationships between mentors and mentees and seek to maximize their positive impact.

References

Augsberger, A., & Swenson, E. (2015). "My worker was there when it really mattered": Foster care youths' perceptions and experiences of their relationships with child welfare workers. *Families in Society, 96*(4), 234–240. https://doi.org/10.1606/1044-3894.2015.96.34

Bell, M. (2002). Promoting children's rights through the use of relationship. *Child & Family Social Work, 7*(1), 1–11. https://doi.org/10.1046/j.1365-2206.2002.00225.x

Bell, T., Romano, E., & Flynn, R. J. (2013). Multilevel correlates of behavioral resilience among children in child welfare. *Child Abuse & Neglect, 37*(11), 1007–1020. https://doi.org/10.1016/j.chiabu.2013.07.005

Bell, T., & Romano, E. (2015). Child resilience in out-of-home care: Child welfare worker perspectives. *Children and Services Review, 48*, 49–59. https://doi.org/10.1016/j.childyouth.2014.12.008

Boivin, M., & Hertzman, C. (Eds.). (2012). *Early childhood development: Adverse experiences and developmental health*. Royal Society of Canada – Canadian Academy of Health Sciences Expert Panel.

Burger, K. (2015). Effective early childhood care and education: Successful approaches and didactic strategies for fostering child development. *European Early Childhood Education Research Journal, 23*(5), 743–760. https://doi.org/10.1080/1350293X.2014.882076

Britner, P. A., Randall, K. G., & Ahrens, K. R. (2014). Youth in foster care. In D. L. DuBois & M. J. Karcher (Eds.), *Handbook of youth mentoring* (pp. 341–353). Sage Publications.

Cheung, C., Goodman, D., Leckie, G., & Jenkins, J. (2011). Understanding contextual effects on externalizing behaviors in children in out-of-home care: Influence of workers and foster families. *Children and Youth Services Review, 33*(10), 2050–2060. https://doi.org/10.1016/j.childyouth.2011.05.036

Cicchetti, D. (2013). Annual research review: Resilient functioning in maltreated children – past, present, and future perspectives. *Journal of Child Psychology and Psychiatry*, 54(4), 402–422. https://doi.org/10.111/j.1469-7610.2012.02608.x

Collins, M. E., Spencer, R., & Ward, R. (2010). Supporting youth in the transition from foster care: Formal and informal connections. *Child Welfare*, 89(1), 125–143.

Daniel, B. (2006). Operationalizing the concept of resilience in child neglect: Case study research. *Child: Care, Health, & Development*, 32(3), 303–309. https://doi.org/10.1111/j.1365-2214.2006.00605.x

Department for Education and Skills. (2007). *Departmental report 2007*. Crown Copyright.

Drapeau, S., Saint-Jacques, M-C., Lepine, R., Begin, G., & Bernard, M. (2007). Processes that contribute to resilience among youth in foster care. *Journal of Adolescence*, 30(6), 977–999. https://doi.org/10.1016/j.adolescence.2007.01.005

Farineau, H. M., Wojciak, A. S., & McWey, L. M. (2013). You matter to me: Important relationships and self-esteem of adolescents in foster care. *Child & Family Social Work*, 18(2), 129–138. https://doi.org/10.1111/j.1365-2206.2011.00808.x

Fernandez, E. (2006). Growing up in care: Resilience and care outcomes. In R. J. Flynn, P. M. Dudding, & J. G. Barber (Eds.), *Promoting resilience in child welfare* (pp.131–156). University of Ottawa Press.

Finlay, J. (2003). *Crossover kids: Care to custody*. Toronto: Office of Child and Family Service Advocacy.

Flynn, R. J., Robitaille, A., & Ghazal, H. (2006). Placement satisfaction of young people living in foster or group homes. In R. J. Flynn, P. M. Dudding, & J. G. Barber (Eds.), *Promoting resilience in child welfare* (pp. 191–205). University of Ottawa Press.

Flynn, R., Vincent, C., & Miller, M. (2011). *User's manual for the AAR-C2-2010*. Centre for Research on Educational and Community Services, University of Ottawa.

Gilligan, R. (2006). Promoting resilience and permanence in child welfare. In R. J. Flynn, P. M. Dudding, & J. G. Barber (Eds.), *Promoting resilience in child welfare* (pp. 18–33). University of Ottawa Press.

Hedin, L., Hojer, I., & Brunnberg, E. (2011). Why one goes to school: What school means to young people entering foster care. *Child & Family Social Work*, 16(1), 43–51. https://doi.org/10.1111/j.1365-22&06.2010.00706.x

Johnson-Garner, M. Y., & Meyers, S. A. (2003). What factors contribute to the resilience of African-American children within kinship care? *Child & Youth Care Forum*, 32, 255–269. https://doi.org/10.1023/A:1025883726991

Legault, L., Anawati, M., & Flynn, R. J. (2006). Factors favoring psychological resilience among fostered young people. *Children and Youth*

Services Review, 28(9), 1024–1038. https://doi.org/10.1016/j.childyouth. 2005.10.006

Luke, N., & Banerjee, R. (2013). Differentiated associations between childhood maltreatment experiences and social understanding: A meta-analysis and systematic review. *Developmental Review,* 33(1), 1–28. https://doi.org/ 10.1016/j.dr.2012.10.001

Luke, N., & Coyne, S. M. (2008). Fostering self-esteem: Exploring adult recollections on the influence of foster parents. *Child & Family Social Work,* 13(4), 402–410. https://doi.org/10.1111/j.1365-2206.2008.00565.x

Masten, A. S. (2006). Promoting resilience in development: A general framework for systems of care. In R. J. Flynn, P. M. Dudding, & J. G. Barber (Eds.), *Promoting resilience in child welfare* (pp. 3–17). University of Ottawa Press.

Masten, A. S., & Shaffer, A. (2006). How families matter in child development: Reflections from research on risk and resilience. In A. Clarke-Stewart & J. Dunn (Eds.), *Families count: Effects on child and adolescent development* (pp. 5–25). Cambridge University Press. https://doi.org/10.1017/ CBO9780511616259.002

McMurray, I., Connolly, H., Preston-Shoot, M., & Wigley, V. (2008). Constructing resilience: Social workers' understandings and practice. *Health and Social Care in the Community,* 16(3), 299–309. https://doi.org/ 10.1111/j.1365-2524.2008.00778.x

McLeod, A. (2010). "A friend and an equal": Do young people in care seek the impossible from their social workers? *British Journal of Social Work,* 40(3), 772–788. https://doi.org/10.1093/bjsw/bcn143

Miller, M., & Flynn, R. (2011). *Looking After Children Ontario provincial report (year 9).* Centre for Research on Educational and Community Services, University of Ottawa.

Miller, M., & Flynn, R. (2011a). *Looking After Children Ontario provincial report (year 10).* Centre for Research on Educational and Community Services, University of Ottawa.

Miller, M., & Flynn, R. (2012). *Looking After Children Ontario provincial report (year 11).* Centre for Research on Educational and Community Services, University of Ottawa.

Miller, M., & Flynn, R. (2013). *Looking After Children Ontario provincial report (year 12).* Centre for Research on Educational and Community Services, University of Ottawa.

Oswald, S. H., Heil, K., & Goldbeck, L. (2010). History of maltreatment and mental health problems in foster children: A review of the literature. *Journal of Pediatric Psychology,* 35(5), 462–472. https://doi.org/10.1093/ jpepsy/jsp114

Poulin, J. E. (1986). Long term foster care, natural family attachment and loyalty conflict. *Journal of Social Service Research,* 9(1), 17–29. https://doi. org/10.1300/J079v09n01_02

Roehlkepartain, E., Pekel, K., Syvertsen, A., Sethi, J., Sullivan, T., & Scales, P. (2017). *Relationships first: Creating connections that help young people thrive.* Search Institute.

Romano, E., Babchishin, L., Marquis, R., & Fréchette, S. (2014). Childhood maltreatment and educational outcomes. *Trauma, Violence, & Abuse,* 16(4), 1–20. https://doi.org/10.1177/1524838014537908

Sanchirico, A., & Jablonka, K. (2000). Keeping foster children connected to their biological parents: The impact of foster parent training and support. *Child and Adolescent Social Work Journal,* 17, 185–203. https://doi.org/10.1023/A:1007583813448

Scales, P. C., Benson, P. L., Oesterle, S., Hill, K. G., Hawkins, D., & Pashak, T. J. (2016). The dimensions of successful young adult development: A conceptual and measurement framework. *Applied Developmental Science,* 20(3), 150–174. https://doi.org/10.1080/10888691.2015.1082429

Schofield, G., & Beek, M. (2009). Growing up in foster care: Providing a secure base through adolescence. *Child & Family Social Work,* 14(3), 255–266. https://doi.org/10.1111/j.1365-2206.2008.00592.x

Sheridan, S. M., Eagle, J. W., & Dowd, S. E. (2013). Families as contexts for children's adaptation. In S. Goldstein & R. B. Brooks (Eds.), *Handbook of resilience in children* (pp. 165–179). Springer.

Shonk, S. M., & Cicchetti, D. (2001). Maltreatment, competency deficits, and risk for academic and behavioral maladjustment. *Developmental Psychology,* 37(1), 3–17. https://doi.org/10.1037/0012-1649.37.1.3

Shuker, L., Sebba, J., & Hojer, I. (2020). Teenagers in foster care: Issues, themes, and debates from and for practice and policy. *Child & Family Social Work,* 24, 349–353. https://doi.org/10.1111/cfs.12650

Singer, E. R., Berzin, S. C., & Hokanson, K. (2013). Voices of former foster youth: Supportive relationships in the transition to adulthood. *Children and Youth Services Review,* 35(12), 2110–2117. https://doi.org/10.1016/j.childyouth.2013.10.019

Storer, H. L., Barkan, S. E., Stenhouse, L. L., Eichenlaub, C., Mallillin, A., & Haggerty, K. P. (2014). In search of connection: The foster youth and caregiver relationship. *Children and Youth Services Review,* 42, 110–117. https://doi.org/10.1016/j.childyouth.2014.04.008

Thomas, M., & Reifel, B. (2010). Child welfare workers' knowledge and use of a resilience approach in out-of-home care. *Advances in Social Work,* 11(1), 17–32. https://doi.org/10.18060/246

Winter, K. (2015, February 20). *Supporting positive relationships for children and young people who have experience of care. Insight 28, Evidence summaries to support social services in Scotland.* Institute for Research and Innovation in Social Sciences (IRISS). http://www.iriss.org.uk/resources/supporting-positive-relationships-children-and-young-people-who-have-experience-care

Assessing Young People's Mental Health from Their Level of Well-Being and Type of Residential Placement

This chapter describes a simple, rapid assessment scheme to determine the mental health status of young people in out-of-home care, based on information readily available in their respective Assessment and Action Records (AAR-C2-2016). We provide data on the validity of the scheme, in terms of its ability to predict four positive and four negative measures of mental health. The assessment scheme, intended for use by child welfare workers, supervisors, or caregivers, is based on answers to just two questions from the AAR. First, does the young person's total score on Keyes' (2006) 14-item measure of well-being fall within the highest, middle, or lowest (i.e., third) tertile of the scores from a large sample of young people in care in Ontario? Second, does the young person currently reside in a residential placement with a higher or lower average level of well-being; that is (in the Ontario context), in a kinship care or foster home (higher well-being) versus an independent living or group home (lower well-being)? As we show, a young person's tertile on Keyes' well-being measure strongly predicts his or her relative status on eight specific AAR measures of mental health. As we also indicate, the type of home in which the young person currently resides adds predictive power on six of the eight specific measures of mental health, even though the type of home is typically a weaker predictor than the well-being tertile.

The main advantage of our 2-variable assessment scheme for workers, supervisors, or caregivers is its simplicity and rapidity, which we hope will facilitate its use in daily clinical practice. From our experience over the last two decades in the Ontario Looking After Children (OnLAC) Project (2000–2021), clinical staff in child welfare agencies almost never use complex, multi-variable assessment methods in daily practice. They tend to view such approaches as overly complicated, technical, and time consuming, for which their prior education and training have rarely prepared them. The scheme that we present here, in contrast, is easy to use, requiring knowledge of only the young person's well-being tertile and type of residential placement. Workers, supervisors, or caregivers know the type of home and can obtain the well-being score from a simple hand calculation from the AAR or from the society's SPSS data set, which is sent to the society routinely upon request. Such an assessment scheme is timely, as the Ontario Ministry of Children, Community and Social Services (MCCSS) is striving to establish more rigorous, empirical, and valid quality standards for the residential services that it licences (MCCSS, 2019). (Child welfare personnel interested in a related but considerably more technical, multi-variable predictive model of the mental health of young people in care, based on a larger number of AAR variables, could consult with and profit from Cullen et al.'s [2021] regression-based approach.)

1. Effects of Child Maltreatment on the Mental Health of Young People in Care

Before addressing our main objective, we first provide a brief overview of research on the mental health of young people in out-of-home care. Previous studies have established that adversity in early childhood, such as maltreatment, is frequently associated with subsequent psychological, emotional, and health problems (Biglan, 2014; Boivin & Hertzman, 2012; Malla et al., 2018). The Expert Panel Report on Early Childhood Development of the Royal Society of Canada and the Canadian Academy of Health Sciences (Boivin & Hertzman, 2012) suggested that child maltreatment is the most severe form of adverse childhood experiences that exists. Child maltreatment may cause poor mental and physical health that lasts into adolescence and young adulthood (Boivin & Hertzman, 2012). Longitudinal studies have found that early adversity stemming from maltreatment, deprivation, disruptions in caregiving, or harsh parenting is typically associated in adolescence and young adulthood with a host of negative consequences, including depression, behaviour problems, anti-social behaviour, delinquency, involvement with the judicial system, substance use disorders, or suicide attempts (Boivin & Hertzman, 2012).

The impact of child maltreatment extends far beyond physical harm, encompassing damage to children's cognitive, behavioural, social, and physical development (Malla et al., 2018; Biglan et al., 2012). Multiple prenatal, environmental, and psychosocial risk factors compound the adverse effects of maltreatment (Oswald et al., 2010), such that by the time children enter the child welfare system, many have already experienced significant trauma (Dorsey et al., 2012). Young people in care are thus likely to have more risk and fewer protective factors than their age peers in the general population (Harpin et al., 2013). Swedish research has shown that young people in care are at greater risk of psychiatric disorders in adolescence and adulthood (Lehmann et al., 2013) and are also more likely to attempt suicide than their age peers in the general population (Vinnerljung et al., 2006).

Each developmental phase in infancy, childhood, and adolescence is important in terms of its potential consequences for healthy functioning and positive outcomes in the cognitive, social-emotional, behavioural, and physical domains (Komro et al., 2011). Childhood maltreatment, in contrast, is associated with negative changes in brain functioning (Ehlert, 2013) and epigenetic processes (i.e., changes in gene expression, as opposed to modifications of the genetic code) that may be transmitted to subsequent generations (Hébert & MacDonald, 2009, p. 453). Indeed, there is accumulating evidence of strong links between epigenetic processes, genetic temperament, and the body's stress-related hormonal and immune systems (Ehlert, 2013). Perry (2009) suggests that the *timing* of developmental experiences is important, with the impact of traumatic (or positive) events possibly differing with age. This is consistent with Masten's (2016) assertion that how an experience influences adaptive systems varies depending on the sensitivity of the system at that time. Known as *plasticity*, this variation in the response to an experience depends upon its context, such that the same "resource or trait or adaptive system could function as a liability in some situations and a protective factor in another" (Masten, 2016, p. 80).

2. Positive Mental Health and Well-Being

According to Keyes (2005; 2006; 2007), *positive mental health* encompasses the capacity to function effectively and the presence of many human strengths, including well-being, maturity, positive emotional balance, socio-emotional intelligence, life satisfaction, and resilience. *Well-being* (a major theme of this volume) consists of three distinguishable components. *Emotional well-being* includes life satisfaction and a balance of positive over negative emotions. *Psychological well-being* encompasses a fully engaged life through self-acceptance, personal growth, autonomy, sense of purpose, sense of mastery, and positive relations with others. *Social well-being* involves the capacity to function effectively within community life (Lamers et al., 2011; Keyes et al., 2015).

International resilience research indicates the importance of protective factors in promoting positive mental health or well-being. At-risk adolescents and young adults who have a positive temperament, self-esteem, good reading skills, and a strong, positive relationship with mentors who provide guidance during the young persons' formative years have better developmental trajectories (Boivin & Hertzman, 2012; Littlefield et al., 2017). Studies of mental health outcomes among young people in out-of-home care have found that high-quality relationships with caregivers are important for well-being (Rayburn et al., 2018; Legault et al., 2006; Dumoulin & Flynn, 2006). The perception of an emotionally secure relationship with a caregiver mediates between a young person's prior exposure to violence and subsequent internalizing, externalizing, or trauma symptoms (Rayburn et al., 2018). Such a relationship has also been shown to be the most consistent predictor of positive psychological outcomes in terms of lower levels of anxiety, more close friends, higher self-esteem (Legault et al., 2006), hope, and active coping skills (Dumoulin & Flynn, 2006). Positive experiences in care, close relationships, and personal development promote positive adaptation and protective processes that enable young people in care to buffer adversity and risk factors (Legault & Moffat, 2006).

Social-emotional skills develop through relationships with significant adults, and young people with greater social and emotional competence tend to have better outcomes (Littlefield et al., 2017). Research on young people in care has generally found that factors promoting emotional and behavioural resilience include internal resources, such as a sense of competency and self-efficacy, intelligence, social skills, academic achievement, and a positive out-look on life. Such factors also include external environments, espe-cially broad and stable social relationships and communities, such as schools, neighbourhoods, extra-curricular organizations, and child welfare workers and agencies. These multiple internal and external influences converge to shape resilient outcomes (Bell et al., 2015; 2013; Bell & Romano, 2015).

3. Negative Mental Health

Young people in care have frequently experienced early adversity, such as family disruption, and often exhibit high rates of cogni-tive, affective, and behavioural difficulties. For instance, the Ontario incidence study of 2008 (Fallon et al., 2010) reported that in 43% of substantiated child maltreatment cases, the investigating worker identified at least one child functioning problem. The most preva-lent issues were academic difficulties (20%), depression, anxiety, or withdrawal (18%), aggression (16%), attachment issues (13%), atten-tion deficit disorder/attention deficit hyperactivity disorder (ADD/ADHD; 11%), and intellectual or developmental disabilities (10%). Similar rates were reported in the United States (Sullivan & van Zyl, 2008) among 2,996 children, aged 0 to 21, residing in care, 44% had an identified emotional need and 32% a diagnosed medical need; older young people were more likely to have an emotional need, whereas those in care for a longer time had more medical needs.

Maltreated young people who are in care tend to have higher rates of behavioural problems compared with those who remain in their homes or youths who have not experienced maltreatment (Berger et al., 2009; Doyle, 2007; 2013; Fernandez, 2006; Keil & Price, 2006; Lawrence et al., 2006; Warburton et al., 2014). In a longitudinal study, Lawrence et al. (2006) found that children placed in care during the early elementary years (grades 1–3) had greater behavioural problems upon exiting care in comparison with those who had been maltreated but had remained in their homes, despite the fact that these two groups did not differ significantly on behavioural measures prior to placement.

3.1. Strengths and Difficulties Questionnaire (SDQ)

The Strengths and Difficulties Questionnaire (SDQ; Goodman 1997) is used internationally to evaluate the behavioural and emotional functioning of young people, including those in care, and has been incorporated into the AAR. It comprises 25 items and, in the AAR context, is completed by caregivers of children or adolescents in care aged 6–17. The SDQ consists of five 5-item sub-scales, four assessing negative mental health (*emotional symptoms, conduct problems, hyperactivity/ inattention,* and *peer problems*) and one assessing positive mental health (*prosocial behaviour*). When summed, the four negative sub-scales form the *Total Difficulties Scale*. The SDQ has been translated into more than 60 languages and is considered a culturally sensitive instrument (Achenbach et al., 2008).

International research with the SDQ has produced important findings. Egelund and Lausten (2009), for example, compared the prevalence of psychiatric diagnoses and mental health problems on the SDQ sub-scales among Danish children living in either foster or residential placements (n = 1,072), children receiving in-home child welfare services (n = 1,457), and non-child-welfare-involved children (n = 71,321). Of the children in care, 20% had a diagnosed mental illness, compared with 21% of those receiving in-homes services but only 3% of those who were non-welfare involved. On the SDQ negative mental health sub-scales (i.e., emotional, conduct, hyperactivity/ inattention, or peer problems), 48% of the children in care, versus 31% of those receiving in-home services and only 5% of the non-welfare-involved children, scored within the abnormal range.

3.2. Research in Ontario with the SDQ, Based on Assessment and Action Record Data

Several OnLAC studies have used the SDQ and AAR data to assess the mental health of young people in care. For example, Marquis and Flynn (2009) compared the functioning of 492 young people in care, aged 11–15, with a normative sample also aged 11–15 from the British general population (used in the absence of Canadian general-population norms). The young people in care in Ontario had significantly higher scores on behavioural problems and lower scores on prosocial behaviour than the British normative sample.

Cheung et al. (2011) assessed externalizing behaviour in a multi-informant study with 1,063 young people in care aged 10–17. Workers reported on whether the young persons had any serious emotional or behavioural problems, caregivers rated them on the SDQ conduct problems scale, and the young people, aged 12–15, self-reported on their own physical aggression and property offences. Multilevel modelling indicated that worker and family effects accounted for a combined 28% of the variance in child externalizing behaviours, highlighting the important influence of contextual factors on young people's behaviour. Worker education, placement type, caregiver ratings of conduct problems, and young people's placement satisfaction were also related to externalizing behaviour.

Bell et al. (2013) also used multilevel modelling to assess the influence of the child, foster family, worker, and child welfare agency on child behavioural outcomes, evaluated by means of the conduct problems, emotional problems, and prosocial behaviour sub-scales of the SDQ. Depending on the outcome in question, 57.1% to 75% of the explained variance was due to children's individual characteristics and experiences, 25% to 42.9% to between-foster-family differences, and 5.9% to between worker and between child welfare agency differences (on conduct problems only). Although the study aimed at identifying resilient children, a considerable proportion were found to be functioning relatively poorly (i.e., below the normal range) on the SDQ sub-scales. Bell et al. (2013) also examined functioning within the domains of peer relationships and academic performance, finding that an even smaller proportion were functioning inside the normal range, which indicated the importance of assessing functioning in a broad, holistic manner.

3.3. Suicidal Behaviour among Young People in Care

Suicide is a significant cause of death among children and adolescents (Keeshan et al., 2017), and young people with a history of abuse or neglect are at an even higher risk of suicidal behaviour than their age peers in the general population (Castellví et al., 2017; Okpych & Courtney, 2018). A meta-analysis of longitudinal studies found that early exposure to violence is a risk factor for both suicide attempts and completions among adolescents and young adults (Castellví et al., 2017). Placement instability, the age at which young people have most recently entered care, placement type, and maltreatment type are all risks for depression, post-traumatic stress disorder (PTSD), and suicide attempts (Okpych & Courtney, 2018). Additional risk factors associated with suicide attempts in the general adolescent population include female sex, a history of psychiatric disorder, substance abuse, and lack of appropriate and timely treatment interventions (Keeshen et al., 2017). The latter study found that, compared to young adults, young children who committed suicide were predominantly male, with high rates of diagnoses of ADHD. Females, on the other hand, were overrepresented among the adolescent age group (12–18 years), compared with young adults (19 and older) and children aged 7–11.

In the Ontario child welfare system, Baiden and Fallon (2018) detected lower than expected rates of referral for mental health services in investigations that had observed self-harming behaviours and suicidal thoughts. They recommended specific training for child welfare workers to identify children in care needing mental health services. By recognizing the symptoms of trauma, depression, anxiety, behavioural problems, and suicide-related behaviour, child welfare workers would be able to make more timely referrals to appropriate mental health services and suicide prevention programs (Baiden & Fallon, 2018; Castellví et al., 2017; Keeshen et al., 2017).

3.4. Mental Health of Indigenous People

Nelson and Wilson (2017) reviewed 223 papers on the mental health of Indigenous people in Canada. They observed that while mental health issues and suicidality were typically higher in the Indigenous than in the general population, there was much variation in rates across different communities. They cited studies documenting the negative physical and mental health outcomes of social inequality, unemployment, poverty and racism, urging caution in formulating conclusions about the prevalence of mental health issues among Indigenous people without considering the impact of intergenerational and individual trauma, such as the association between residential schools and suicide.

Nelson and Wilson (2017) identified barriers to addressing the physical and mental health needs of Indigenous people and made a number of recommendations:

- Address colonial perspectives within health services, to counteract racism and discrimination;
- Integrate Indigenous cultural practices and healing methods into mental health services to make them more accessible and promote community wellness through strengthening cultural identity and pride;

- Conduct research into which integrated and culturally adapted community-based mental health interventions are most effective for different Indigenous people in different environments (e.g., on reserve vs. off-reserve);
- Understand the importance of cultural safety in addressing societal power imbalances and the impact of social determinants of health on the well-being of individuals and their overall communities;
- Realize that focusing research on substance abuse and suicide may have the unintended consequences of perpetuating stereotypes of substance abuse and unhealthy behaviours and diverting attention from the resolution of structural issues facing Indigenous people in Canada;
- Appreciate that the underrepresentation of urban Inuit, Métis, or First Nations communities may promote over-generalizations regarding Indigenous mental health problems and neglect unique issues.

4. Method in the Present Assessment Study

4.1. Level of Well-Being and Type of Current Residential Placement as Predictors of Specific Mental Health Indicators in Young People in Care in Ontario

As we stated at the outset, our main objective in this chapter is to provide workers and supervisors with a simple, rapid, and valid, albeit preliminary, means of assessing the mental health of young people in care, based on AAR data. This initial insight into a young person's mental health status hinges on answers to just two questions that can be posed regarding information in the young person's AAR: Does the young person's total score on Keyes' (2006) 14-item self-report measure of positive well-being fall within the highest, middle, or lowest tertile of the distribution of total scores of young people in care in Ontario? And, does the young person currently reside in a relatively higher-well-being home (i.e., a kinship care or foster home) or in a relatively lower-well-being-home (i.e., an independent living or group home)? As we will show, a young person's tertile (highest, middle, or lowest) on Keyes' measure of general well-being strongly predicts the favourableness of his or her standing on eight specific AAR measures of mental health, four positive and four negative. The type of home in which the young person currently resides provides added predictive power in the case of six of the eight specific indicators of mental health. As a predictor, the effect size of the type of home is smaller, compared with that of the well-being tertile, in the case of four of the eight mental health indicators, and about equal in the case of the other four indicators (see the effect-size column in Table 8.4, below).

4.2. Keyes' 14-Item Measure of Well-Being

Keyes' measure of well-being (a term which in the present context we view as a synonym for positive mental health) is displayed in Table 8.1. The first three items assess emotional well-being, items 4–8 assess social well-being, and items 9–14 assess psychological well-being. We sought to validate Keyes' measure as a consistent predictor of eight specific indicators of mental health that, like Keyes' well-being measure, form part of the current version of the AAR (AAR-C2-2016). Four are indicators of positive mental health: the quality of the young person's relationship with the main caregiver and his or her level of hope, developmental assets, and placement satisfaction. Four are indicators of negative mental health: the young person's level of behavioural difficulties, stress symptoms, soft drug use, and suicidal behaviour. We also wanted to discover whether the relatively higher or lower well-being type of home where the young person was living added any predictive power and assessment value to the young person's well-being tertile, in relation to our eight specific mental health indicators.

4.3. Participants: Young Persons in Care in Ontario

We used AAR data from 2017 from the OnLAC Project database. The data included 2,114 young people in care who, in calendar year 2017, were 10–17 years of age and had a completed AAR for 2017. There were 1,117 males (52.8%), 997 females (47.2%), and one intersex young person (0.1%). As noted in Table 8.1, the mean total score on Keyes' 14-item measure of well-being was 53.54 (median = 56.0, SD = 13.92). The young persons responded to the items listed in Table 8.1 on a 6-point scale (Every day = 5; Almost every day = 4; Two or three times a week = 3; About once a week = 2; Once or twice a month = 1; and Never = 0). The internal consistency (alpha coefficient) of the instrument was excellent (.93).

Table 8.1. Means and standard deviations on Keyes' (2006) 14-item measure of well-being (N = 2,115)

Item	Mean	SD
During the past MONTH, how often did you feel:		
1. Happy?	4.04	.95
2. Interested in life?	4.14	1.10
3. Satisfied?	4.05	1.12
4. That you had something important to contribute to society?	3.40	1.60
5. That you belonged to a community (like a social group, your school, or your neighbourhood)?	3.84	1.49
6. That our society is becoming a better place for people like you?	3.26	1.72
7. That people are basically good?	3.63	1.45
8. That the way our society works made sense to you?	3.21	1.72
9. That you liked most parts of your personality?	4.15	1.17
10. Good at managing the responsibilities of your daily life?	3.99	1.11
11. That you had warm and trusting relationships with other children/youth?	3.99	1.31
12. That you had experiences that challenged you to grow and become a better person?	3.83	1.37
13. Confident to think or express your own ideas and opinions?	4.13	1.17
14. That your life has a sense of direction or meaning to it?	3.89	1.39
Total score:	53.54	13.92

Note. Items 1–3 measure emotional well-being, items 3–8 social well-being, and items 9–14 psychological well-being. Response options for all items: 5 = Every day; 4 = Almost every day; 3 = Two or three times a week; 2 = About once a week; 1 = Once or twice a month; 0 = Never. *Source:* Ontario Looking After Children Project data from 2017.

4.4. Highest, Middle, and Lowest Well-Being Tertiles

Based on the total scores on Keyes' 14-item measure of well-being, as well as on natural breaks in the distribution of total scores, we classified the young people in care into approximate tertiles (i.e., thirds). The 673 young people whose total scores fell between 62 and 70 constituted the highest well-being tertile (31.8%); the 730 whose total scores fell between 50 and 62 (34.5%) formed the middle tertile; and the 712 whose total scores were between 0 and 50 (33.7%) made up the lowest tertile. That Keyes' well-being measure and our eight mental health indicators can all be viewed as mental health measures is supported by the moderate to strong and uniformly statistically significant correlations between them in Table 8.2, below. Accordingly, we

Table 8.2. Means and standard deviations on Keyes' (2006) 14-item well-being measure of the young people in care residing in each type of home

Type of Placement	Mean	SD	n
Higher Well-Being Homes			
Kinship Care Home	57.26	10.79	205
Foster Home	55.27	13.10	1305
Lower Well-Being Homes			
Independent Living Home	50.34	13.65	105
Group Home	47.48	15.43	349

Note. A one-way ANOVA, followed by a Tukey HSD test, revealed that the four types of homes formed two homogeneous and significantly different clusters ($p < .05$). The clusters comprised, respectively, "higher well-being homes" (i.e., kinship care and foster homes, the difference between whose means was not significant, $p = .11$), and "lower well-being homes" (i.e., independent living and group homes, the difference between whose means was also not significant, $p = .40$).
Source: Ontario Looking After Children Project data from 2017.

expected that those in the highest well-being tertile would also score most favourably on all eight of our specific mental health indicators, those in the middle well-being tertile would score moderately favourably and those in the lowest well-being tertile would score poorly. (As will be seen, these expectations were confirmed in our data analyses, suggesting that the young people in the lowest well-being tertile should receive the most immediate assistance from clinicians to improve their mental health, followed by those in the middle tertile and then, as needed, those in the highest tertile.)

In a previous study based on AAR data (Flynn, Miller, & Vincent, 2012), we had found that a young person's tertile in terms of developmental assets was a good predictor of several educational outcomes. We had also observed that workers found it clinically meaningful to think in terms of highest, middle, and lowest asset tertiles and the gradient they formed in relation to educational outcomes. The asset tertiles conveyed two key ideas. First, a young person's asset tertile communicated immediate information about his or her likely position on a range of educational outcomes. Second, the idea of the young person's progressing from a lower to a higher asset tertile, or at least from a lower to a higher position within his or her current tertile, presented the young person, worker, and caregiver with a concrete and motivating goal. We anticipated similar advantages from using tertiles in the present mental-health context.

4.5. Higher and Lower Well-Being Homes

We classified the four types of homes in which the young people in care had been placed in terms of the total scores on Keyes' (2006) 14-item well-being measure of the young people currently living in each type of home: kinship care, foster, independent living, and group homes. Table 8.3 displays the number of young people residing in each type of home and their respective means and standard deviations on Keyes' well-being measure. We carried out a one-way analysis of variance (ANOVA) on the four types of homes ($F[3] = 38.19$, $p < .001$). A follow-up Tukey Honestly Significant Difference (HSD) test revealed that the four types of homes clustered into two homogeneous sub-types,

Table 8.3. Means, standard deviations, correlations with Keyes' (2006) 14-item measure of well-being, alpha, range, and skew of indicators of positive and negative mental health

Mental Health Indicators	N	Mean	SD	Correlation with Keyes' 14-Item Measure of Well-Being	Alpha	Range	Skew
Indicators of Positive MH							
Relationship with Main Caregiver Scale	1891	6.51	1.95	.42*	.87	0–8	-1.36
Hope Scale	1704	13.13	4.03	.59*	.86	0–18	-.52
Total Developmental Assets Scale	1964	26.76	8.28	.30*	.80	0–40	-1.01
Placement Satisfaction Scale	1861	10.12	2.80	.45*	.89	0–12	-1.54
Indicators of Negative MH							
SDQ Total Difficulties Scale	1783	12.97	7.61	-.37*	.86	0–40	.34
Stress Symptoms Scale	1749	3.31	3.34	-.33*	.67	0–16	1.10
Soft Drug Use Scale	1905	1.58	2.45	-.28*	.87	0–9	1.37
Suicidal Risk Scale	1683	.77	1.09	-.32*	.76	0–4	1.51

Note. MH = Mental Health. *$p < .001$
Source: Ontario Looking After Children Project data from 2017.

which we labelled *higher-well-being homes* (kinship care and foster homes) and *lower-well-being homes* (independent living and group homes). The two sub-types or clusters were significantly different from one another ($p < .05$). The kinship care and foster homes had the highest mean well-being scores (57.26 and 55.27, respectively, which were not significantly different, $p = .11$). The independent living and group homes had the lowest mean well-being scores (50.34 and 47.48, which were also not significantly different, $p = .40$).

We speculate that the differences between the two clusters of homes might have been due in part to selection or program effects or both. *Selection effects* could have resulted from a tendency of the child welfare system to place young people with higher levels of well-being in kinship care or foster homes and those experiencing lower levels of well-being in independent living or group homes. *Program effects* may have stemmed from organizational elements such as a basic difference in staff models, with kinship care and foster homes yielding higher well-being among young people in care because of the presence of live-in adult caregivers, whereas independent living and group homes were marked by lower well-being because of the absence of live-in caregivers.

4.6. Working Hypotheses

Our first working hypothesis was that on the four indicators of *positive* mental health, the mean of the young people in the highest well-being tertile (calculated based on Keyes' 14-item measure) would be significantly *higher* than the mean of the middle tertile, which in turn would be significantly *higher* than the mean of the lowest tertile. Conversely, on the four indicators of *negative* mental health, we predicted that the mean of the highest well-being tertile would be significantly *lower* than that of the middle tertile, which in turn would be significantly *lower* than the mean of the lowest tertile.

Our second working hypothesis was that on each of the four indicators of *positive* mental health, young people residing in the higher well-being homes (i.e., foster or kinship care homes) would report *higher* mean scores than those living in the lower well-being homes (i.e., independent living or group homes). Conversely, on the four indicators of *negative* mental health, the young people residing in the higher well-being (kinship care or foster) homes would report *lower* mean scores than those living in the lower well-being (independent living or group homes). (The eight indicators of mental health, all incorporated into the AAR-C2-2016, are described in greater detail in the *User's Manual for the AAR-C2-2016* [Miller et al., 2017].)

4.7. Indicators of Positive Mental Health

To test our two working hypotheses, we chose four measures of positive mental health and four of negative mental health from those available in the 2017 OnLAC data set. The positive and negative indicators are defined briefly in Table 8.3, together with their internal consistency (alpha) coefficients, correlations with Keyes' 14-item measure of well-being, and other characteristics.

- Quality of Young Person's Relationship with Primary Caregiver Scale: a 4-item scale that the young person uses to rate the quality of his or her relationship with the main caregiver (who in most cases is female), in terms of the caregiver's understanding, fairness, and affection, and the overall closeness of the relationship. (Response options: "A great deal" = 2, "Some" = 1, "Very little" = 0.)
- Children's Hope Scale (Snyder et al., 1997): a 6-item self-report measure of the young person's perception that they can meet their goals. Sample item: "When I have a problem, I can come up with lots of ways to solve it." (Response options: "Most of the time" = 3 to "Never" = 0.)
- Total Developmental Assets Scale: a 40-item scale, completed by the child welfare worker. It covers 20 external assets of the young person in care, in four areas: support, empowerment, boundaries and expectations, and constructive use of time. It also covers 20 internal assets, in four areas: commitment to learning, positive values, social competencies, and positive identity.
- Placement Satisfaction Scale: a 6-item self-report scale measuring the young person's level of satisfaction with his or her current home. Sample item: "Overall, would you say that you are satisfied with your current living situation here?" (Response options: "A great deal" = 2; "Some" = 1; "Very little" = 0.)

4.8. Indicators of Negative Mental Health

- SDQ Total Difficulties Scale: a 20-item scale that the caregiver uses to rate the behavioural difficulties of the young person in care (Goodman, 1997). It includes four 5-item sub-scales, covering emotional symptoms, conduct problems, hyperactivity/inattention, and peer problems. (Response options: "True" = 2, "Somewhat true" = 1, and "Not true" = 0).
- Stress Symptoms Scale: A 4-item scale on which the young person reports the frequency during the past six months of headache, stomach ache, backache, or difficulties in getting to sleep. (Response options: "Seldom/never" = 0 to "Most days" = 4.)
- Soft Drug Use Scale: A 3-item measure in which the young person reports the frequency of use of cigarettes or other tobacco products, alcohol, or marijuana or cannabis products in the past 12 months. (Response options: "Daily" = 0 to "Not at all" = 3.)
- Suicidal Risk Scale: A 3-item measure on which the young person reports whether, in the past 12 months, they attempted to hurt themselves, seriously considered suicide, or attempted suicide. (Response options: "Yes" = 1, "No" = 0.)

4.9. Data Analysis

To test our working hypotheses, we carried out a two-way analysis of variance (i.e., three well-being tertiles × two types of homes ANOVAs), one for each of the eight mental health indicators. We followed up each ANOVA with Tukey HSDT tests for the multiple comparisons among the tertile means.

5. Results

Table 8.4 displays the tertile and type-of-home sub-group sizes for the eight indicators of positive or negative mental health and, from the two-way ANOVAs, the F-tests for the well-being tertile and type-of-home factors and the tertile-by-type-of-home interactions. On the eight mental health indicators, the F-tests for the tertiles were all statistically significant at the $p < .001$ level, and virtually all the multiple comparisons among the tertile means (conducted with Tukey HSD

Table 8.4. Group sizes, F-tests, and effect sizes from factorial ANOVAs conducted on the eight mental health indicators, for the tertile and type-of-home factors and their interaction

Mental Health Indicators	Group sizes for the H-Highest, M-Middle, & L-Lowest Well-Being Tertiles	Group sizes for the H-Higher & L-Lower Well-Being Types of Homes	F(df) For the Tertile Factor	F(df) for the Type-of-Home Factor	F(df) for the Tertile-by-Type-of Home Interaction	Effect size (ES=partial eta squared) for: T=Tertiles, H=Type-of-Home, & I=Interaction
Relationship with Main Caregiver Scale	H - 583 M - 620 L - 571	H - 1418 L - 356	F(2,1768) =64.37***	F(1,1768) = 24.16***	F(2,1768) = 0.05 (ns)	T - .068*** H - .013*** I - .000 ns
Hope Scale	H - 542 M - 592 L - 570	H - 1293 L - 411	F(2,1698) =234.13***	F(1,1698) = 2.92ᵃ	F(2,1698) = 0.47 (ns)	T - .216*** H - .002 ns I - .001 ns
Total Developmental Assets Scale	H - 636 M - 683 L - 645	H - 1510 L - 454	F(2,1958) = 69.59***	F(1,1958) =170.17***	F(2,1958) = 0.58 (ns)	T - .066*** H - .080*** I - .001 ns
Placement Satisfaction Scale	H - 615 M - 648 L - 604	H - 1455 L - 412	F(2,1861) = 94.52***	F(1,1861) =184.05***	F(2,1861) = 3.61*	T - .092*** H- .090*** I - .004*
SDQ Total Difficulties Scale	H - 578 M - 623 L - 582	H - 1408 L - 375	F(2,1777) = 55.04***	F(1,1777) = 99.92***	F(2,1777) = 0.30 (ns)	T - .058*** H - .053*** I - .000 ns
Stress Symptoms Scale	H - 559 M - 610 L - 580	H - 1334 L - 415	F(2,1743) = 73.58***	F(1,1743) = 32.05***	F(2,1743) = 0.31 (ns)	T - .078*** H- .018*** I - .000 ns
Soft Drug Use Scale	H - 613 M - 668 L - 624	H - 1463 L - 442	F(2, 1899) =46.00***	F(1,1899) = 72.16***	F(2,1899) = 4.74**	T - .046*** H - .037*** I - .005**
Suicidal Risk Scale	H - 538 M - 576 L - 569	H - 1280 L - 403	F(2,1677) = 40.04***	F(1,1677) = 13.87***	F(2, 1677) = 0.16 (ns)	T - .046*** H - .008*** I - .000 ns

Note. ES = effect size = partial eta squared; ns = not significant. Here, ES = the proportion of the total variance in a given mental health indicator associated with membership in the different levels of the tertile or type-of-home independent variables, with the effects of the other independent variable and interaction partialled out. In the case of the interaction, ES = the proportion of the total variance associated with the interaction, with the effects of the tertile and type-of-home independent variables partialled out (Richardson 2011). Small, medium, and large values of partial eta squared are, respectively, .01, .06, and .14.
*p < .05, **p < .01, ***p < .001, ᵃp = .09
Source: Ontario Looking After Children Project data from 2017.

tests) were also significant at the $p < .001$ level, with only two significant at either the $p < .002$ or $p < .003$ level. These results were in close agreement with our first working hypothesis.

Seven of the eight F-tests for the type-of-home factor were also statistically significant at the $p < .001$ level, in good agreement with our second working hypothesis. Only the F-test for the type-of-home factor on the Hope Scale was not statistically significant ($p > .05$). Finally, six of the eight interaction F-tests (about which we had not formulated any working hypotheses) were not statistically significant.

Overall, these results were supportive of our two working hypotheses. In presenting Figures 8.1–8.8 now, we describe visually the results of the pairwise comparisons among the highest, middle, and lowest well-being tertiles and the contrasts between the two types of homes. We also include (in the last column in Table 8.4) the size of the effects, expressed as *partial eta squared,* associated with the tertile and type-of-home factors and their interactions, respectively, for the eight mental health indicators. Partial eta squared is equal to the proportion of the total variance in a dependent variable that is associated with the membership of different groups defined by a particular independent variable, with the effects of other independent variables and interactions partialled out (Richardson, 2011). Small, medium, and large partial eta squared effect sizes are, respectively, .01, .06, and .14.

5.1. Association of Well-Being Tertiles and Types of Homes with Four Indicators of Positive Mental Health

5.1.1. Quality of Young Person's Relationship with the Main Caregiver Scale

Figure 8.1 displays the mean scores for the two types of homes within each of the three well-being tertiles, on the first indicator of positive mental health, namely, the quality of the young person's relationship with the main caregiver scale. As can be seen from Figure 8.1, within the highest well-being tertile, the mean quality-of-relationship score reported by the young people in the combined kinship and foster care home category was 7.4 (out of a maximum of 8.0), compared with 6.9 for the young people in the combined independent-living and group home category. Similarly, within the middle well-being tertile, the mean scores for youths in the two categories of homes were 6.7 versus 6.1, respectively, and within the lowest well-being tertile, 5.9 versus 5.3, respectively. As hypothesized, Tukey's HSD test indicated that the young people in the highest well-being tertile rated the quality of their relationships with their main caregivers more highly than did those in the middle tertile ($p < .001$), who in turn rated their relationships with their caregivers more highly than did those in the lowest tertile ($p < .001$). Also, as hypothesized, those residing in higher-well-being homes (i.e., kinship care or foster care homes) rated their relationships with their caregivers as being of higher quality ($p < .001$), on average, than those in lower-well-being placements (independent living or group homes).

In Figure 8.1, the virtually parallel lines indicate that the tertile-by-placement-type interaction was far from statistically significant ($p = .95$). Thus, the tertile and type-of-home factors affected the quality of the relationship with the main caregiver independently (i.e., additively), without the influence of one factor being conditional on the influence of the other. The effect on the quality of the youth–caregiver relationship due to tertiles (partial eta-squared = .068, $p < .001$) was of medium size, more than five times as large as the small effect due to type-of-home (.013, $p < .001$). (Figures 8.2–8.8 are to be interpreted in

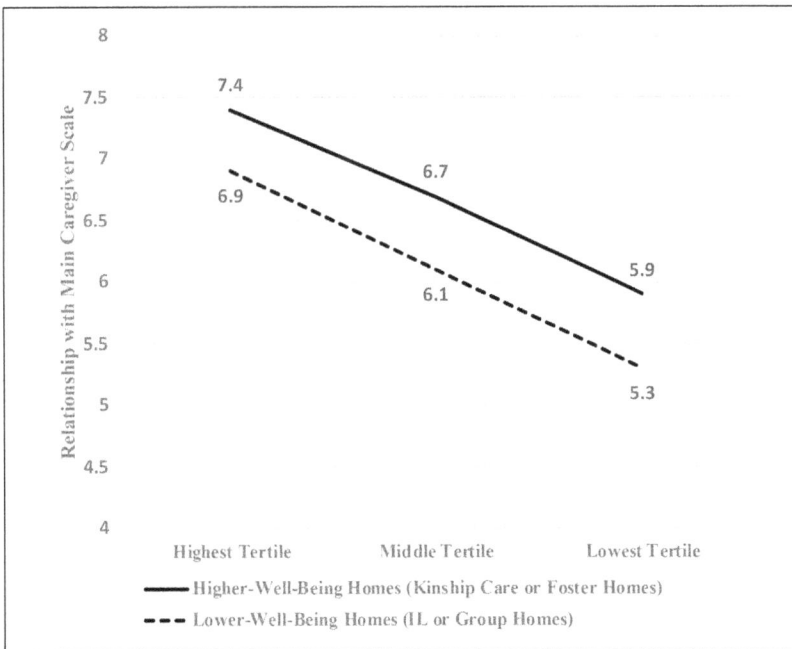

Figure 8.1. Mean scores of young people in care on Quality of Relationship with Main Caregiver, by well-being tertile and type of home ($N = 1774$).

Source: Ontario Looking After Children Project data from 2017.

a fashion similar to the way we have interpreted Figure 8.1, with due allowance made for obvious differences in findings.)

We note that the positive link we found here between the young person's well-being and the quality of his or her relationship with the main caregiver is consistent with the results of the meta-analysis by Chodura et al. (2021). These authors found that caregivers' functional parenting was positively related to the social-emotional development and adaptive functioning of the children in their care.

5.1.2. Hope Scale

Figure 8.2 displays the findings for the Hope Scale, the second indicator of positive mental health. The effect size of the well-being tertile factor was very large on the young persons' level of hope (ES = .216, $p < .001$), and Tukey's HSD test indicated that the three pairwise comparisons on hope between the highest, middle, and lowest well-being tertiles were all significantly different from one another, in that order ($p < .001$). The effect of type-of-home on hope, on the contrary, was

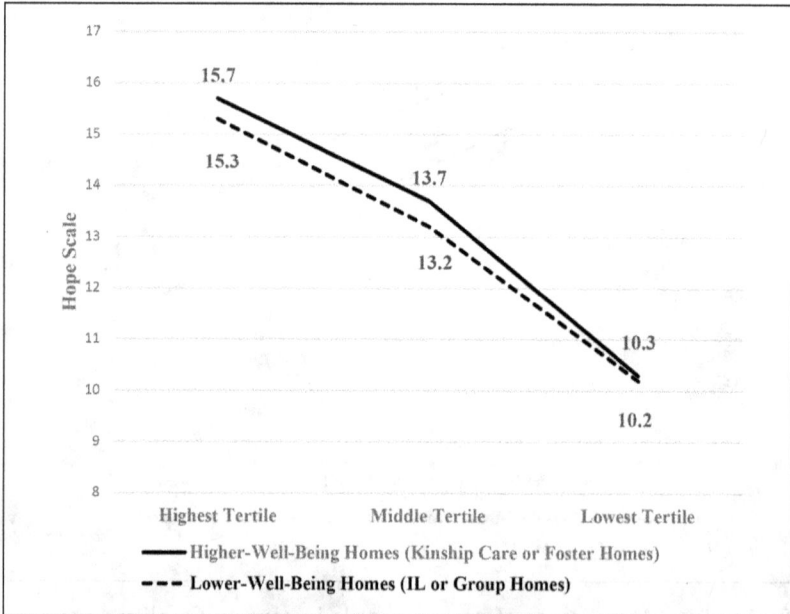

Figure 8.2. Mean scores of young people in care on Hope Scale, by well-being tertile and type of home ($N = 1704$).

Source: Ontario Looking After Children Project data from 2017.

very small (.002) and not significantly different from zero, as indicated by the closeness of the solid and broken lines in Figure 8.2. The tertiles-by-type-of-home interaction was also non-significant, as suggested by the near-parallelism of the two lines in Figure 8.2.

5.1.3. Total Developmental Assets Scale

A young person's total developmental assets are the sum of his or her external (or environmental) assets and internal (or acquired) assets. In our past OnLAC Project research, we have found that these assets are among the best predictors of positive development and resilience that we have in the AAR instrument. In Figure 8.3, the effect on total assets of the well-being tertiles factor was of medium size, with the pairwise comparisons among the highest-, middle-, and lowest-asset tertile means all significantly different from one another ($p < .001$), in the projected order. The effect of the young person's type of home, however, on his or her total developmental assets was even larger.

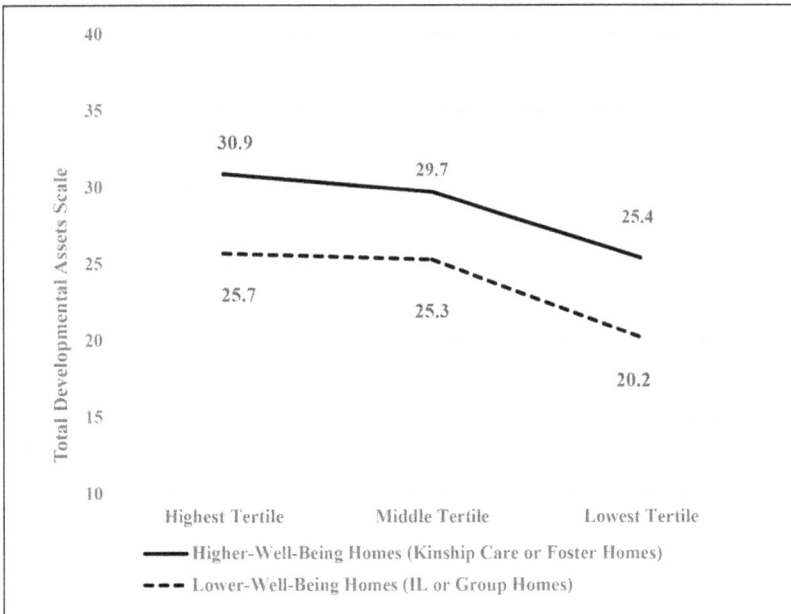

Figure 8.3. Mean scores of young people in care on Total Developmental Assets Scale, by well-being tertile and type of home ($N = 1964$).

Source: Ontario Looking After Children Project data from 2017.

As we suggested earlier, this may indicate the operation of a selection or program effect, or both, in which some young people in care are chosen to live in higher well-being homes or are shaped by them. Similarly, lower well-being youths may be selected or shaped by lower-well-being homes. The tertiles-by-type-of-homes interaction was not significant.

5.1.4. Placement Satisfaction Scale

On the fourth indicator of positive mental health, placement satisfaction, the effects of the well-being tertile and type-of-home factors were moderately large, equal in size (between medium and large), and statistically significant ($p < .001$) in accounting for placement satisfaction. Although small, the interaction effect was also significant ($p < .05$), as indicated by the somewhat non-parallel lines in Figure 8.4. Tukey HSD tests showed that the pairwise comparisons among the placement satisfaction means, among the highest, middle, and lowest

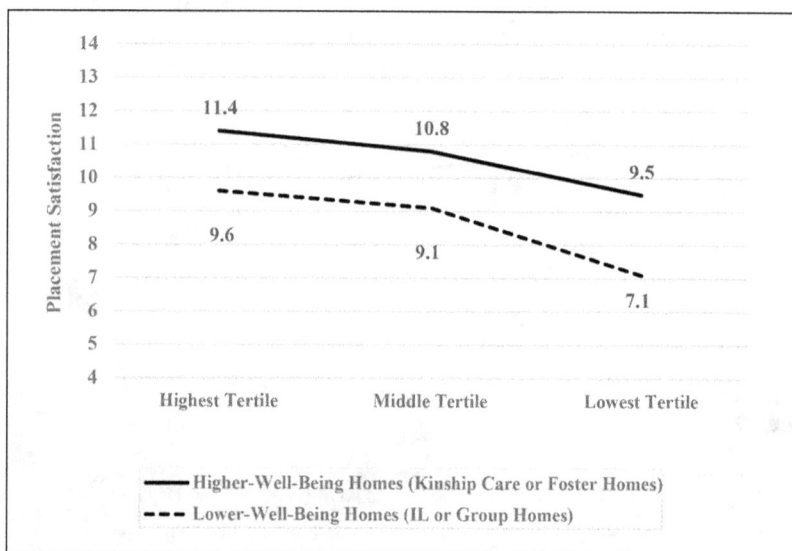

Figure 8.4. Mean scores of young people in care on Placement Satisfaction Scale, by well-being tertile and type of home ($N = 1867$).

Source: Ontario Looking After Children Project data from 2017.

well-being tertiles, were all significant at the $p < .001$ level.

5.2. Association of Well-Being Tertiles and Types of Homes with Four Indicators of Negative Mental Health

5.2.1. SDQ Total Difficulties Scale

On the first indicator of negative mental health, the SDQ Total Difficulties Scale, the tertile and placement-type factors were both close to medium in size (.058 and .053, respectively), and statistically significant ($p < .001$). The interaction effect was not statistically significant, as suggested by the nearly parallel lines in Figure 8.5. A Tukey test revealed that the pairwise comparisons on the Total Difficulties Scale, among the highest, middle, and lowest well-being tertiles, were all significant at the $p < .001$ level.

5.2.2. Stress Symptoms

On the Stress Symptoms Scale (Figure 8.6), the effect due to the well-being tertiles (.078) was considerably larger than that due to the type-of-home factor (.018), although both were statistically significant ($p < .001$). The interaction effect was not significant, and Tukey HSD

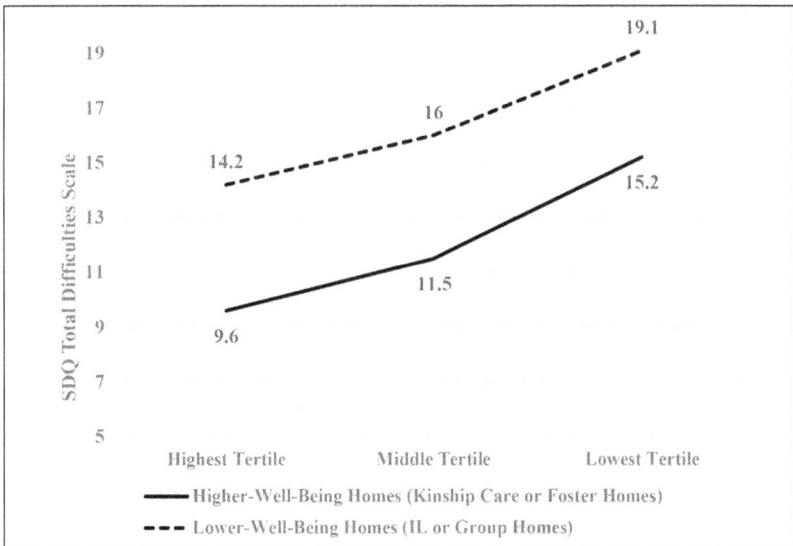

Figure 8.5. Mean scores of young people in care on Strengths and Difficulties Questionnaire Total Difficulties Scale, by well-being tertile and type of home ($N = 1783$).

Source: Ontario Looking After Children Project data from 2017.

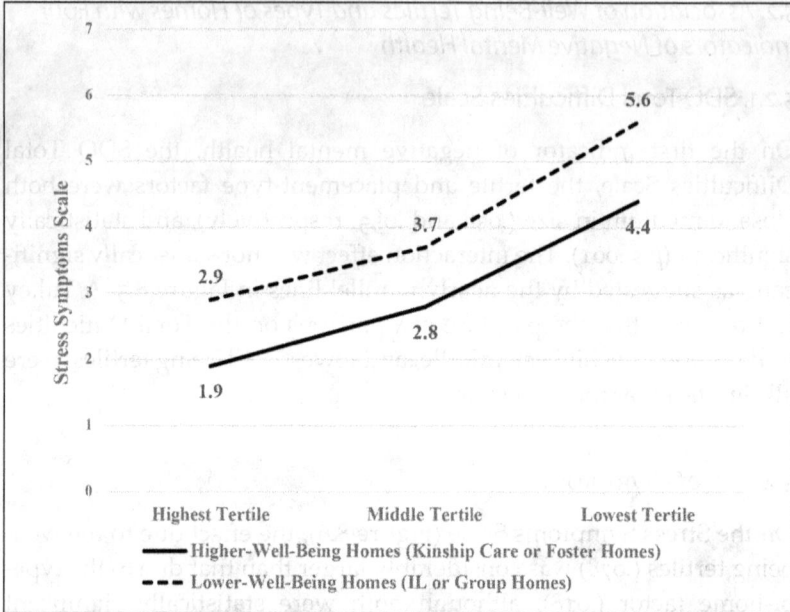

Figure 8.6. Mean scores of young people in care on Stress Symptoms Scale, by well-being tertile and type of home ($N = 1749$).

Source: Ontario Looking After Children Project data from 2017.

tests showed that the pairwise comparisons among the tertiles on the Stress Symptoms Scale were all significant at the .001 level, in the predicted order.

5.2.3. Soft Drug Scale

The well-being tertile and type-of-home effects were both small to medium in size and statistically significant ($p < .001$). The interaction was also significant ($p < .01$), as indicated by the non-parallel lines at the level of the lowest tertile in Figure 8.7. Tukey HSD tests revealed that the pairwise comparisons on the Soft Drug Scale among the highest, middle, and lowest well-being tertiles were all statistically significant ($p < .001$), in the expected order.

5.2.4. Suicidal Risk Scale

On this final negative mental health indicator, the well-being tertile effect was in the moderate range, while the type-of-home effect was

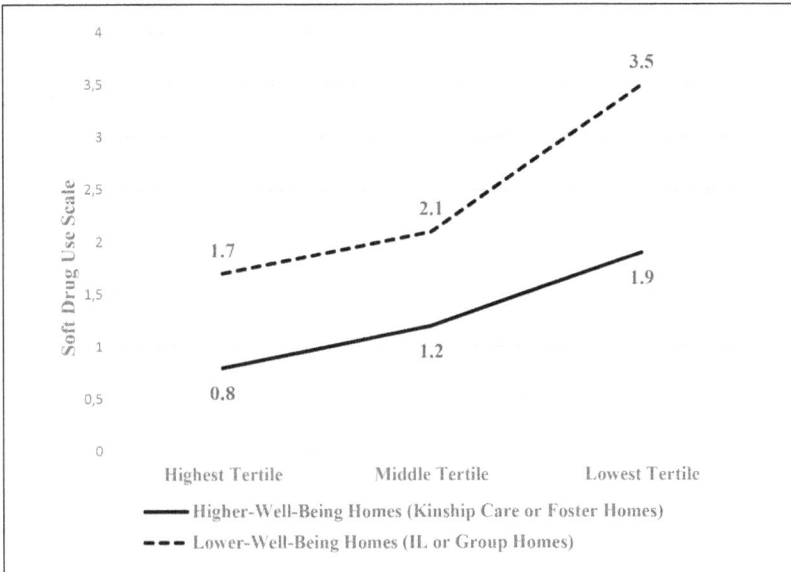

Figure 8.7. Mean scores of young people in care on Soft Drug Use Scale, by well-being tertile and type of home (*N* = 1905).

Source: Ontario Looking After Children Project data from 2017.

small, although both were statistically significant (*p* < .001). The interaction was not significant (Figure 8.8). Tukey tests showed that the pairwise comparisons on the Suicidal Risk Scale among the three well-being tertiles were all significant at the *p* < .002 level or lower. Suicidal risk was lowest in the young people in the highest well-being tertile, intermediate among those in the middle tertile, and highest among those in the lowest well-being tertile. Also, the fact that suicidal risk was significantly higher among the young people residing in lower well-being homes (i.e., in independent living or group homes) was consistent with Anderson's (2011) results: among youths aged 7 to 15 placed in group homes, suicidal ideation was higher than among those placed in kinship or foster homes.

6. Conclusion

In the present chapter, we have used a correlational research design, such that any inferences that we may be tempted to draw about causality require a great deal of caution. Nevertheless, we look upon our results as certainly suggestive. Rather than relying mainly on clinical

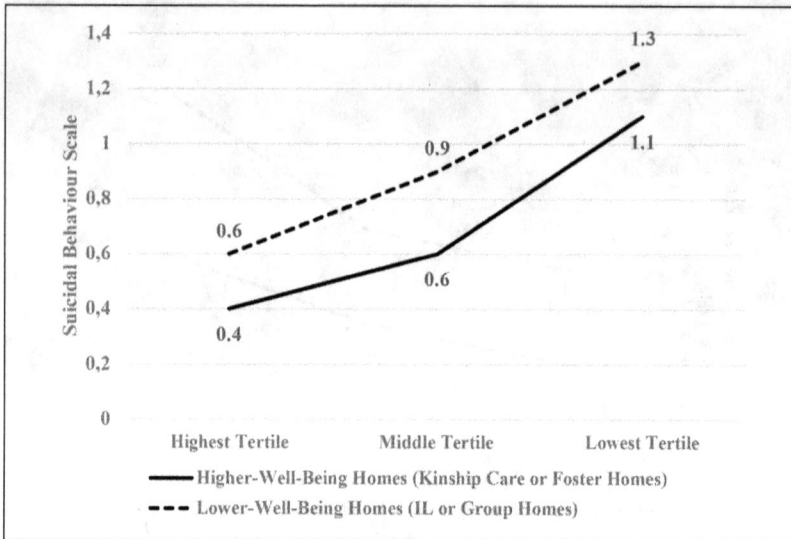

Figure 8.8. Mean scores of young people in care on Suicidal Behaviour Scale, by well-being tertile and type of home (*N* = 1683).

Source: Ontario Looking After Children Project data from 2017.

impressions or intuition to draw conclusions, we recommend that workers, supervisors, or caregivers use our outcome-based assessment approach. In beginning to work with a young person in care whom they do not know well, they can fruitfully begin by answering just two questions related to mental health: from the young person's most recent AAR, what is his or her self-reported total score on Keyes' 14-item well-being measure (and in what well-being tertile does this total score place the young person: in the highest tertile, 62–70; middle tertile, 50–62; or lowest tertile, 0–50)? And, in what kind of home is the young person currently living? Child welfare personnel and caregivers can be assured that Keyes' well-being measure has excellent construct validity in assessing mental health because, without exception, we found that a young person's total score and tertile on Keyes' well-being measure predicted the young person's score in the high, moderate, or low favourableness range on eight positive or negative indicators of mental health. After an initial understanding has been obtained of the young person's mental health status, more complex and detailed assessments can be made later. However, we suspect that in many cases they will not be needed, as the worker, supervisor, or caregiver get to know the young person better and learn to make better use of the rich information in the young person's recent AAR.

In sum, we have shown in this chapter that Keyes' 14-item well-being measure has wide applicability as a fundamental mental health measure in child welfare. The young person who scores favourably or unfavourably on Keyes' instrument will almost certainly score favourably or unfavourably on the kind of instruments often used in child welfare to assess mental health, of which we have offered eight specific examples here. In addition, from a policy perspective, our results suggest that kinship care or foster homes are more likely to promote young people's well-being successfully than are independent living or group homes.

References

Achenbach, T. M., Becker, A., Dopfner, M., Heiervang, E., Roessner, V., Steinhausen, H.-C., & Rothenberger, A. (2008). Multicultural assessment of child and adolescent psychopathology with ASEBA and SDQ instruments: research findings, applications, and future directions. *Journal of Child Psychology and Psychiatry, 49*(3), 251–275. https://doi.org/10.1111/j.1469-7610.2007.01867.x

Anderson, H. D. (2011). Suicide ideation, depressive symptoms, and out-of-home placement among youth in the U. S. child welfare system. *Journal of Clinical Child and Adolescent Psychology, 40*(6), 790–796. https://doi.org/10.1080/15374416.2011.614588

Baiden, P. & Fallon, B. (2018). Examining the association between suicidal behaviors and referral for mental health services among children involved in the child welfare system in Ontario, Canada. *Child Abuse & Neglect, 79*, 115–124. https://doi.org/10.1016/j.chiabu.2018.01.027

Bell, T., & Romano, E. (2015). Child resilience in out-of-home care: Child welfare worker perspectives. *Children and Youth Services Review, 48*, 49–59. https://doi.org/10.1016/j.childyouth.2014.12.008

Bell, T., Romano, E., & Flynn, R. J. (2013). Multilevel correlates of behavioral resilience among children in child welfare. *Child Abuse & Neglect, 37*(11), 1007–1020. https://doi.org/10.1016/j.chiabu.2013.07.005

Bell, T., Romano, E., & Flynn, R. J. (2015). Profiles and predictors of behavioral resilience among children in child welfare. *Child Abuse & Neglect, 48*, 92–103. https://doi.org/10.1016/j.chiabu.2015.04.018

Berger, L. M., Bruch, S. K., James, S., Johnson, E. I., & Rubin, D. (2009). Estimating the "impact" of out-of-home placement on child well-being: Approaching the problem of selection bias. *Child Development, 80*(6), 1856–1876. https://doi.org/10.1111/j.14678624.2009.01372.x

Biglan, A. (2014). *A comprehensive framework for nurturing the well-being of children and adolescents.* [Integrating Safety, Permanency and Well-being Series, Paltech Inc. under the Technical Support and Product Development for the Children's Bureau and its Grantees, contract number HHSP23320095648WC]. The U.S. Department of Health and Human Services.

Boivin, M. & Hertzman, C. (Eds.). (2012). *Early childhood development: Adverse experiences and developmental health.* Royal Society of Canada – Canadian Academy of Health Sciences Expert Panel.

Castellví, P., Miranda-Mendizabal, A., Pares-Badell, O., Almenara, J., Alonso, I., Blasco, M. J., Cebria, A, Gabilondo, A., Gili, M., Lagares, C., Piqueras, J. A., Roca, M., Rodriguez-Marin, J., Rodriguez-Jimenez, T., Soto-Sanz, V., & Alonso, J. (2017). Exposure to violence, a risk for suicide in youths and young adults. A meta-analysis of longitudinal studies. *Acta Psychiatrica Scandinavica,* 135(3), 195–211. https://doi.org/10.1111/acps.12679

Cheung, C., Goodman, D., Leckie, G., & Jenkins, J. (2011). Understanding contextual effects on externalizing behaviors in children in out-of-home care: Influence of workers and foster families. *Children and Youth Services Review,* 33(10), 2050–2060. https://doi.org/10.1016/j.childyouth.2011.05.036

Chodura, S., Lohaus, A., Symanzik, T., Heinrichs, N., & Konrad, K. (2021). Foster parents' parenting and the social-emotional development and adaptive functioning of children in foster care: A PRISMA-guided literature review and meta-analysis. *Clinical Child and Family Psychology Review,* 24(2), 326–347. https://doi.org/10.1007/s10567-020-00336-y

Cullen, G. J., Yule, C., Walters, D., & O'Grady, W. (2021). Mental health outcomes of youth in care: Investigating the effect of general strain and self-control theories. *Child and Adolescent Social Work Journal,* 39, 409–423. https://doi.org/10.1007/ws10560-021-00748-x

Dorsey, S., Burns, B. J., Southerland, D. G., Cox, J. R., Wagner, J. R., & Farmer, M. Z. (2012). Prior trauma exposure for youth in treatment foster care. *Journal of Child and Family Studies,* 21, 816–824. https://doi.org/10.1007/s10826-011-9542-4

Doyle, J. J. (2007). Child protection and child outcomes: Measuring the effects of foster care. *The American Economic Review,* 97(5), 1583–1610. https://doi.org/10.1257/aer.97.5.1583

Dumoulin, A., & Flynn, R. J. (2006). Hope in young people in care: Role of active coping and other predictors. In R. J. Flynn, P. M. Dudding, & J. G. Barber (Eds.), *Promoting resilience in child welfare* (pp. 206–215). University of Ottawa Press.

Egelund, T., & Lausten, M. (2009). Prevalence of mental health problems among children placed in out-of-home care in Denmark. *Child & Family Social Work,* 14(2), 156–165. https://doi.org/10.1111/j.1365-2206.2009.00620.x

Ehlert, U. (2013). Enduring psychobiological effects of childhood adversity. *Psychoneuroendocrinology*, 38(9), 1850–1857. https://doi.org/10.1016/j.psyneuen.2013.06.007

Fallon, B., Trocmé, N., MacLaurin, B., Sinha, V., Black, T., Felstiner, C., Schumaker K., Van Wert, M., Herbert, A., Petrowski, N., Daciuk, J., Lee, B., DuRoss, C., & Johnston, A. (2010). *Ontario incidence study of reported child abuse and neglect – 2008 (OIS-2008)*. Canadian Child Welfare Research Portal.

Fernandez, E. (2006). Growing up in care: Resilience and care outcomes. In R. J. Flynn, P. M. Dudding, & J. G. Barber (eds.), *Promoting resilience in child welfare* (pp. 131–156). University of Ottawa Press.

Flynn, R. J., Miller, M. L., & Vincent, C. C. (2012). Levels of developmental assets and educational outcomes in young people in transitional living in Canada. *Diskurs Kindheits-und Jugendforschung*, 3, 277–290.

Goodman, R. (1997). The Strengths and Difficulties Questionnaire: A research note. *Journal of Child Psychology and Psychiatry*, 38(5), 581–586. https://doi.org/10.1111/j.14697610.1997.tb01545.x

Harpin, S., Kenyon, D. B., Kools, S., Bearinger, L. H., & Ireland, M. (2013). Correlates of emotional distress in out-of-home youth. *Journal of Child and Adolescent Psychiatric Nursing*, 26(2), 110–118. doi.org/10.1111/jcap.12030

Hébert, P. C., & MacDonald, N. (2009). Health care for foster kids: Fix the system, save a child. *Canadian Medical Association Journal*, 181(8), 453. https://doi.org/10.1503/cmaj.091627

Keeshen, B. R., Gray, D., Zhang, C., Presson, A. P., & Coon, H. (2017). Youth suicide deaths: Investigation of clinical predictors in a statewide sample. *Suicide and Life-Threatening Behavior*, 48(5), 601–612. https://doi.org/10.1111/sltb.12386

Keil, V., & Price, J. M. (2006). Externalizing behavior disorders in child welfare settings: Definition, prevalence, and implications for assessment and treatment. *Children and Youth Services Review*, 28(7), 761–779. https://doi.org/10.1016/j.childyouth.2005.08.006

Keyes, C. L. M. (2005). Mental illness and/or mental health? Investigating axioms of the complete state model of health. *Journal of Consulting and Clinical Psychology*, 73(3), 539–548. https://doi.org/10.1037/0022-006X.73.3.539

Keyes, C. L. M. (2006). Mental health in adolescence: Is America's youth flourishing? *American Journal of Orthopsychiatry*, 76(3), 395–402. https://doi.org/10.1037/00029432.76.3.395

Keyes, C. L. M. (2007). Promoting and protecting mental health as flourishing: A complementary strategy for improving national mental health. *American Psychologist*, 62(2), 95–108. https://doi.org/10.1037/0003-066X.62.2.95

Keyes, C. L., Kendler, K. S., Myers, J. M., & Martin, C. C. (2015). The genetic overlap and distinctiveness of flourishing and the Big Five Personality Traits. *Journal of Happiness Studies*, 16, 655–668. https://doi.org/10.1007/s10902-014-9527-2

Komro, K. A., Flay, B. R., Biglan, A., & the Promise Neighborhoods Research Consortium. (2011). Creating nurturing environments: A science-based framework for promoting child health and development within high poverty neighborhoods. *Clinical Child and Family Psychology Review, 14*, 111–134. https://doi.org/10.1007/s10567-011-0095-2

Lamers, S. M. A., Westerhof, G. J., Bohlmeijer, E. T., ten Klooster, P. M., & Keyes, C. L. M. (2011). Evaluating the psychometric properties of the Mental Health Continuum-Short Form (MHC-SF). *Journal of Clinical Psychology, 67*(1), 99–110. https://doi.org/10.1002/jclp.20741

Lawrence, C. R., Carlson, E. A., & Egeland, B. (2006). The impact of foster care on development. *Development and Psychopathology, 18*, 57–76. https://doi.org/10.1017/S0954579406060044

Legault, L., Anawati, M., & Flynn, R. (2006). Factors favoring psychological resilience among fostered young people. *Children and Youth Services Review, 28*(9), 1024–1038. https://doi.org/10.1016/j.childyouth.2005.10.006

Legault, L., & Moffat, S. (2006). Positive life experiences that promote resilience in young people in care. In R. J. Flynn, P. M. Dudding, & J. G. Barber (Eds.), *Promoting resilience in child welfare* (pp. 206–215). University of Ottawa Press.

Lehmann, S., Havik, O. E., Havik, T., & Heiervang, E. R. (2013). Mental disorders in foster children: A study of prevalence, comorbidity and risk factors. *Child and Adolescent Psychiatry and Mental Health, 7*(39), 1–23. https://doi.org/10.1186/1753-2000-7-39

Littlefield L., Cavanagh S., Knapp R., & O'Grady L. (2017). KidsMatter: Building the capacity of Australian primary schools and early childhood services to foster children's social and emotional skills and promote children's mental health. In E. Frydenberg, A. Martin, & R. Collie (Eds.), *Social and emotional learning in Australia and the Asia-Pacific* (pp. 293–311). Springer.

Malla, A., Shah, J., Iyer, S., Boksa, P., Joober, R., Andersson, N., Lal, S., & Fuhrer, R. (2018). Youth mental health should be a top priority for health care in Canada. *Canadian Journal of Psychiatry/Revue canadienne de psychiatrie, 63*(4), 216–222. https://doi.org/10.1177/0706743718758968

Marquis, R. A., & Flynn, R. J. (2009). The SDQ as a mental health measurement tool in a Canadian sample of looked-after young people. *Vulnerable Children and Youth Studies, 4*(2), 114–121. https://doi.org/10.1080/17450120902887392

Masten, A. S. (2016). Resilience in developing systems: the promise of integrated approaches. *European Journal of Developmental Psychology, 13*(3), 297–312.

McCrystal, P., & McAloney, K. (2010). Assessing the mental health needs of young people living in state care using the Strengths and Difficulties Questionnaire. *Child Care in Practice, 16*(3), 215–226. https://doi.org/10.1080/13575271003755969

Miller, M., Vincent, C., & Flynn, R. (2017). *User's manual for the AAR-C2-2016.* Centre for Research on Educational and Community Services, University of Ottawa.

Nelson, S. E., & Wilson, K. (2017). The mental health of Indigenous peoples in Canada: A critical review of research. *Social Science & Medicine, 176,* 93–112. https://doi.org/10.1016/j.socscimed.2017.01.021

Okpych, N. J., & Courtney, M. E. (2018). Characteristics of foster care history as risk factors for psychiatric disorders among youth in care. *American Journal of Orthopsychiatry, 88*(3), 269–281. https://doi.org/10.1037/ort0000259

Ontario Ministry of Children, Community and Social Services. (2019). *Developing a quality standards framework for licensed residential services in Ontario: Discussion guide.*

Oswald, S. H., Heil, K., & Goldbeck, L. (2010). History of maltreatment and mental health problems in foster children: A review of the literature. *Journal of Pediatric Psychology, 35*(5), 462–472. https://doi.org/10.1093/jpepsy/jsp114

Perry, B. D. (2009). Examining child maltreatment through a neurodevelopmental lens: Clinical applications of the Neurosequential Models of Therapeutics. *Journal of Loss and Trauma, 14*(4), 240–255. https://doi.org/10.1080/15325020903004350

Rayburn, A. D., Withers, M. C., & McWey, L. M. (2018). The importance of the caregiver and adolescent relationship for mental health outcomes among youth in foster care. *Journal of Family Violence, 33,* 43–52. https://doi.org/10.1007/s10896-017-9933-4

Richardson, J. T. E. (2011). Eta squared and partial eta squared as measures of effect size in educational research. *Educational Research Review, 6*(2), 135–147. https://doi.org/10.1016/j.edurev.2010.12.001

Snyder, C. R., Hoza, B., Pelham, W. E., Rapoff, M., Ware, L., Danovsky, M., Highberger, L., Ribinstein, H., & Stahl, K. J. (1997). The development and validation of the Children's Hope Scale. *Journal of Pediatric Psychology, 22*(3), 399–421. https://doi.org/10.1093/jpepsy/22.3.399

Sullivan, D. J., & van Zyl, M. A. (2008). The well-being of children in foster care: Exploring physical and mental health needs. *Children and Youth Services Review, 30*(7), 774–786. https://doi.org/10.1016/j.childyouth.2007.12.005

Vinnerljung, B., Hjern, A., & Lindblad, F. (2006). Suicide attempts and severe psychiatric morbidity among former child welfare clients – a national cohort study. *Journal of Child Psychology and Psychiatry, 47*(7), 723–733. https://doi.org/10.1111/j.1469-7610.2005.01530.x

Warburton, W. P., Warburton, R. N., Sweetman, A., & Hertzman, C. (2014). The impact of placing adolescent males into foster care on education, income assistance, and convictions. *Canadian Journal of Economics, 47*(1), 35–69. https://doi.org/10.1111/caje.12064

Norms for the Canadian Casey Life Skills Assessment, Based on Assessment and Action Record Data for Ontario Young People in Care

This chapter aims to provide norms for scales and individual items on the Canadian version of the Casey Life Skills Assessment (referred to hereafter as "the Casey") and we also include some recent international and Canadian research on transitions from care and the needs of care leavers. The Casey is an assessment tool intended to measure and increase the readiness of young people in out-of-home care to become aware of and meet the challenges of independent living in the community. We embedded a slightly adapted version of the U.S. Casey within the current version of the Assessment and Action Record (AAR-C2-2016) when we last revised the AAR. Our Canadian Casey consists of 112 unduplicated items, grouped into 8 scales: Permanency (20 items), Daily Living (15), Self-Care (15), Relationships and Communication (11), Housing and Money Management (19), Work and Study (18), Career and Education Planning (6), and Looking Forward (8). A young person's scores on these eight scales can be summed to form the Casey total scale score. The norms presented here compare Casey scale and item means by sex (female vs. male), age (16- vs. 17-year-olds), current residential placement (independent living home vs. kinship, foster, or group home), and well-being tertile (highest vs. middle vs. lowest).

At present, there is little high-quality research available on the Casey, including the often-used U.S. version. We thus still need to determine in future study whether young people's self-reported scores on the Casey while they are still in care actually predict better outcomes when they are living in the community, or whether gains in their Casey scores really reflect meaningful improvements in important dimensions of their lives after leaving care. We hope that making these norms available here will encourage greater clinical use of (and predictive research on) the Canadian Casey, by at least three audiences:

- First, individual young people in care preparing for the day when they will leave care, and their caregivers and child welfare workers, during discussions of the opportunities and challenges of community living and the range of life skills needed for greater success and satisfaction in doing so;
- Second, quality assurance personnel responsible for evaluating the effectiveness of local society interventions aimed at improving the young people's transitions from care to independent living; and,
- Third, researchers collaborating with local societies to discover whether and how well care leavers' pre-transition Casey scale scores predict their post-transition outcomes in areas such as social support, mental health, housing, education, or employment.

1. The Canadian Version of the Casey Life Skills Assessment Compared with the U.S. Version

The Casey tool (formerly known as the Ansell-Casey Life Skills Assessment) was originally created in the United States in response to the U.S. federal requirement in the Independent Living Initiative of 1986 that young people in care be assessed in terms of their level of life skills by the age of 16 (Nollan et al., 2000). The intent was to allow problems to be identified and addressed before the young person left care. The U.S. version of the Casey is viewed as usable with virtually all young people aged 14 to 21, whether they live in foster homes, group homes, their families of origin, or elsewhere. The Canadian Casey, on the other hand, currently targets young people in care who are 16 years of age or older. (Like the U.S. version, however, it could probably be employed with a broader range of young people, but supportive research is necessary.)

The U.S. and Canadian versions of the Casey have the same eight scales, composed of virtually the same items, except for the adaptation to the Ontario or Canadian context needed for a few items (e.g., those mentioning programs such as the Ontario Student Assistance Program [OSAP]). The AAR version of the Casey has 112 items, whereas the U.S. version has 113. The items in the Canadian version that compose the eight Casey scales are interwoven throughout the Looking After Children developmental dimensions of the AAR (e.g., health, education, identity, etc.). In responding to each Casey item, the young person assigns a rating to his or her self-perceived familiarity, understanding, or proficiency with the life-skill issue discussed in the item.

2. Norming Sample from the AAR Data Set for the Canadian Version of the Casey

In our analyses in the present chapter on the Casey scales and items, we used an Ontario Looking After Children (OnLAC) Project sample composed of young people aged 16 or 17 and residing in out-of-home care in Ontario. We established norms for the sample as a whole, which included 1,858 unduplicated young people who had been in care in Ontario in calendar years 2016, 2017, 2018, or 2019. They had complete data on the 112 Canadian Casey items, the 8 Casey scales, and the total Casey scale (see Tables 9.1–9.9, below). We also derived from the same sample sub-group norms for young people in care on four background variables. These were sex (911 females and 945 males), age (1,265 youths, 16 years of age, and 593 youths, 17 years of age), type of residential placement (183 living in an independent living home and 1,510 in a kinship, foster, or group home), and well-being tertile (550 in the highest vs. 660 in the middle vs. 638 in the lowest tertile; see Tables 9.10–9.13, below).

3. Canadian Casey Scales

We now introduce the eight Canadian Casey scales, including the broad life-skill areas that each is intended to assess. We also list the items included in each scale in Tables 9.1–9.8, a careful reading of which will permit a good grasp of the content of the scale in question. This will enable a child welfare worker or caregiver to compare their perceptions of the life skills of a particular young person in care with the latter's self-reports on the Casey items or scales.

Permanency Scale (Casey items 1–20): assesses a young person's relationships with trusted adults, connections, and a supportive community (Table 9.1).

Table 9.1. Canadian Casey Permanency scale (20 items, nos. 1–20; N = 1858)

Name	Item	Mean	SD
cls1	I know at least one adult, other than my worker, who would take my call in the middle of the night if I had an emergency.	4.63	.91
cls2	An adult I trust, other than my worker, checks in with me regularly.	4.59	.88
cls3	I have at least one trusted adult who would visit me if I were in the hospital.	4.79	.62
cls4	There is at least one adult I trust who would be legally allowed to make medical decisions for me and advocate for me if I was unable to speak for myself.	4.71	.78
cls5	I am part of a family and we care about each other.	4.47	1.01
cls6	I can get in touch with at least one family member when I want to.	4.70	.75
cls7	I have friends or family to spend time with on holidays and special occasions.	4.63	.86
cls8	I know at least one adult I can depend on when I exit care.	4.58	.95
cls9	I know an adult who could be a grandparent, aunt or uncle to my children now or my future children.	4.49	1.06
cls10	I know what my permanency goal is.	4.21	1.27
cls11	I have information about my family members.	4.47	.95
cls12	I know an adult who would help me if I had a financial emergency.	4.52	.97
cls13	I know an adult I could live with for a few days or weeks if I needed to.	4.47	1.06
cls14	There is at least one adult I have regular contact with, other than my child welfare worker, who lives in stable and safe housing.	4.64	.89
cls15	I know an adult I can go to for financial advice.	4.67	.80
cls16	I know an adult who will go with me if I need to change schools.	4.87	.54
cls17	I have an adult in my life who cares about how I am doing at school or work.	4.87	.47
cls18	I have recently talked to an adult who works in a job I would like to have.	3.15	1.74
cls19	I have talked about my education plans with an adult who cares about me.	4.53	1.01
cls20	I know an adult who will help me apply for training or education after high school.	4.62	.89

Note. The response options to the CLS items in Tables 9.1–9.8 correspond to the following 5-point scale: "Yes" (= 5); "Mostly yes" (= 4); "Somewhat" (= 3); "Mostly no" (= 2); "No" (= 1).
SD = Standard Deviation, in Tables 9.1–9.13.
Source: Ontario Looking After Children Project data, 2016–2019.

Daily Living Scale (Casey items 21–35): covers the topics of meal planning and preparation, food storage, home cleaning and maintenance, and the basics of computer use (Table 9.2).

Table 9.2. Canadian Casey Daily Living scale (15 items, nos. 21–35; N = 1858)

Name	Item	Mean	SD
cls21	I know how to use my email account.	4.74	.82
cls22	I can create, save, print, and send computer documents.	4.68	.87
cls23	I know the risks of meeting someone in person that I met online.	4.76	.71
cls24	I would not post pictures or messages if I thought it would hurt someone's feelings.	4.20	1.25
cls25	If someone sent me a message online that made me feel bad or scared, I would know what to do or who to tell.	4.61	.85
cls26	When I shop for food, I take a list and I compare prices.	3.23	1.59
cls27	I can make meals with or without using a recipe.	4.08	1.22
cls28	I think about what I eat and how it impacts my health.	3.38	1.38
cls29	I understand how to read food product labels to see how much fat, sugar, salt, and calories the food has.	4.29	1.16
cls30	I know how to do my own laundry.	4.64	.87
cls31	I keep my living space clean.	4.10	1.05
cls32	I know the products to use when cleaning the bathroom and kitchen.	4.55	.91
cls33	I know how to use a fire extinguisher.	3.80	1.52
cls34	I know where to go to get on the Internet.	4.87	.52
cls35	I can find what I need on the Internet.	4.83	.58

Source: Ontario Looking After Children Project data, 2016–2019.

Self-Care Scale (Casey items 36–50): assesses healthy physical and emotional development, including personal hygiene, taking care of one's health and pregnancy prevention (Table 9.3).

Table 9.3. Canadian Casey Self-Care scale (15 items, nos. 36–50; N = 1858)

Name	Item	Mean	SD
cls36	I can take care of my own minor injuries and illnesses.	4.44	.92
cls37	I can get medical and dental care when I need it.	4.70	.76
cls38	I know how to make my own medical and dental appointments.	3.65	1.48
cls39	I know when I should go to the emergency room instead of the doctor's office.	4.34	1.10
cls40	I know my family medical history.	2.90	1.41
cls41	I know how to get health insurance when I am older than 18.	2.64	1.59
cls42	I know how to get the benefits I am eligible for (such as RESP, OCBe, OSAP, bursaries, Victim's Compensation, CCSY, funds from FNMI Band/Community, ODSP, Aftercare Benefits Initiative, Living and Learning Grants, etc.).	3.02	1.55
cls43	I bathe (wash up) daily.	4.66	.73
cls44	I brush my teeth daily.	4.61	.83
cls45	I know how to get myself away from harmful situations.	4.49	.86
cls46	I have a place to go when I feel unsafe.	4.68	.78
cls47	I can turn down a sexual advance.	4.66	.78
cls48	I know ways to protect myself from sexually transmitted diseases (STDs).	4.65	.87
cls49	I know how to prevent getting pregnant or getting someone else pregnant.	4.74	.77
cls50	I know where to go to get information on sex and pregnancy.	4.67	.84

Source: Ontario Looking After Children Project data, 2016–2019.

Relationships and Communication Scale (Casey items 51–61): measures the development and maintaining of healthy relationships and permanent connections with caring adults (Table 9.4).

Table 9.4. Canadian Casey Relationships and Communication scale (11 items, nos. 51–61; *N* = 1858)

Name	Item	Mean	SD
cls51	I can speak up for myself.	4.63	.75
cls52	I know how to act in social or professional situations.	4.53	.82
cls53	I know how to show respect to people with different beliefs, opinions, and cultures.	4.70	.70
cls54	I can describe my racial and ethic identity.	4.46	.98
cls55	I can explain the difference between sexual orientation and gender identity.	4.26	1.15
cls56	I have friends I like to be with who help me feel valued and worthwhile.	4.57	.89
cls57	My relationships are free from hitting, slapping, shoving, being made fun of, or name calling.	4.62	.79
cls58	I know the signs of an abusive relationship.	4.64	.77
cls59	I think about how my choices impact others	3.91	1.10
cls60	I can deal with anger without hurting others or damaging things.	4.11	1.06
cls61	I show others that I care about them.	4.40	.84

Source: Ontario Looking After Children Project data, 2016–2019.

Housing and Money Management Scale (Casey items 62–80): covers the skills of banking, establishing credit, locating and retaining affordable housing, budgeting, and living within one's means (Table 9.5).

Table 9.5. Canadian Casey Housing and Money Management scale (19 items, nos. 62–80; N = 1858)

Name	Item	Mean	SD
cls62	I understand how interest rates work on loans or credit purchases.	3.08	1.59
cls63	I understand the disadvantages of making purchases with my credit card.	3.70	1.52
cls64	I know the importance of a good credit score.	3.63	1.57
cls65	I know how to balance my bank account.	3.56	1.52
cls66	I put money in my savings account when I can.	3.33	1.65
cls67	I use online banking to keep track of my money.	2.81	1.79
cls68	I know the advantages and disadvantages of using a cheque cashing or payday loan store.	3.25	1.68
cls69	I know how to find safe and affordable housing.	3.12	1.55
cls70	I can figure out the costs to move to a new place, such as deposits, rents, utilities, and furniture.	3.14	1.60
cls71	I know how to fill out an apartment rental application.	2.49	1.54
cls72	I know how to get emergency help to pay for water, electricity, and gas bills.	2.51	1.56
cls73	I know what can happen if I break my rental lease.	2.90	1.65
cls74	I can explain why people need renter's or homeowner's insurance.	2.82	1.62
cls75	I plan for expenses that I must pay each month.	3.02	1.65
cls76	I keep records of the money I am paid and the bills I pay.	2.55	1.62
cls77	I know what happens in my province if I am caught driving without car insurance or a driver's license.	4.11	1.35
cls78	I can explain how to get and renew a driver's license or Ontario Photo Card.	3.31	1.62
cls79	I can figure out all the costs of car ownership, such as registration, repairs, insurance, and gas.	2.89	1.56
cls80	I know how to use public transportation to get where I need to go.	4.23	1.29

Source: Ontario Looking After Children Project data, 2016–2019.

Work and Study Scale (Casey items 81–98): assesses skills related to employment, legal questions, study skills, and management of one's time (Table 9.6).

Table 9.6. Canadian Casey Work and Study scale (18 items, nos. 81–98; $N = 1858$)

Name	Item	Mean	SD
cls81	I know how to develop a resume.	4.30	1.19
cls82	I know how to fill out a job application.	4.23	1.26
cls83	I know how to prepare for a job interview.	4.16	1.25
cls84	I know what the information on a paystub means.	3.19	1.64
cls85	I can fill out the necessary payroll forms when I get a job.	3.25	1.61
cls86	I know what employee benefits are.	3.49	1.57
cls87	I know what sexual harassment and discrimination are.	4.57	.92
cls88	I know the reasons why my personal contacts are important for finding a job.	4.28	1.19
cls89	I know how to get the documents I need for work, such as my Social Insurance Number card and birth certificate.	3.94	1.43
cls90	I know how and when I can see my child welfare records.	3.40	1.60
cls91	I know how to get help from my school's mental health services.	4.05	1.36
cls92	I know where I can get help with an income tax form.	2.85	1.67
cls93	I can take criticism and direction at school or work without losing my temper.	4.05	1.07
cls94	I know how to prepare for exams and/or presentations.	4.30	1.13
cls95	I know where I can get tutoring or other help with school work.	4.43	1.07
cls96	I look over my work for mistakes.	3.61	1.32
cls97	I get to school or work on time.	4.20	1.22
cls98	I get my work done and turned in on time.	3.79	1.15

Source: Ontario Looking After Children Project data, 2016–2019.

Career and Education Planning Scale (Casey items 99–104): assesses the young person's planning of his or her own post-secondary education and career, of special relevance to older youths who are preparing for their eventual transition from care (Table 9.7).

Table 9.7. Canadian Casey Career and Education Planning scale (6 items, nos. 99–104; *N* = 1858)

Name	Item	Mean	SD
cls99	I know how to find work-related internships/co-ops.	3.27	1.59
cls100	I know where to find information about job training.	3.53	1.52
cls101	I can explain the benefits of doing volunteer work.	4.26	1.17
cls102	I know what type of education (e.g., college, trade school, university) I need for the work I want to do.	3.95	1.37
cls103	I know how to get into the school, training, or job I want after high school.	3.77	1.39
cls104	I know how to find financial aid to help pay for my education or training.	3.40	1.51

Source: Ontario Looking After Children Project data, 2016–2019.

Looking Forward Scale (Casey items 105–112): assesses the young people's sense of control over their lives and their level of confidence in the future (Table 9.8).

Table 9.8. Canadian Casey Looking Forward scale (8 items, nos. 105–112; *N* = 1858)

Name	Item	Mean	SD
cls105	I believe I can influence how my life will turn out.	4.28	.97
cls106	I can describe my vision for myself as a successful adult.	4.09	1.13
cls107	I have a good relationship with a trusted adult I like and respect.	4.80	.60
cls108	I would like to use my experience to help other youth.	3.79	1.36
cls109	I believe my relationships with others will help me succeed.	4.22	1.02
cls110	I feel I am ready for the next phase of my life.	3.86	1.23
cls111	Most days, I am proud of the way I am living my life.	4.08	1.10
cls112	Most days, I feel I have control of how my life will turn out.	4.03	1.10

Source: Ontario Looking After Children Project data, 2016–2019.

Total Casey Scale is calculated as the sum of the 8 Casey scales (or their 112 constituent items). Table 9.9 presents the means, standard deviations, and internal consistency (alpha) coefficients of the individual Casey scales and the total scale, as well as their inter-correlations. The alpha coefficient for the individual scales ranged between good (.79) and excellent (.91), with an alpha of .88 (good) in the case of the total scale. These results suggest that the individual Casey scales, as well as the total scale, can be treated as internally consistent measures.

Table 9.9. Means, standard deviations, internal consistency (alpha) coefficients, and inter-correlations of the eight Canadian Casey scales and total scale (N = 1858)

Casey Scale	Mean	SD	Alpha	1.	2.	3.	4.	5.	6.	7.	8.
1. Permanency (20 items)	90.62[1] 4.53[2]	10.60	.88	–							
2. Daily Living (15 items)	64.79 4.32	8.57	.82	41	–						
3. Self-Care (15 items)	62.87 4.19	8.76	.83	44	77	–					
4. Relationships and Communications (11 items)	48.82 4.44	5.70	.79	54	71	70	–				
5. Housing and Money Management (19 items)	60.45 3.18	21.01	.94	26	63	73	52	–			
6. Work and Study (18 items)	70.09 3.89	14.88	.91	41	73	80	68	82	–		
7. Career and Education Planning (6 items)	22.17 3.70	6.46	.85	44	66	73	62	76	83	–	
8. Looking Forward (8 items)	33.14 4.14	6.20	.86	56	51	51	67	41	54	55	–
9. Casey Total Scale (112 items; sum of 8 scales)	452.95 4.04	67.10	.88[3]	46[4]	77	84	75	74	88	84	62

Note. Decimals omitted from correlations. Unlike the US Casey, the Canadian (AAR) Casey has no item overlap between scales because each of the 112 items was used in only one scale.

[1] The scale mean.

[2] The average item mean, calculated by dividing the scale mean by the number of scale items.

[3] The internal consistency (alpha) coefficient for the total Casey scale was .88 when the 8 CLS scales were entered as items in the reliability analysis.

[4] The correlations of the scales with the total scale were corrected for scale-total redundancy.

Source: Ontario Looking After Children Project data, 2016–2019.

The good internal consistency of the total scale was supported by a principal components analysis that we carried out on the total scores of the eight scales (N = 1858 for all analyses). With an oblimin rotation and the extraction limited to a single component, we accounted for 66% of the overall variance, with substantial loadings of all eight scales on the single component.

In a second principal components analysis, again with an oblimin rotation, we extracted two components that had eigenvalues of 5.29 and 1.01, respectively, and were quite highly correlated. This result suggested that for certain purposes (e.g., to evaluate a program aimed at assessing young people's apparent readiness to transition from care), an evaluator could also envision a model composed of two correlated Casey dimensions. In this two-dimensional model, which accounted for 79% of the total variance, the Housing and Money Management, Work and Study, Career and Education Planning, Self-Care, and Daily Living scales constituted a primary dimension that grouped the five Casey scales that assess relatively concrete and practical life skills. A secondary dimension was composed of the three scales, Permanency, Looking Forward, and Relationships and Communication, that assess more relationship-oriented life skills that measure supportive or friendship relationships between young people and people in their families or social circles. The internal consistency (alpha) coefficients of the primary and secondary dimensions were, respectively, .88 and .76, and the correlation between the two dimensions was a substantial .60 (95% confidence interval = .57 and .63).

4. Comparing Local Society AAR Data with the Results in Tables 9.1–9.9

Originally, when the OnLAC Project team established the SPSS codes for each of the 112 items in the Canadian version of the Casey, we coded the five possible responses from which the young person in care chooses the response that best matches his or her own opinion: "Yes" (4); "Mostly yes" (3); "Somewhat" (2); "Mostly no" (1); and "No" (0). We discovered later, however, that the U.S. Casey Life Skills Assessment codes the items on a 5–1 rather than a 4–0 basis, namely: "Yes" (5); "Mostly yes" (4); "Somewhat" (3); "Mostly no" (2); and "No" (1). Therefore, in the present chapter, we have added a constant of one unit to each item, converting the 4–0 coding scheme in the SPSS

OnLAC data to a 5–1 coding scheme. Doing so did not change at all the item standard deviations, the item inter-correlations, or the item correlations with other variables, such as sex, age, developmental assets, etc.

In this chapter, we have also eliminated the item overlap that the creators of the U.S. Casey built into the tool (*Casey Life Skills Practice Guide*; Casey Family Programs, 2021). This overlap resulted from the repetition in the U.S. Casey of Permanency scale items in other Casey scales and was also adopted in the version of the Casey found in the *User's Manual for the AAR-C2-2016* (Miller et al., 2017, pp. 135–153). This repetition and overlap of items produced an artificial inflation of the inter-correlations among the Casey scales and of the internal consistency (alpha) coefficients of the various scales. Such item over-lap may not be problematic for purely clinical purposes and makes little difference in the item (rather than scale) means presented in the AAR *User's Manual*. However, in the present chapter we wanted to avoid the inflation of results stemming from item overlap. Instead, we wanted our results to reflect the "true" (uninflated) correlations of the Casey scales with each other and with external variables, such as the young people's sex or age, and the uninflated internal consistency coefficients of the Casey scales. We recommend that local society data analysts follow our practice in this chapter, and we will revise the AAR *User's Manual* accordingly. (Local society data analysts should remember to add a constant of one unit to each of the Casey items ["cls1," "cls2," "cls3," etc., up to "cls112"] in their own OnLAC SPSS data, which they receive from the OnLAC Project. This will ensure that the Casey items in their own SPSS OnLAC data follow the same 5–1 rather than 4–0 coding scheme that we have used in the present chapter.)

5. Research on Transitions of Young People from Care

Before going on to present additional norms for the Canadian Casey, based on comparisons between sample sub-groups based on sex, age, type of residential placement, and well-being tertiles (see Tables 9.10–9.13), we consider selected research findings in areas of child welfare to which the Casey seems especially pertinent. These areas include interventions to improve transitions from care, recent research in Canada on transitions, and research on the U.S. Casey itself.

5.1. A Systematic Review of Scientific Studies of Interventions on Transitions

Gunawardena and Stich (2021), from McGill University, in Montréal, authored what is apparently the first systematic review of scientific studies of interventions aimed at enhancing the transitions of young persons aging out of the child welfare system. These interventions took place at either the micro level, involving individuals, families, or small groups, or the macro level, involving community organizing, policy, or administration. Using Preferred Reporting Items for Systematic Reviews and Meta-Analyses (PRISMA) criteria (BMJ, 2021), Gunawardena and Stich (2021) initially screened 2,802 studies, analyzing a final sample of 30 interventions: 23 from the United States, 2 from the United Kingdom, 2 from Australia, and 1 each from Canada, Denmark, and Israel.

Of the 30 interventions, 12 (40%) promoted independent living readiness (sometimes known as transitional living programs). The most frequent type of intervention in the scientific literature, these programs aimed to increase self-sufficiency and independence in young people's transition from care. (This is an area in which controlled research is neither easy nor frequent, as the first randomized controlled trial of independent living services was published only in 2015 [Greeson et al., 2015].) These independent living readiness programs sought to improve young people's social, educational, housing, employment, health, mental health, or related outcomes. Some interventions provided housing or independent living in apartments, some furnished additional health or wellness services or life-skills training, and several referred young people to community programs. A number of the programs were limited to 18-to-25-year-olds, others served 13-to-21-year-olds, and still others served both age groups.

The results of the independent living interventions were mixed. Regarding education, some independent living programs were associated with more frequent high school graduation or college attendance, whereas others had no positive effect. With respect to employment, some interventions saw improved outcomes, while others did not. Positive outcomes included improved housing stability, less involvement with the legal system, and lower rates of mental health difficulties. On the other hand, some participants reported problems with employment, education, and mental health, despite support and stable housing. Staff restrictions or lack of knowledge, especially related to housing or mental health, sometimes impeded young people's growth in independence. Loneliness and isolation from living alone in apartments, or roommates, who did not respect rules, also rendered transitions more difficult.

Four of the 30 interventions (13%) consisted of policy changes that allowed young people to stay in care after the age of majority. Three studies from the U.S. Midwest Evaluation of the Adult Functioning of Former Foster Youth found that extending care was effective in lowering young women's involvement with the criminal justice system, but not young men's. Women still in care at the age of 19 had fewer arrests, convictions, incarcerations, and property crimes than those who had left care before age 19, and for both women and men, leaving care between the ages of 18 and 19 was associated with a higher risk of being arrested during the first year out of care. In terms of educational outcomes, young people who stayed in care past the age of 20 were more likely to finish high school and complete at least one year of college. On the other hand, in Denmark it was found that a new law in 2001 allowing young people to stay in care or receive other types of services until the age of 23 seemed to reduce their labour market efforts and had little or no effect on their educational outcomes.

Mentoring was the subject of 3 of the 30 interventions (10%). Care-leaving youths were matched with adult mentors, who were often volunteers. The mentors taught basic life skills and acted as positive role models, while providing social and emotional support. Young people who took part in the study had a higher level of employment and a lower risk of incarceration, homelessness, and addiction than youths in transition who did not participate in mentoring. Also, two qualitative studies indicated that youths in transition confided more readily in their mentors than in child welfare staff. The mentors provided emotional support, basic life-skills training, and practical support, such as transportation to school and employment.

Art or mindfulness interventions were evaluated in 3 of the 30 studies (10%). Mindfulness training, although associated with lower stress and improved sleep, was not shown to be effective. However, a phenomenological study suggested that 10 three-hour sessions of group mindfulness, combined with drawing and painting, had a positive effect on the self-awareness, acceptance, optimism, emotion regulation, and sleep of young people aging out of child welfare services. A second phenomenological study discovered that youths within two years of aging out of care who engaged in a drama-based intervention for six hours a month over six to eight months reported a more positive self-image, higher self-efficacy, less loneliness, greater healing, and increased confidence in relation to their future goals.

Two of the 30 studies (7%) evaluated interventions aimed at increasing participation and success in post-secondary education of young people with a care background. States with statewide programs of tuition waivers, fee waivers, competitive scholarships, and support initiatives were found to have higher levels of post-secondary enrollments, with considerable variability, however, in the nature and effects of the state interventions. Another evaluation, of a university campus-based intervention that included housing, financial, academic, and life-coaching support for young people who had previously been in care, had a six-year graduation rate of 30%. This was higher than the national average for students who had been in care but lower than the graduation rate of a comparable population of students. The students from care said that financial support, housing, and campus coaches were the three most significant types of support, while specific life-skills activities and instruments to assess them and heighten skills awareness were rated as moderately helpful.

Two of the 30 interventions (7%) had a focus on employment. One study, a randomized trial of individual job-search counselling and preparation, enrolled young people in out-of-home care, on probation, or in subsidized guardianship. The evaluation found no difference between the experimental and control groups in terms of employment or self-sufficiency outcomes but did confirm that many youths transitioning from care experience poverty-level incomes. On the other hand, another employment-related intervention had greater success. The five-year project promoted career readiness by offering a combination of group and individual support as well as practical work experience. Use of a randomized pre-post design indicated that participation in the program resulted, during the first post-enrollment year, in an increase in greater exploration, work readiness, and work retention activities. Also, greater engagement in program activities and career readiness was associated with a higher likelihood of employment at follow-up. Moreover, the researchers stressed the importance of both work and relational skills in the overall career preparedness and employment process.

Two other studies (7%) assessed the role of psychological self-empowerment or self-determination in the transition from care process. The first intervention consisted of the participation by young people in decision-making roles (e.g., in committees, boards, staff positions, work groups, or councils), while benefiting from the tutelage of a supportive adult of older youth leader. With controls for relevant confounds, participation in the intervention predicted higher levels of perceived control, motivation to influence, sociopolitical skills, and participatory behaviour (effects sizes varied between .25 and .59). The second intervention involved young persons' involvement in one-on-one weekly or biweekly coaching to assist them in identifying and seeking to attain goals that they valued. Also, they took part in peer-mentoring workshops in which they discussed topics related to transition and received support from successful "near peers" and adults. The results indicated that young people who took part in the program were able to express themselves, increase their confidence, make progress on future goals, and benefit from meaningful relationships.

Finally, the last two studies examined the effect on young people in transition from care of extracurricular activities, such as sports, drama or chess club, band, or student government, or educational accomplishments such as high school graduation, passing the General Educational Development (GED) test, or beginning college. The evaluation found that among young people who took part in extracurricular activities, receipt of a high school diploma was twice as likely but unrelated to receipt of a GED or beginning college by age 19.

Overall, Gunawardena and Stich's (2021) systematic review suggested that independent living programs, especially, appeared promising in their ability to support care leavers, on several levels. We thus hope that some of the Casey scales presented in the present chapter prove useful in identifying those life-skill domains clearly and which seem particularly useful for youths in their quest for successful transitions. The Casey may also help in efforts by child welfare organizations to evaluate the effects of new policy innovations, such as Courtney and Hook's (2017) discovery in the Midwest study of former foster youths that extending the age at which young people could stay in care was associated with improved educational attainment. In concluding their review, Gunawardena and Stich (2021) placed special emphasis on enabling young people to stay in care longer and on recognizing that education and employment have a special role to play in interventions that attempt to reduce the economic and related disparities that confront many youths on leaving care.

5.2. Recent Research in Canada on the Needs of Care Leavers

The findings and recommendations of two recent Canadian needs-assessment and outcome reports align well with the results and primary message of Gunawardena and Stich (2021). Jane Kovarikova, a former care leaver herself who is currently pursuing PhD studies in political science at Western University in Ontario, is the founder of the Child Welfare Political Action Committee Canada (Child Welfare PAC). This organization, Child Welfare PAC, has become an influential source of advocacy in promoting the interests of young people in Canada with a care background. Child Welfare PAC has made important gains on policy issues affecting care leavers, especially related to the issue of tuition waivers from colleges and universities across Canada.

Kovarikova (2017) provided a report to the Ontario Provincial Advocate for Children and Youth that explored the service needs and outcomes of young people who had transitioned or aged out of the child protection system in Ontario or elsewhere. She synthesized the international literature on transitions from care from several sources: academic, peer-reviewed papers; "grey" literature (i.e., reports in the media or by professionals in the field); and 17 informal interviews with staff members of Ontario organizations serving youths in care. Kovarikova's findings on young people who have transitioned from care echoed the results of many other international reports:

- Academic outcomes are often poor, with youth in care in Ontario and elsewhere often struggling to complete high school or gain access to post-secondary education.
- Unemployment and underemployment are frequent whether in Canada, the United States, the United Kingdom, or Australia, as a result of low academic achievement and its attendant risks of poverty, early pregnancy, and criminal convictions.
- Homelessness, housing insecurity, and moves are frequent among former youths in care, particularly in the first six months after transition, with particular vulnerability among young people with special needs, including mental health, behavioural, or substance abuse difficulties.
- Early pregnancy (e.g., by age 19) and parenthood occur at relatively high rates among young women who age out of care and are associated with psychiatric difficulties, substance use

disorders, or delinquency. Conversely, attachment to caregivers and educational achievement are associated with delays in pregnancy.

- Health and mental health outcomes are worse among youths who have aged out of care than among other young people, with many reporting special needs, post-traumatic stress, or reliance on psychotropic medication.
- Loneliness, as well as isolation and stigma, is reported by young people who have aged out of care, with negative effects on their educational and career outcomes.

In light of these persistent problems, Kovarikova (2017) made several pertinent suggestions for improving the effectiveness of child welfare policies for care leavers in Ontario. She suggested the launching of a longitudinal study of young people aging out of care in Ontario, with a focus on the main sub-groups of care leavers, including those whose post-transition trajectories have been positive. Also, there needs to be a commitment to collecting and publishing data on how young people fare *after* leaving care, in order to evaluate the effectiveness of new policies and reforms. In addition, the wisdom and experience of former young people in care need to be tapped when new child welfare policies or structural changes are introduced (such as during the current redesign of child welfare services in Ontario). Child Welfare PAC noted that as of August 2021, 18 post-secondary institutions in 5 of Canada's 10 provinces had created more than 140 placements with tuition waivers for young people with a care background (Christensen, 2021). More colleges and universities were expected to initiate tuition waivers in the future.

In light of the obvious importance of college and university education in improving the transitions and career prospects of care leavers, as also attested by Gunawardena and Stich (2021) and Kovarikova (2017) (see also Chapter 4 on education in the present volume), we now examine a recent Canadian needs-assessment study conducted at the University of Ottawa (Lamborn & Aubry, 2021). This project resulted in the adoption and initial implementation of a three-year pilot program of tuition waivers and other supports for young people with a care background. We believe the report, *University of Ottawa Students with Extended Society Care Status: A Needs Assessment*, may provide a useful model for those considering similar initiatives at other Canadian universities or colleges.

Lamborn and Aubry (2021) undertook their needs assessment with the twin goals of understanding whether a tuition-support program would be beneficial for youth with a care background at the University of Ottawa and what other supports (e.g., mentoring or navigational) would also be needed. Recommendations were to be made to the administration of the University of Ottawa, the Children's Aid Society of Ottawa, and the Children's Aid Foundation of Ottawa. Semi-structured interviews were conducted with six current University of Ottawa students, aged 18–22, who had care backgrounds; three University of Ottawa alumni with care backgrounds, aged 21–29; two Ottawa Society informants, and one University of Ottawa informant. (The evaluation questions and interview protocols used with each type of respondent—students, alumni/alumnae, or informants—have been included in appendices of the report, for use by interested parties.)

The students reported a range of obstacles in pursuing their studies at the University of Ottawa, in commerce, psychology, chemistry, human kinetics, and other fields:

- Financial obstacles: Trying to make ends meet by pulling together various income sources; stress from aging out of the CAS system, often with the loss of monthly support payments in the middle of their degree programs; stress from grants from the Ontario Student Assistance Program (OSAP) turning into repayable loans if they were unable to maintain a full-time course load.
- Academic obstacles: Difficulty in navigating the online portal used to register in courses; difficulty in time management, self-direction, and handling the workload and other demands of university; for some, paying for the assessments needed to document disabilities and to access needed academic accommodations.
- Social obstacles: Many students said they lacked social support, with no one they knew who had attended university and could offer guidance; difficulty in meeting and forming friendships with new people or knowing how much to share about their care background; awareness that their family lives differed from those of other students, especially during holidays or when moving into residence.
- Other obstacles: All the students said that mental health was a challenge while at the University of Ottawa, including

anxiety, depression, low motivation, and attentional problems; also challenging were times of transition, such as moving to Ottawa or aging out of their continuing care agreements
when they reached the age of 21.

Despite their needs for support and knowledge of some of the
services available on campus, few students had used these services.
They cited reports of long waiting lists, being turned away when late
for appointments, or having experienced a lack of fit with services
that they had previously accessed.

Lamborn and Aubry (2021) formulated several recommendations aimed at improving the situation at the University of Ottawa of
students with a care background:

- Financial and navigational/human support: students' financial needs should be evaluated on an individual basis, to
  make sure that additional funds would not negatively influence their government-provided funding; also, students in
  financial need should receive additional funds through a
  well-defined bursary program, with no limit on the student's
  age or the time required to complete a degree program.
- Support availability: the University of Ottawa should assist
  students from the beginning of their studies and make it easy
  for students aged 21 and older to access support; information
  about bursary and navigational support should be simple to
  find on the university website; and students should be able to
  identify themselves as having a care background.
- Outcome tracking and program evaluation: the University
  of Ottawa should evaluate the bursary and navigational
  programs, and the Children's Aid Foundation of Ottawa
  should develop procedures that enable it to track the educational outcomes of young people who have received its
  bursaries.
- Funding for psychoeducational assessments: the Children's
  Aid Society of Ottawa, the Children's Aid Foundation
  of Ottawa, and the University of Ottawa should investigate available options that would allow students to document their disabilities and thereby access needed academic
  accommodations.

The needs-assessment study by Lamborn and Aubry (2021) identified two primary gaps confronting students with a care background
who pursue their studies at the University of Ottawa: funding to help
cover the cost of tuition, and help with navigating a large and complex
university. As a result of their study and meetings with administrative leaders at the University of Ottawa, a three-year trial of a bursary and individualized mentoring support program was approved.
Implementation of the trial began in the fall of 2021, with monitoring
to ensure that the problems identified have been effectively addressed.

5.3. Use of the Casey Life Skills Assessment as a Practice Tool

The U.S. Casey has been used in the United States mainly as a tool in
clinical child welfare services, with little peer-reviewed and published
research completed to date. Despite this, we had included in the AAR-
C2-2016 the items and scales comprising the Canadian Casey and
shown Tables 9.1–9.9 because they struck us as having good content
validity, were an improvement over the transition-related items in
the AAR-C2-2010, and seemed likely to facilitate useful conversations
about transitions among young people in care, caregivers, and child
welfare workers. We also hoped that making norms on the Canadian
Casey available in the present chapter would facilitate needed predictive validity studies. Such research is especially urgent in Canada,
as a recent meta-analysis of the impact of transitional programs on
outcomes among care leavers (Heerde et al., 2018) found that of the
19 studies that met the inclusion criteria, all 19 were from the United
States. This result is similar to one reported by Gunawardena and
Stich (2021) in their systematic review of scientific studies of interventions on transitions (summarized earlier in the chapter), namely, that
only 1 of the 30 studies reviewed had been conducted in Canada.

Local society staff can use the items in Tables 9.1–9.8 to recon-
struct a young person's or group's scores on the eight Casey scales
and total scale (see Table 9.9). They can do so from the OnLAC SPSS
data that their society receives each year from the OnLAC Project staff
at the University of Ottawa. More simply, individual child welfare
workers or caregivers can use Tables 9.1–9.9 to conduct life-skills conversations or assessments with the young persons in their charge. The
Casey Life Skills Practice Guide (Casey Family Programs, 2021) suggests
a process to follow in conducting such conversations or assessments
to maximize their impact:

- Motivate the young person in care to take part in the life-skills assessment;
- Review the results with the young person;
- Invite caregivers to take part, to share their insights;
- Engage the young person in a conversation about the results; and
- Use *the Casey Life Skills Resource Guide* (Casey Family Programs, 2012) to help the young person to develop a learning plan, with suggested goals and activities.

Also, Evidence-Based Associates (n.d.) provides a useful example of how a community program uses the U.S. Casey to develop an individualized program for a young person.

5.4. Research on the U.S. Casey Life Skills Assessment

Casey et al. (2010) evaluated young people's transition skills (including but going beyond life skills) that they expected would be related to successful transitions among young people who had left residential care. The sample was composed of 104 youths who were leaving the Boys Town Treatment Family Home residential program. The perceptions of the young people and their house parents were compared on two of the Ansell-Casey Life Skills Assessment scales (as the U.S. Casey was formerly known), namely, the Daily Living and Housing and Money Management scales. There were no statistically significant differences between the mean scores of the young people and those of their house parents on either the Daily Living or Housing and Money Management scales. This provides some but limited support for the validity of young people's self-reported scores, but more research of this kind is obviously required.

In a cross-sectional sample of 294 youths in out-of-home care, aged 15–18, Trejos-Castillo et al. (2015) used the U.S. Ansell-Casey Life Skills Assessment to study the relationship between independent living skills and economic well-being. The young people were preparing for transition by completing the Texas-mandated Preparation for Adult Living program. Life skills were measured with the Daily Living, Self-Care, Relationships and Communications, Work and Study, Career and Education Planning, and Looking Forward scales. Economic well-being was assessed by dividing the items in the Housing and Money Management scale into two indicators: Financial

Literacy (11 items) and Housing (8 items). Internal consistency (alpha) coefficients for the various measures ranged between .79 and .91. In hierarchical regression of the two economic well-being indicators on the six life-skills scales—Career and Education Planning, and Work and Study—were statistically significant predictors of both Financial Literacy and Housing. The Self-Care also predicted Housing. Trejos-Castillo et al. (2015) suggested that their quantitative results indicated that financial literacy and housing-related knowledge merit greater attention in preparing young people for transition. Moreover, from qualitative data gathered in focus groups with 15 young people who were already living independently, the researchers found that the two main themes that emerged—economic struggles and financial planning—both corroborated their quantitative findings and were highly relevant to successful transitions from care. More research of this nature is needed, with attention, however, to more independent measures of economic well-being. In the research by Trejos-Castillo et al. (2015), method variance no doubt accounted for a sizable portion of the substantial correlations found between the predictor and dependent variables, all of which were drawn from the Ansell-Casey scales.

Researchers from Finland (Häggman et al., 2019) published a systematic review and synthesis of 13 international quantitative studies published in English between 2010 and 2017 that had been assessed as being of good quality and had focused on the subjective perceptions and experiences of young people with a care background regarding their independent living during their transition to adulthood. The young people viewed themselves as adults and were hopeful and confident about the future, although they confronted problems often reported in the literature: pursuing their education, securing employment, and finding a person upon whom they could rely. They also stated that they were not always highly involved in fashioning their transitions, and professionals were not always supportive. The young people said their need for support lay especially in forming relationships, physical health, managing money, and pursuing secondary and post-secondary education. Regarding coping strategies, the importance of adequate material resources was clear. Stable housing and employment were likely to improve the ability of care leavers to cope. Häggman et al. (2019) remarked, however, that many care leavers had "remarkable" difficulty in completing a high school diploma, without which post-secondary education was typically beyond reach.

Of particular interest to the present chapter, Häggman et al. (2019, p. 658) insisted that past research has taken little account of care leavers' individuality or strengths and has produced "little" knowledge of their "realistic perceptions of their identity, abilities, emotions and future wishes." Accordingly, the authors recommended the use of tools such as the Casey Life Skills Assessment, widely used in the United States, to identify and meet a range of possible support needs in different cultures, as well as potential female–male differences in felt needs.

6. Norms for Sub-Groups of Young People in Care on the Canadian Casey: Mean Differences by Sex, Age, Type of Residential Placement, and Level of Well-Being

Despite the relative lack of research on the Casey Life Skills Assessment, we formulated several working hypotheses about the kind of sub-group differences that we were likely to find on the Casey scales. In our sample of young people in care, we expected to observe greater readiness for transition and independent living (and thus higher mean scores on the Casey scales) among females rather than males, older rather than younger young people, those already living in independent living rather than other types of homes, and those displaying higher rather than lower levels of well-being. If our results were reasonably consistent with our working hypotheses, we felt that we would be able to recommend the Casey scales as measures of the preparedness of a young person or group of young persons in care for transition and independent living, or to evaluate the short-term outcomes of a program preparing young people for transition.

On the other hand, we did not want to have this recommendation seen as an endorsement of classroom-based life-skills training. Courtney et al. (2008) evaluated such a program in Los Angeles County, California. The curriculum lasted five weeks, composed of 10 three-hour classes held twice a week in 19 community colleges throughout Los Angeles County. The program included seven competency skills areas: education, employment, daily living skills, survival skills, choices and consequences, interpersonal/social skills, and computer/internet skills. Outreach advisors assessed the care leavers with the Ansell-Casey assessment instrument before and after the classroom modules. Of the sample of 482 young people in the sample, 234 had been assigned to the life-skills training (treatment) group and

248 to the control group. The researchers' control over who actually received the life-skills training was imperfect, such that almost 23% of the control group ended up graduating from the program. Overall, the impact evaluation found little or no evidence of the added effectiveness of classroom-based life-skills training. According to young people leaving care, much of the help they had received with independent living had come from biological parents, other family members, teachers and schools, caregivers, caseworkers, or independent living programs.

6.1. Mean Differences on the Canadian Casey by Sex

Table 9.10 shows that on all the Casey scales except Permanency and Looking Forward, females had higher mean scores than males. This was in accordance with our working hypothesis, based on female adolescents' usually greater social maturity, compared with males of the same age. In terms of effect sizes (Cohen's d), the statistically significant mean differences were in the small range, between .22 for Career and Education Planning and .09 for Housing and Money Management. The fact that the mean differences were not significant on either Permanency ($d = .03$, ns) or Looking Forward ($d = .07$, ns) may reflect the relatively generic, versus concrete and specific, content of the respective scale items.

In Tables 9.10–9.13 we have provided not only the scale means but also the average item means for each of the scales, calculated by dividing the scale mean (e.g., for females or males, in Table 9.10) by the number of items in the scale (e.g., 20 in the case of the Permanency scale). On some of the scales, the item means are around 4.5, not far from the maximum possible of 5.0. As a result, it should be noted that on these scales (e.g., Permanency and Relationships and Communications, in Table 9.10), a ceiling effect may be encountered, thereby limiting the possibility of finding any pre-test/post-test gains. This will obviously be less of a problem on scales with lower average item means (e.g., Career and Education Planning, in Table 9.10).

6.2. Mean Differences on the Canadian Casey by Age

Table 9.11 presents the mean differences for 16-year-olds versus 17-year-olds in care. Our working hypothesis was that older youths would display a somewhat higher average level of preparedness for

Table 9.10. Means, standard deviations, *t*-tests, and effect sizes from comparisons of means of female versus male youths in care on eight Canadian Casey scales and total scale

Casey Scale	Females (*n* = 911)		Males (*n* = 945)		*t* (1854)	Effect Size (Cohen's *d*)
	Mean	SD	Mean	SD		
Permanency (Item level)	90.47[1] (4.52)[2]	11.13	90.78[1] (4.54)[2]	10.08	.64 *ns*	.03
Daily Living (Item level)	65.61 (4.37)	7.84	63.99 (4.27)	9.15	4.09***	.19
Self-Care (Item level)	63.73 (4.25)	8.35	62.04 (4.14)	9.07	4.17***	.19
Relationships and Communications (Item level)	49.23 (4.48)	5.31	48.42 (4.40)	6.03	3.08**	.14
Housing and Money Management (Item level)	61.45 (3.23)	21.21	59.50 (3.13)	20.77	2.01*	.09
Work and Study (Item level)	71.47 (3.97)	14.36	68.78 (3.82)	15.26	3.92***	.18
Career and Education Planning (Item level)	22.90 (3.82)	6.22	21.47 (3.58)	6.60	4.79***	.22
Looking Forward (Item level)	33.36 (4.17)	6.21	32.93 (4.12)	6.18	1.52 *ns*	.07
Total Casey Scale (Item level)	458.22 (4.09)	64.89	447.90 (4.00)	68.88	3.32***	.15

Note. ns = Not significant. *$p < .05$, **$p < .002$, ***$p < .001$
1 The scale mean.
2 The average item mean for females or males, calculated by dividing their respective means on the Permanency scale (i.e., 90.47 and 90.78) by 20, the number of items in the scale. Comparisons can be made with the individual item means on the Permanency scale for the combined sample (see Table 9.1), and similar comparisons of item means can be made with the other Casey scales in Tables 9.2–9.8.
Source: Ontario Looking After Children Project data, 2016–2019.

transition and independent living, given that transition was likely to be a more pressing concern for them than for their younger peers. As Table 9.11 shows, this was borne out for all the scales except Relationships and Communications ($d = .06$, *ns*) and Looking Forward ($d = .08$, *ns*). The effect sizes of the statistically significant differences in means were again in the small range of roughly .20, except for the small-to-moderate *d* of .33 for Housing and Money Management.

Table 9.11. Means, standard deviations, *t*-tests, and effect sizes from comparisons of 16- versus 17-year-old youths in care on eight Canadian Casey scales and total scale

Casey Scale	16-year-olds (n = 1265)		17-year-olds (n = 593)		t (1856)	Effect Size (Cohen's d)
	Mean	SD	Mean	SD		
Permanency (Item level)	90.231 (4.51)2	10.78	91.47[1] (4.57)[2]	10.16	2.35*	.12
Daily Living (Item level)	64.34 (4.29)	8.61	65.73 (4.38)	8.40	3.25**	.16
Self-Care (Item level)	62.34 (4.16)	8.62	64.01 (4.27)	8.93	3.85**	.19
Relationships and Commuications (Item level)	48.72 (4.43)	5.69	49.03 (4.46)	5.73	1.12 ns	.06
Housing and Money Management (Item level)	58.27 (3.07)	20.87	65.10 (3.43)	20.56	6.60**	.33
Work and Study (Item level)	68.98 (3.83)	14.87	72.47 (4.03)	14.63	4.74**	.24
Career and Education Planning (Item level)	21.77 (3.63)	6.47	23.01 (3.84)	6.37	3.87**	.19
Looking Forward (Item level)	32.98 (4.12)	6.23	33.50 (4.19)	6.11	1.68 ns	.08
Total Casey Scale (Item level)	447.63 (4.00)	66.48	464.31 (4.15)	67.07	5.03**	.25

Note. ns = Not significant. *p < .05, **p < .001
1 The scale mean.
2 The average item mean for 16- and 17-year-olds, calculated by dividing their respective means on the Permanency scale (i.e., 90.23 and 91.47) by 20, the number of items in the scale. Comparisons can be made with the individual item means on the Permanency scale for the combined sample (see Table 9.1), and similar comparisons of item means can be made with the other Casey scales in Tables 9.2–9.8.

6.3. Mean Differences on the Canadian Casey by Current Type of Residential Placement

Our working hypothesis was that young people in care who were currently residing in independent-living homes would score higher on the Casey measures than those living in kinship care, foster care, or group care homes. We reasoned that the daily experience of independent living, in which the youths would not have adult caregivers to guide them on a daily basis and would have to take greater personal responsibility for their lives, would generate greater awareness of the realities of transition and independence. As Table 9.12 shows, this was indeed the case. Except for the Permanency ($d = .00$, ns) and Looking Forward ($d = .10$, ns) scales, the means of the young people residing in independent-living

Table 9.12. Means, standard deviations, *t*-tests, and effect sizes from comparisons of means of youths in care living in independent living homes versus kinship care, foster, or group homes on eight Canadian Casey scales and total scale

Casey Scale	Youths in Independent Living Homes ($n = 183$)		Youths in Kinship, Foster, or Group Homes ($n = 1510$)		t (1691)	Effect Size (Cohen's d)
	Mean	SD	Mean	SD		
Permanency (Item level)	90.80[1] (4.54)[2]	10.01	90.82 (4.54)	10.48	.02 ns	.00
Daily Living (Item level)	67.75 (4.52)	6.01	64.38 (4.29)	8.86	5.01***	.39
Self-Care (Item level)	66.97 (4.46)	6.49	62.32 (4.15)	8.97	6.81***	.53
Relationships and Communications (Item level)	49.81 (4.53)	4.88	48.77 (4.43)	5.79	2.33*	.18
Housing and Money Management (Item level)	75.20 (3.96)	16.35	58.64 (3.08)	20.77	10.40***	.81
Work and Study (Item level)	76.11 (4.23)	11.68	69.58 (3.87)	15.00	5.68***	.45
Career and Education Planning (Item level)	24.52 (4.09)	5.32	21.95 (3.66)	6.52	5.13***	.40
Looking Forward (Item level)	33.79 (4.22)	5.79	33.18 (4.15)	6.21	1.27 ns	.10
Total Casey Scale (Item level)	484.96 (4.33)	53.18	449.63 (4.01)	67.69	6.81***	.53

Note. ns = Not significant. *$p < .05$, ***$p < .001$
[1] The scale mean.
[2] The average item mean for youths in care living in IL versus other types of homes, calculated by dividing their respective means on the Permanency scale (i.e., 90.80 and 90.82) by 20, the number of items in the scale. Comparisons can be made with the individual item means on the Permanency scale for the combined sample (see Table 9.1), and similar comparisons of item means can be made with the other Casey scales in Tables 9.2–9.8.
Source: Ontario Looking After Children Project data, 2016–2019.

homes were significantly higher on all the Casey scales than the means of their peers in other types of homes. Moreover, the effect sizes associated with the type of home tended to be quite a bit larger than those associated with sex or age. They ranged from large ($d = .81$ for Housing and Money Management), through medium ($d = .53$ on Self-Care, $d = .45$ on Work and Study Life, and $d = .53$ on the Total Casey scale), to small ($d = .18$ for Relationships and Communications).

6.4. Mean Differences on the Canadian Casey by Well-Being Tertile

Our last comparison was between the means on the Casey scales of the young people in care who scored in the highest, middle, and lowest well-being tertiles (i.e., thirds) on Keyes' (2006) 14-item measure of well-being, of which we made extensive use in Chapter 8 of the present volume. We wanted to know whether young persons, who were experiencing different levels of well-being, would score at different levels on each of the Casey scales. If so, this would suggest that a youth's level of emotional, psychological, and social well-being (i.e., positive mental health), along with factors such as sex, age, or type of home, is associated with—and thus may influence—his or her perceived level of knowledge or performance on the Casey scales. Our working hypothesis was that young people reporting higher levels of well-being would also score more favourably on the Casey scales (as they had scored more favourably on our eight measures of positive or negative of mental health in Chapter 8).

As shown in Table 9.13, the young persons in the highest well-being tertile had the highest means on all the Casey scales, followed by those in the middle tertile, and then by those in the lowest tertile. All the between-groups F-tests were statistically significant at the $p < .001$ level, with the well-being tertiles accounting for 5% to 38% of the variance in the Casey scales. Benchmarks for small-, medium-, or large-effect sizes have yet to be established for eta-squared (Richardson, 2011); however, the fact that 5% to 38% of the variance in the youths' perceived life-skills knowledge and performance was accounted for by their level of well-being indicates that the relationship is an important one. This was especially true for the three Casey scales that, as we noted earlier, comprise a statistical dimension that is focused more on young people's relationships and friendships and less on concrete and specific life skills: Looking Forward (eta-squared = .38), Relationships and Communications (.22), and Permanency (.15).

Table 9.13. Means, standard deviations, F-tests, and effect sizes comparing the means of youths in care in the lowest, middle, and highest well-being tertiles on eight Canadian Casey scales and total scale

Casey Scale	Highest Well-Being Tertile (n = 550)		Middle Well-Being Tertile (n = 660)		Lowest Well-Being Tertile (n = 638)		$F(2,1845)$	Effect Size (Eta-Squared)
	Mean	SD	Mean	SD	Mean	SD		
Permanency (Item level)	94.84[1] (4.74)[2]	6.48	92.39 (4.62)	8.18	85.19 (4.26)	13.10	160.46*	.15
Daily Living (Item level)	67.57 (4.50)	7.54	65.68 (4.79)	7.00	61.57 (4.10)	9.69	85.42*	.09
Self-Care (Item level)	65.54 (4.37)	7.74	64.08 (4.27)	7.37	59.42 (3.96)	9.70	89.46*	.09
Relationships and Communications (Item level)	51.89 (4.72)	3.80	49.66 (4.51)	4.45	45.40 (4.13)	6.07	261.64*	.22
Housing and Money Management (Item level)	66.04 (3.48)	20.95	61.76 (3.25)	20.25	54.58 (2.87)	20.25	48.13*	.05
Work and Study (Item level)	75.39 (4.19)	13.59	71.69 (3.98)	13.14	64.08 (3.56)	15.40	101.29*	.10
Career and Education Planning (Item level)	24.41 (4.07)	5.92	22.94 (3.82)	5.88	19.53 (3.26)	6.49	101.81*	.10
Looking Forward (Item level)	37.47 (4.68)	3.40	34.42 (4.30)	4.45	28.17 (3.52)	6.12	574.33*	.38
Total Casey Scale (Item level)	483.16 (4.31)	57.37	462.63 (4.13)	56.03	417.93 (3.73)	69.18	179.32*	.16

Note. Eta-squared = proportion of total variance in Y (here, a given Casey scale) associated with membership of different groups in X (here, well-being tertiles) (Richardson 2011). *$p < .001$
1 The scale mean.
2 The average item mean for youths in care who were in the highest versus the middle or lowest well-being tertiles, calculated by dividing their respective means on the Permanency scale by 20, the number of items in the scale. Comparisons can be made with the individual item means on the Permanency scale for the combined sample (see Table 9.1), and similar comparisons of item means can be made with the other Casey scales in Tables 9.2–9.8.
Source: Ontario Looking After Children Project data, 2016–2019.

7. Summary and Conclusion

In the present chapter, we made available overall and sub-group norms for the Canadian Casey Life Skills Assessment. We recommend its use with individual young people aged 16–17 who are preparing to leave care, to make them aware of the many life skills involved in living independently in the community. The instrument can also be used as a source of items for evaluating changes in youths' self-rated life skills as the date of leaving care approaches. We also summarized two noteworthy Canadian publications on transitions. First was the first systematic review of scientific studies of transition (Gunawardena and Stich, 2021); second was a report on the needs of care leavers by the founder of the Child Welfare PAC (Kovarikova, 2017). We also provided a summary of Lamborn and Aubry's (2021) recent assessment of the support needs of young people in care who choose to pursue a university education. This model may serve as a useful guide for other communities seeking to establish a similar university support program for former young people in care.

References

BMJ. (2021, March 29). The PRISMA 2020 statement: An updated guideline for reporting systematic reviews. *BMJ*, 372(71). https://doi.org/10.1136/bmj.n71

Casey Family Programs. (2012). *Casey life skills resource guide*. http://www.itsmymove.org/docs/CLSA/CLSResourcestoInspire2012.pdf

Casey Family Programs. (2021). *Casey life skills practice guide*. https://www.casey.org/media/CLS_Project_PracticeGuide.pdf

Christensen, S. (2021, August 10). Communication from the Child Welfare PAC Canada.

Courtney, M., & Hook, J. (2017). The potential educational benefits of extending foster care to young adults: Findings from a natural experiment. *Children and Youth Services Review*, 72, 124–132. https://doi.org/10.1016/j.childyouth.2016.09.030

Courtney, M. E., Zinn, A., Zielewski, W. H., Bess, R. J., Malm, K. E., Stagner, M., & Pergamit, M. (2008, July). *Evaluation of the life skills training program, Los Angeles Country, California: Final report*. Prepared by The Urban Institute, Washington, D.C.; Chapin Hall Center for Children, University of Chicago, Chicago, IL; and National Opinion Research Center, University of Chicago, Chicago, IL.

Evidence-Based Associates. (n.d.). *Casey life skills (CLS)*. [PowerPoint of the logic model of a community-based service program based on the Casey Life Skills Assessment]. https://evidencebasedassociates.com/wp-content/uploads/2019/11/Casey-Life-Skills-Logic-Model_EBA.pdf

Greeson, J. K. P., Garcia, A. R., Kim, M., & Courtney, M. E. (2015). Foster youth and social support: The first RCT of independent living services.

Research in Social Work Practice, 25(3), 349–357. https://doi.org/10.1177/1049731514534900

Gunawardena, N., & Stich, C. (2021). Interventions for young people aging out of the child welfare system: A systematic literature review. *Children and Youth Services Review,* 127, Article 106076.

Häggman-Laitila, A., Salokekkilä, P., & Karki, S. (2019). Young people's pre-paredness for adult life and coping after foster care: A systematic review of perceptions and experiences in the transition period. *Child and Youth Care Forum,* 48, 633–661. https://doi.org/10.1007/s10566-019-09499-4

Heerde, J. A., Hemphill, A. A., & Scholes-Balog, K. E. (2018). The impact of transitional programmes on post-transition outcomes for youth leaving out-of-home care: A meta-analysis. *Health and Social Care,* 26(1), e15–e30.

Kovarikova, J. (2017, April 24). *Exploring youth outcomes after aging-out of care.* Ontario Office of the Provincial Advocate for Children and Youth. https://cwrp.ca/sites/default/files/publications/report-exploring-youth-outcomes.pdf

Lamborn, P., & Aubry, T. (2021, August). *Assessment of the needs of University of Ottawa students with extended society care status - Final report.* Centre for Research on Educational and Community Services, University of Ottawa.

Miller, M., Vincent, C., & Flynn, R. (2017, August). *User's manual for the AAR-C2-2016.* Centre for Research on Educational and Community Services, University of Ottawa. https://ruor.uottawa.ca/handle/10393/37843

Nollan, K. A., Wolf, M., Ansell, D., Burns, J., Barr, J., Copeland, W., & Paddock, G. (2000). Ready or not: Assessing youths' preparedness for indepen-dent living. *Child Welfare,* 79(2), 159–176.

Richardson, J. T. E. (2011). Eta squared and partial eta squared as measures of effect size in educational research. *Educational Research Review,* 6(2), 135–147.

Squires, J., Bricker, D., & Twombly, E. (2003). *The ASQ:SE user's guide for the Ages and Stages Questionnaires: Social-Emotional.* Paul H. Brookes.

Squires, J., Twombly, E., Bricker, D., & Potter, L. (2009). *ASQ-3 user's guide: Ages and Stages Questionnaire, Third Edition.* Paul H. Brookes.

Trejos-Castillo, E., Davis, G., & Hipps, T. (2015). Economic well-being and independent living in foster youth: Paving the road to effective transi-tioning out of care. *Child Welfare,* 94(1), 53–71.

Lessons from the Ontario Looking After Children Project for Improving the Outcomes and Well-Being of Young People in Care

Since its inception in 2000, the Ontario Looking After Children (OnLAC) Project has sought to collaborate with people in the field of child welfare in Ontario and elsewhere to improve the outcomes and well-being of young people in care. Identifying the key service needs of the young person during the forthcoming 12 months, coupled with examining the young person's progress during the past 12 months, is at the heart of the conversational interview carried out each year with the Action and Assessment Record (AAR). In the OnLAC model, the three-way information-gathering and clinical discussion among the young people in care (if aged 10 or older), the caregiver, and the child welfare worker are essential for creating or revising the young person's annual plan of care. The youth's service needs and outcomes belong to one of eight OnLAC outcome dimensions: health, education, identity, family and social relationships, social presentation, emotional and behavioural development, self-care skills, and developmental assets. Each of these contributes to the young person's overall well-being.

This last chapter distills eight major lessons from the many learning opportunities that we have experienced during the first 22 years of the OnLAC Project (2000–2022). We hope that action, based on these lessons by local societies, the Ontario Association of Children's Aid Societies (OACAS), and the Ministry of Children, Community and Social Services (MCCSS) will benefit young people in care and their families, caregivers, workers, and supervisors, as well as others. We have divided the "lessons of OnLAC" somewhat arbitrarily into two types.

The first set of four lessons are related closely to building capacity in the local society to achieve improved services through better care planning, outcome monitoring, and program evaluation. Lesson 1 is about the needed renewal of OnLAC and AAR training. Lesson 2 suggests how AAR data can be used for planning, monitoring, and evaluation purposes. Lesson 3 provides more general information on program development and evaluation that is intended to be of use beyond AAR data. Finally, lesson 4 provides a concrete case study of how one Ontario society used AAR data to improve the relationship between young people in care and its caregivers.

The second set of lessons from OnLAC is related primarily to the idea of innovation, which we see as timely and aligned with the encouraging "modernization and re-design" effort that is taking place at present in child welfare in Ontario. Lesson 5 makes the case for prevention, in the form of high-quality early childhood education and care for pre-K children and high-impact tutoring for those of primary-school age. Lesson 6 advocates that MCCSS should consider implementing a new "OnLAC-2" program that would follow up a random sample of care leavers each year, partly to see how effective child welfare preparation programs are and partly to see how "permanent" permanency in the province actually is. Lesson 7 argues that a special child welfare research fund would be extremely useful, with goals similar to those of the applied research programs of the ministries of health and education. Lastly, lesson 8 concludes the chapter with a plea for a renewed OnLAC Project partnership among the University of Ottawa, OACAS, and MCCSS.

1. OnLAC Project Lesson 1: High-Quality and Readily Available OnLAC and AAR Training for New and Veteran Caregivers, Workers, Supervisors, Quality-Assurance Staff, and Others Is Urgently Needed

As described in Chapter 1, the OnLAC Project is based theoretically and philosophically on two major developmental frameworks. The first is Looking After Children, of U.K. origin, with its eight outcome dimensions—health, education, identity, family and social relationships, social presentation, emotional and behavioural development, self-care skills, and developmental assets. The second is the Child Well-Being framework, of U.S. origin, with its four broad outcome domains—physical development; cognitive development; psychological, emotional, and behavioural development; and social development. In a long-standing, 22-year (and counting) initiative such as the OnLAC Project, it is inevitable that the enthusiasm and high-fidelity practice of the early-adopting societies, caregivers, and staff would decline over time and need to be renewed on a regular basis. The main vehicle for such renewal is high-quality, early available, and interesting training. Unfortunately, as many people in the field have told us, OnLAC training has become very rare in Ontario. The result is that many new and veteran society staff and caregivers currently have little or no accurate, up-to-date knowledge of the purpose or use of OnLAC or the AAR, whether on the level of the young person in care, the society in which they work, or the province as a whole. There is an urgent need for updated and widely available training, presented in formats adapted to the needs of different groups. The members of the OnLAC team need to have a significant role in preparing and delivering the revised OnLAC training, given their many years of contact with people in the field, including OACAS and MCCSS, their role in previous revisions of the AAR, and their in-depth expertise and experience with on OnLAC practice and research.

A central tenet of Looking After Children, since its beginning more than three decades ago in the United Kingdom and more than two decades ago in Canada, has been the importance of the annual face-to-face AAR interview, which brings together three key people: the young person in care, the caregiver, and the child welfare worker. The purpose of the AAR dialogue is to accomplish two essential tasks needed for preparing the best possible plan of care to guide the care of the young person over the next 12 months. First, the three participants must gather and record up-to-date and accurate information on the young person's experiences during the past year, to enable monitoring of the progress made. Second, the participants must listen to one another to distill and incorporate in the plan of care for the coming year the most important implications of the information that they have shared during the AAR conversation. That is, what are the young person's most pressing needs? What outcomes require the greatest improvement? What services can be put in place to produce these outcomes?

The foregoing paragraph expresses, in a nutshell, what the OnLAC team views as expected, high-fidelity OnLAC and AAR practice. Anything less is not acceptable, except in exceptional circumstances (e.g., in situations where the worker is located at a great distance from the caregiver and young person and a meeting via Zoom or Microsoft Teams is not feasible). Unfortunately, in the absence of high-quality and accessible training over the last decade, some child welfare workers (whose job it is to oversee the annual AAR interview) have replaced the essential face-to-face, three-way clinical discussion with the simple expedient of "dropping off" a copy of the AAR with the caregiver, with a request that the caregiver (and perhaps the young person) "fill it out" on their own. This low-fidelity practice eliminates the raison d'être of OnLAC and the AAR, namely, the clinical, face-to-face discussion in which collaborative, high-quality plans of care are crafted, specifying the most important outcomes that the young persons need to attain over the next year and the services that are likely to produce these benefits.

We also want to emphasize that the quality of training and frequency of use of the AAR in supervision are important components of high-fidelity practice with the AAR. Pantin, Flynn, and Runnels (2006) found in a sample of 125 supervisors and child welfare workers in Ontario societies that these two factors shape clinicians' perceptions of the utility of the AAR in helping them do their jobs better. First, when workers or supervisors perceived more positively the quality of the OnLAC training they had received, they rated the utility of the AAR more highly. Second, the more frequently they discussed information from the AAR in supervision, the more useful they rated the tool. Those who discussed information from the AAR "often or always" rated the tool as having high utility; those who discussed AAR information in supervision "from time to time" saw the instrument as having average utility; and those who "rarely or never" discussed AAR information in supervision saw the tool as having low utility.

Overall, between two thirds and three quarters of the workers and supervisors rated the AAR as "very useful" or "useful" in helping them carry out the following aspects of their jobs (Pantin et al., 2006), toward:

- understanding the needs of the young person in care;
- collaborating with the caregiver in implementing the young person's plan of care;
- preparing useful plans of care;
- assisting young people in planning their futures;

- carrying out clinical or supervisory work;
- having targeted discussions with young people in care; and
- becoming more aware of the young person's progress.

Besides mandatory training for caregivers and society personnel, we also recommend that OACAS and MCCSS program analysts receive relevant training to enable them to use OnLAC publications and AAR data to improve provincial services and policies. Such use has been very rare to date at OACAS or MCCSS.

Romano et al. (2020) studied the use of data in child welfare service planning and found that training needs to focus especially on using the AAR to prepare the plan of care and on promoting evidence-informed practice throughout the sector. Romano et al. (2020, p. 7) stated that "training content should focus on enhancing practitioners' skills with integrating OnLAC data into their plans of care through repeated practice exercises and continued support for data use by supervisors." When practitioners were given thorough OnLAC and AAR training, Romano et al. (2020, p. 5) observed that there were significant positive changes in knowledge and attitudes regarding both the AAR and evidence-informed practice. High-quality training will also promote the basic resilience framework that, with its evidence-based risk and protective factors, remains the foundation of effective clinical services, policies, and improved outcomes.

As an example of the contribution that the OnLAC team could make to vastly improved training, in 2018 the team worked with the OACAS Child and Youth Caring Council to create an e-learning module on understanding and applying the Developmental Assets, an AAR measure that is a consistently good predictor of young people's success on many resilience-related outcomes. If provided with the needed training resources, the OnLAC team would be very interested in creating and teaching similar learning modules on other key AAR measures or dimensions. For example, young people in care, caregivers, workers, and supervisors would benefit from learning how to apply the Casey Life Skills (see Chapter 9) to assess preparedness for community living and planning transitions.

2. OnLAC Project Lesson 2: OnLAC Information and AAR Data Need to be Used Routinely for Clinical Service Planning, Outcome Monitoring, and Program Evaluation by Local Societies, OACAS, and MCCSS

The OnLAC database contains annual cross-sections of AAR data covering the period 2001–2022, as of the time of writing. This data also becomes longitudinal when young people complete two or more AARs. It forms a unique treasure trove of information on the services received and outcomes experienced by approximately 35,000 young people in care served by Ontario societies that will continue to grow. At the clinical level, the AAR provides a yearly voice for young people in care, with the information gained during the conversational interview enabling child welfare workers, caregivers, and supervisors to attain a precise and detailed picture of individual young persons' strengths, preferences, needs, outcomes, and year-over-year progress. If used regularly and strategically, which has been the exception rather than the rule in the province, aggregated AAR data and OnLAC reports and publications could help societies, OACAS, and MCCSS understand much better the children and young people they serve, tailor practices and policies much more closely to age-appropriate needs, and significantly improve the effectiveness of the services provided.

After the Ontario government mandated in 2006 that societies in the province were to use the AAR on an annual basis with all young persons who had been in care for one year or more, the workload of the OnLAC team at the University of Ottawa grew quickly but with no increase in staff resources. Not surprisingly, this caused a delay in the ability of the OnLAC team to provide local societies with their AAR data on a timely basis. Since 2010, however, the OnLAC team has had sufficient personnel to be able to provide societies with their cleaned, up-to-date data within two weeks of requesting them, as well as forwarding to each society its cleaned database from the previous year.

We recognize, however, that societies face ongoing challenges to making strategic and regular use of their OnLAC data. Such usage varies greatly, depending on local staff expertise in data analysis and other resources. Until now, the only province-wide use of OnLAC data has occurred in the child welfare performance indicators (PI) project. The AAR has been the source of yearly data for three well-being indicators

(Miller, 2021a) that form part of the MCCSS accountability framework: PI-14 (Developmental Assets); PI-15 (Relationship of Young Person in Care with Primary Caregiver); and PI-16 (Performance in School in Reading and Math). Some local societies, especially larger ones, have robust quality-assurance departments and staff adept at data analysis and interpretation, while other societies make no use of AAR data at all. Overall, systematic use of AAR data has been lacking.

Over the past two decades, the OnLAC team has offered consultation on a one-off basis to societies wanting to use their AAR data to improve their performance in particular domains. In addition, between 2008 and 2014, the OnLAC team provided semi-annual data analysis workshops in the computer labs at the University of Ottawa to help society and OACAS staff understand the structure of the OnLAC database and learn how to use SPSS to run basic descriptive, correlational, and predictive analyses. These workshops were well attended, until competing demands on the time of society staff—especially the mandated rollout across the province of the new Child Protection Information Network (CPIN)—led to a decline in enrollment and the end of the workshops. More recently, the OnLAC team has developed an Education Snapshot (described in Chapter 5), together with staff training in its use. The Education Snapshot uses OnLAC data to help young people, caregivers, and workers evaluate educational progress and guide service planning.

Overall, the Ontario child welfare sector would greatly benefit from high-quality training on how to use AAR data to improve local clinical services. Such use would build on society knowledge of contextual factors at play in the local community and complement available administrative service data. The regular, even routine, use of AAR data and OnLAC reports and publications would enlighten and empower societies, OACAS, and MCCSS in their assessments of individual, local, and provincial priorities. It would also help them gain a firmer grasp of burning issues such as the disproportionality and disparity experienced by Black and Indigenous young people in care. A role for the Association of Native Child and Family Services Agencies of Ontario (ANCFSAO) should no doubt be explored, especially in relation to assisting the seven Indigenous societies (out of a total of 13 in the province) to make better use of OnLAC/AAR and similar data to improve their service planning, clinical interventions, and program evaluations. A discussion on the same topic would likely be fruitful also with the First Nations Information Governance Centre (FNIGC), although FNIGC has a federal and national rather than Ontario focus, unlike ANCFSAO.

One of the most important innovations introduced by the International Looking After Children Initiative in the United Kingdom in the 1990s was a new and long-overdue emphasis on measuring the outcomes (i.e., benefits) that young people in care and their families actually derive from their experience of care. Knowledge of outcomes and of service processes were viewed as a precondition of their improvement. For example, until Looking After Children was launched, it was not known that a surprising number of young people in care of school age were not attending school. In launching the OnLAC Project in 2000, in partnership with OACAS and the United Kingdom's international initiative, we made the assessment of outcomes a priority and have maintained it ever since. Moreover, we constructed the AAR as a structured interview guide with demographic, psychometric, and quantitative strengths in order to be able to turn the results of the AAR conversations rapidly into computer-readable form. This was the only feasible way of gathering and analyzing the outcomes of large numbers of young people in care each year, on the individual, society, and provincial levels. A mainly qualitative tool would have required a prohibitive number of data analysts to accomplish the same objective, which is why the OnLAC Project has outlived those projects that took a primarily qualitative approach.

The OnLAC AAR has incorporated from the beginning, in the initial version of 2001 and the major revisions of 2006, 2010, and 2016, a number of standardized psychometric instruments of very good reliability and validity, mainly to measure key outcomes. Some of these measures originated in the National Longitudinal Survey of Children and Youth of Statistics Canada, which served as the early template for the AAR (Michaud, 2001). Over the years, we have incorporated other standardized tools into revised versions of the AAR. These measures assess a wide range of outcomes within the eight OnLAC development domains, including the young person's emotional, psychological, and social well-being as well as more specific outcomes such as his or her placement satisfaction, health status, educational success in reading and math, identity and self-esteem, relationships with caregivers, level of hope, mental health, and number of developmental assets. The AAR also assesses some negative outcomes, including the young person's behavioural difficulties, stress symptoms, soft and hard drug use, and suicidal behaviour. We describe these outcomes, both positive and negative, in the annual public (non-confidential) report that we produce each year for a widespread audience, including local societies, OACAS, and MCCSS (see Miller, 2021b, for an example). We also forward confidential reports annually to each of the 44 societies that submit AAR data each year to the OnLAC Project.

In the course of the OnLAC Project, some quality assurance or other staff in local societies have made good use of their own AAR data and our confidential reports to evaluate and improve their services and outcomes (see lesson 4 in this chapter for a good example). This is encouraging and in keeping with the original intent of the International Looking After Children Initiative and the OnLAC Project itself. However, such use of the data has been the exception, and OACAS and MCCSS themselves made little or no in-house use of the AAR data to answer their own practice or policy questions (e.g., related to enhancing services for Indigenous or Black young people and their families). Key contributing factors have included a relative lack of staff familiarity with quantitative data analysis, too little knowledge of the OnLAC model and the AAR, and a lack of training in outcome monitoring and program evaluation. The OnLAC Project staff did offer introductory training in AAR data analysis via SPSS between 2008 and 2014 but ultimately was forced to stop because of the demands on society time from the introduction in local societies of CPIN.

In order to make outcome monitoring and program evaluation regular and integral components of service delivery and improvement in Ontario, we propose that the scope of the OnLAC team's mandate be broadened to include a training and evaluation function, and that a training and evaluation specialist be added to the team. Under the guidance of this individual, members of the OnLAC team could then offer AAR-based monitoring and evaluation training on a regular basis, both on line and in person, to child welfare personnel from local societies, OACAS, and MCCSS. Child welfare in Ontario cannot hope to achieve its current ambitious goal of a modernized, redesigned, and more effective service system without the capacity at the local and provincial levels of monitoring young people's outcomes and evaluating its own services on a routine basis.

What kind of skills would child welfare personnel require in order to put into practice outcome monitoring and program evaluation? Child welfare is a complex, knowledge-dependent field of service and research, and it needs to function as such. Thus, it needs quality assurance and related staff who, as much as possible, already possess when hired basic data analysis skills on which more specialized monitoring and evaluation training can build. We suggest that each local society provide opportunities for training to two or more individual staff members, to facilitate sharing of skills on the job and help ensure that these new skills will not be lost if trained staff accept employment elsewhere or retire.

Basic familiarity with descriptive and inferential statistics is a prerequisite to carrying out straightforward descriptive or other basic analyses of AAR data. Such skills should be acquired, as much as possible, at the bachelor's or master's levels. McGill University, for example, requires training in statistics for undergraduate students in social work, which allows them to collaborate in applied research when employed in the field. For interested and motivated staff, there are now online courses in basic statistics and data analysis. For example, the company Udemy offers an inexpensive online course entitled Data Analysis and Statistics: Practical Course for Beginners (https://www.udemy.com/course/data-analysis-statistics/). For trainees with this kind of basic preparation, the OnLAC Project could offer several short courses each year on the analysis of local society AAR data, whether online to reduce costs or in person.

Udemy also offers introductory and inexpensive online courses on monitoring and evaluation (https://www.udemy.com/course/monitoring-and-evaluation/), as well as more advanced online offerings in program logic models, theories of action, and monitoring and evaluation. For selected society, OACAS, or MCCSS staff members who already have basic skills in data analysis, monitoring, and evaluation, the OnLAC team could furnish online or in-person short courses on the use of AAR data to answer specific monitoring and evaluation questions.

As mentioned earlier, with a modest increase in its mandate and training resources, the OnLAC Project team could help child welfare Ontario—local societies, OACAS, and MCCSS—to realize a key goal of the Looking After Children approach, namely, regular measurement and ongoing improvement in the benefits experienced by young people in care and their families. It is time to move the system to this new and more ambitious level.

3. OnLAC Project Lesson 3: Local Societies, OACAS, and MCCSS Need Greater Knowledge and Capacity than They Have at Present to Be Able to Construct and Evaluate Effective Programs

Lesson 3 goes well beyond the OnLAC and AAR focus of the previous lesson. Rather, after more than 20 years of witnessing new child welfare policies being created and launched in the province (e.g., for care leavers), often in a top-down fashion with little or no obvious local or regional experimentation, we believe that a more effective strategy of program development and evaluation is called for. What is required is a more viable blueprint for constructing new programs in a patient, evolutionary, phase-by-phase way. Here, we are able only to point towards a feasible solution to this endemic and costly problem, in both government ministries and voluntary organizations, which frequently results in the creation of programs or policies of unknown efficacy that are displaced only by the arrival on the scene of the next program or policy of equally dubious effectiveness. The OnLAC team would welcome the opportunity in future to provide training in program development and evaluation to the field.

William Trochim of Cornell University is a renowned research methods, evaluation, public health, and health services thinker and practitioner. A former president of the American Evaluation Association, he is currently a professor of policy analysis and management, evaluation, and health services research at Cornell University. He received his PhD from the Department of Psychology at Northwestern University, in its highly regarded doctoral training program in methodology and evaluation research. His research focuses on the use of evaluation and applied social research methods to better manage and improve social and health service systems. Trochim and two colleagues published a notable article in 2014, with the title "Evolutionary Evaluation: Implications for Evaluators, Researchers, Practitioners, Funders and the Evidence-Based Program Mandate" (Brown Urban et al., 2014). We believe their paper holds out the promise of a much more systematic, thorough, and successful strategy of program development and evaluation by local societies, OACAS, and MCCSS. Thus, we summarize the paper here.

Brown Urban et al. (2014) start from the position that the basic idea of evolution is at the root not only of the biological sciences but also of the development of knowledge, including our knowledge of social interventions and programs (e.g., in a complex field such as child welfare). Thus, programs develop according to the evolutionary principles of ontogeny (individual development), phylogeny (species development), natural selection, and the trial-and-error cycle of variation and selective retention. Programs, like individual people, develop in phases over the course of a program life course. These multiple phases are directly similar to those involved in pharmaceutical research, in which a new molecule (e.g., to combat COVID-19) is first created and studied, then subjected to a number of mainly qualitative tests. If sufficiently promising, the molecule is evaluated in the third phase with one or a series of randomized controlled trials, and, in the final phase, followed up in the field to evaluate its longer-term performance and safety. Only about 25% of new molecules survive this rigorous evolutionary process of development and evaluation.

The heart of the argument of Trochim and his colleagues is that the phases of social program development and evaluation should be "in sync," that is, "aligned." Programs in phase 1 (Initiation) are in their beginning phase, and the focus on program development should be on the feasibility of implementation. The program may be completely new, or it may be an adaptation of an already-existing one. The program has been tried out but is still undergoing important changes or adaptations. In this first stage, the evaluation of the program is post-only, centred on issues of process and response. The major concerns are implementation-related, especially the reaction and satisfaction of program participants. The evaluation should also look for the presence or absence of anticipated outcomes and attend to the internal consistency (reliability) of measures.

In phase 2 (Development), program revisions are more minor. Elements of the program, which is still evolving, are implemented with growing consistency. The evaluation studies the link of the program with outcomes at the group level, and then at the group or individual level. Both qualitative and quantitative methods are employed to assess change, with an increasing focus on the reliability and validity of the measures used.

In phase 3 (Stability), the program is implemented with consistency. A curriculum has been written for the program, such that participants experience the program in much the same way in different implementation settings. Written procedures or protocols enable new trainers to implement the program in a stable and consistent fashion. In this phase, the evaluation assesses the effectiveness of the now mature and stable program, using the formal methods of statistical control and, increasingly, randomized controlled trials or regression-discontinuity designs.

Finally, in phase 4 (Dissemination), the program is implemented in a range of different sites. A formal protocol is used to implement the program consistently and widely. The evaluation focuses on the effectiveness of the programs in producing desired outcomes in a wide range of implementation contexts. Systematic reviews and meta-analyses are used to assess these cross-context outcomes.

In this evolutionary perspective, even social programs that prove, on evaluation, to be unsuccessful or of only limited effectiveness, can serve a purpose, namely, by revealing adaptations that may be needed to achieve success. Trochim and his colleagues also make the point that their evolutionary model of programs and evaluation makes room for both top-down programs (e.g., originating with MCCSS) and bottom-up programs (e.g., suggested by practitioners in a local society, based on their first-hand experience). Moreover, the evolutionary model cautions decision makers to avoid premature pressure on practitioners to furnish proof of effectiveness before programs have achieved a needed stage of stability and maturity, especially when the practitioners do not have the required resources to evaluate programs in the various phases sketched above. Practitioners need to be consulted at the key program design and implementation stages.

4. OnLAC Project Lesson 4: A Case Study of How Local Societies Can Use Their AAR Data to Improve Their Delivery of Services

This fourth lesson is based on an actual example of how quality assurance personnel in an Ontario society used its own AAR data to improve an important aspect of its overall services, namely, the quality of the relationships between its caregivers and young people in care. This case study illustrates that service improvement was one of the main reasons that the OnLAC Project was founded. We thank the society in question for allowing us to include this example in this "lessons of OnLAC" chapter. The information was originally presented several years ago at a meeting among MCCSS, OACAS, individual societies, and the OnLAC Project team to review OnLAC findings from the field, based on AAR data.

The caregiver–youth in care relationship is critical, as caregivers provide both practical and emotional support that can buffer the negative effects of previous adverse life experiences. The best data we have on the quality of caregiver–youth relationships comes from the AAR. Young people, aged 10–17, respond to four questions during the annual AAR conversational interview:

1. How well do you feel they [caregivers] understand you?
2. How much fairness do you receive from them?
3. How much affection do you receive from them?
4. Overall, how would you describe your relationship with them?

In order to improve the average relationship between its caregivers and young people in care, the society decided to identify factors that would predict the strength of the relationship. For purposes of future service planning, the quality-assurance staff reviewed the relevant literature and analyzed its own AAR data to identify factors associated with higher and lower quality of the caregiver–youth relationship (as rated by the young person in care). In a sample of 191 youths, aged 10–17 (53.9% boys), taken from a one-year period of the society's AAR data set, the following variables were found to be statistically significantly correlated with *higher* quality of the caregiver–youth relationship (note that a correlation of $r = .10$ is considered to be small, one of .30 is seen as medium, and one of .50 is seen as large; Cohen, 1977):

- Satisfaction with the current placement ($r = .66$);
- Attachment to caregiver ($r = .44$);
- Greater external assets ($r = .23$);
- Greater internal assets ($r = .22$).

Conversely, the following variables were statistically significantly related to *lower* quality of the caregiver–youth relationship:

- Youth alcohol use ($r = -.23$);
- A greater number of changes in caregivers since birth ($r = -.20$);
- Youth drug use ($r = -.19$);
- Older age at first placement ($r = -.16$).

When statistical controls had been introduced for other background youth or placement variables (e.g., the young person's sex, age, placement type, or past-year adversities, or the total number of children in the home besides the young person, the caregiver–youth ethnic match, or the caregiver's sex), the following variables remained or became significantly *positively* related to the quality of the caregiver–young person relationship: placement satisfaction, continuity of care, attachment to the caregiver, a greater number of internal and external developmental assets, and greater caregiver–youth shared activities. Also, as expected, a greater number of changes in caregivers since birth and alcohol use by the young person were *negatively* associated with the quality of the caregiver–young person relationship.

In a final step in its service-improvement initiative, the quality-assurance personnel carried out a number of interviews with society caregivers, young persons, and workers. The final report contained several recommendations aimed at bolstering the quality of caregiver–youth relationships:

- Workers were encouraged to continue checking in with caregivers and youths regarding the quality of their relationships, as seen especially by the young people;
- Society personnel were to remind workers and caregivers from time to time about the positive role played by the caregiver relationship on youths' overall satisfaction and well-being in the placement;
- Society personnel were to offer parenting support to caregivers who had young people in their care who had challenging behavioural issues;
- Current information sharing processes between the society and caregivers were to be reviewed and improved, if needed, in terms of issues such as placement planning;
- Young people were to be consulted as much as possible in placement decisions and planning;
- The society was to continue supporting the development of relationships between caregivers and biological parents; and
- Young people were to be encouraged to be reflective when answering questions on the AAR.

5. OnLAC Project Lesson 5: Ontario Needs to Provide Universal Access to High-Quality Early Childhood Education and Care for Young Children in Out-of-Home Care

The Canadian federal budget of 2021 had as its centrepiece the promise of greatly expanded and affordable early childhood education and care (ECEC) over the next five years. This is a signal opportunity for most young children and their families across Canada, but especially for young children who have known early adversity in life. In Chapter 4, we reviewed the scientific evidence concerning the impact of early childhood education programs on child development, and on the need for ECEC for young children in care, for whom we have OnLAC Project data (see also Cameron et al., 2020). Suffice it to make three points here.

First, OnLAC data indicate that young children in care are in urgent need of high-quality ECEC. In a sample of 520 children in foster homes in Ontario, aged 12–47 months, the median score on a standardized measure of motor, social, and cognitive development was only 89, compared with a median of 100 for children in the general U.S. population. This placed the Ontario children in care at only the 23rd percentile for their ages. They were already 0.75 standard deviations below the general population level even though they were still too young to start junior kindergarten.

Second, Cleveland's (2018) comprehensive report on ECEC in Ontario, *Affordable for All: Making Licensed Child Care Affordable in Ontario*, provides a phased strategy for achieving affordable and available child care in the province. Cleveland advocated the immediate implementation of free child care for children aged 30 months to kindergarten age, with affordable care to be introduced over a period of several years for infants and toddlers. The emphasis on ECEC in the 2021 federal budget makes this plan considerably more financially feasible than when Cleveland proposed it. We know that Ontario has fewer ECEC and child care arrangements than the average of the provinces and territories, 53.6% versus 59.9% of the population aged 0 to 5. Unfortunately, we have not been able to find publicly available data on the proportion of young children in care (or still in their families under society supervision) who are served by ECEC programs. Even in Sweden and the United Kingdom, where ECEC is more plentiful, evidence of attendance by children in state care is sparse (Cameron et al., 2020). Regardless, improved accessibility of effective ECEC for children in the general population would no doubt also increase its availability for children in child welfare.

Third, in Chapter 4, we showed that with the current (2016) version of the OnLAC AAR, societies are able to screen their young children in terms of overall child development with the Ages and Stages Questionnaire, Third Edition (ASQ-3), and monitor their social-emotional status with the Ages and Stages Questionnaire: Social-Emotional (ASQ-SE). The results we presented in Chapter 4 suggested that 15%–30% of our OnLAC young children in care required further assessment on the ASQ-3 and possible referral to community intervention programs. Similarly, on the ASQ:SE, as many as 40% were seen as meriting closer monitoring and possible referral to community programs. (We caution that these estimates are only approximate and may be underestimates. We are currently collaborating with other users of the ASQ in trying to establish more definitive Canadian norms for the ASQ for use with young children in care. However, while awaiting these further refinements, we encourage local societies, OACAS, and MCCSS to make the best albeit tentative use of the measures we already have.)

Beyond the foregoing, we want to emphasize two other aspects of ECEC: the long-term effects of ECEC, and the potentially modifiable relationship between higher levels of teacher quality and the ECEC environment. The long-term effects of ECEC programs are important because of a persistent worry that while they may have positive short-term effects, their benefits may diminish or even disappear over time. In this regard, a recent report by Bai et al. (2020) is noteworthy. The authors described findings from two large-scale early childhood intervention programs implemented on a large scale in the U.S. state of North Carolina. The first program, Smart Start, began in 1993 and was established in all 100 North Carolina counties by 1998. Its mission was to improve ECEC for children from birth to age 4 so that they would begin school in good health and ready to learn. The program offered subsidies to children and an education-based salary supplement to teachers. The second program, More at Four, was initiated in 2001 to provide high-quality ECEC and promote school readiness for disadvantaged 4-year-olds. The two programs were theoretically based on a framework of multistage, cumulative, long-term skill formation. Basic skills were seen as leading to the acquisition of more advanced skills, such that early intervention effects do not fade out but instead grow. In extensive analyses based on a sample of some 900,000 students who had been followed up through the end of middle school (grade 8), Bai et al. (2020) found that both ECEC programs were associated with positive outcomes in reading and math, with no evidence that the size of the effects had been reduced between grades 3 and 8. In fact, More at Four displayed the opposite trend, with growing effect sizes across grade levels. In a word, these programs in North Carolina could serve as a promising model for expanded ECEC programs in Ontario, as the latter receive increased financial support from the federal and provincial governments over the next few years.

On the second topic, the quality of teachers and that of quality of the ECEC environment, Manning et al. (2019) completed a meta-analysis of centre-based settings that served infants, toddlers, preschool, and kindergarten children. There were a total of 49 studies with 83 independent samples, carried out between 1980 and 2015. Encouragingly, Manning et al. (2019) found that the teachers' level of education was positively and significantly associated with overall ECEC quality, as measured by an environmental rating scale. Moreover, teacher education was positively and significantly associated with all seven sub-scales of the environmental rating instrument: activities, parents and staff, language reasoning, interactions, program structure, space and furnishings, and personal care routine. According to Manning et al. (2019), viable means of improving service quality in the ECEC sector would include greater government investment in enhanced training and education for ECEC teachers and higher payments to programs with more qualified staff.

6. OnLAC Project Lesson 6: Permanency, and the Need for OnLAC-2

In 2018, the OnLAC Project team and the OACAS Child and Youth Caring Council-Community of Practice discussed the issue of just how "permanent" permanency really was in Ontario's child welfare services. To help answer this question, the OnLAC team reviewed the relevant literature and produced a working document, *Permanency: Definition, Measurement, and Outcomes* (Greenberg et al., 2018). In writing this report, it became clear that answering our question about permanency required a research project to track what happens to young people who leave care in the province. Currently, we have an abundance of anecdotes but little or no reliable and valid data on the longitudinal experiences of young people after they have left care.

In a nutshell, thanks to the investments made in the OnLAC Project, we now have a great deal of rich information on young people's outcomes and well-being while they are in care. What is needed is an additional project, which we have come to call OnLAC-2—one that will extend the reach of OnLAC to post-care outcomes by following samples of care leavers over an extended period of time (a point to which we return).

A good example of innovation in this area of research in Canada has been provided for the last few years by Professor Martin Goyette of the École nationale d'administration publique in Quebec. Goyette and his colleagues have gathered three waves of data to date in their *Étude longitudinale sur le devenir des jeunes placés au Québec et en France*. Their most recent report was published in June 2022, with the title *Itinérance, judiciarisation et marginalisation des jeunes ex-placés au Québec* (Homelessness, use of the courts and police, and marginalization of youth formerly placed in out-of-home care in Quebec). The researchers found that more than a third of the young people who had spent an extended period in the child welfare system had also experienced at least one episode of homelessness during the first few years after leaving care. Moreover, 53% of those who had experienced homelessness at least once also experienced mental health difficulties, compared to 33% who had experienced residential stability. On a more positive note, placement in family foster care proved to be an important protective and stabilizing factor: only 18.5% of those placed in family foster care had been homeless since leaving care, compared with 44.3% of those in other types of placements. Finally, 44% of the young people who had been homeless during wave 3 of the longitudinal study had been stopped by the police, compared with 25% of those in stable residential placements. Also, 21.4% of those who had been homeless during wave 3 reported having gone to prison since leaving care, versus only 8% and 6%, respectively, for those in unstable or stable residential settings. Overall, Goyette et his colleagues concluded that a system of prolonged support up to age 25 was needed to ensure that young people who had been in the youth protection system for an extended period could make a harmonious transition towards adult autonomy.

A primary goal of permanency in child welfare is often to reunite children with their families of origin. Evidence, however, suggests that permanent reunification is not always possible. Our review of the literature suggested, in fact, that "permanency" may often be a misleading and unattainable goal. Instead, the provision of a *stable*

environment should be the priority, together with the enduring relationships with caring adults and well-being that stable environments
promote (Font, Sattler, & Gershoff, 2018; Salazar et al., 2018; Walsh,
2015; Strijker, Knorth, & Knot-Dickscheit, 2008; Schofield & Beek,
2005; Allen & Bissell, 2004; Goldsmith, Oppenheim, & Wanlass, 2004;
Jones, 2004; Rubin et al., 1995).

Researchers have also found that outcomes associated with permanency, as traditionally understood, may in fact be negative, with
aging out of care sometimes associated with better educational outcomes than reunification with the family of origin. Font et al. (2018),
for example, found that many young people in care experience what
they termed "non-progress moves" into riskier settings upon leaving
care. To avoid this, the researchers felt that much more assessment,
planning, and follow-up was required. Ensuring access to services
and support was viewed as a key component of successful reunifica-
tions with families.

Overall, the literature indicates that many barriers to successful reunification exist, including the inability of families of origin to
procure needed supports and services. Systemic factors at play that
prevent young people from being reunited with their families include
poverty, homelessness, and deteriorating housing. The child welfare
system cannot address these issues by itself and must act in conjunction with relevant governmental organizations (D'Andrade &
Nguyen, 2014; Anderson, 1997). Concurrent planning helps address
the time lags often associated with sequential planning (Tilbury &
Osmond, 2006).

Earlier, we suggested that a new project (OnLAC-2) is needed
to follow up samples of young people after they have left care. At
present, the AAR is not mandated by MCCSS for young people aged
18 and older, with the result that data collection for this age group is
limited to perhaps 5% of eligible young people. For those who have
left care, we have no precise idea of their outcomes simply because
we do not track them. Only by doing so can we know how "permanent" permanency really is in Ontario and, ultimately, how successful the care system is in raising the developmental trajectories of
young people who have often known severe adversity early in life.
Jane Kovarikova (2017), creator of the Child Welfare Political Action
Committee Canada (Child Welfare PAC), has voiced this same concern, that no provincial or federal government body tracks young
people once they become "adults." As Treleaven (2019) noted, "For

Kovarikova, the bottom line is this: the state needs to care more about what happens to the children it raises. And one way to do that is by changing its perception of foster kids as damaged goods, unlikely to thrive regardless of intervention."

We hereby propose to OACAS and MCCSS that the OnLAC Project team be mandated to launch OnLAC-2, in partnership with OACAS and an advisory board comprising representatives of Ontario care leavers, caregivers, and local societies. OnLAC-2 would follow up a random sample of 1,000 young people who leave care in Ontario in the course of a given calendar year. Just as OnLAC teaches us a great deal about how young people fare while in care, OnLAC-2 would instruct us about the stability and well-being they experience after they have left care. Knowing how permanent our permanency options actually are for care leavers and how successful their transitions are to family reunification, independent living, post-secondary education, and relationships with caring adults would enable us, finally, to evaluate the ultimate success of our in-care and post-care intervention programs.

7. OnLAC Project Lesson 7: A Child Welfare Research Fund Is Needed in Ontario, Reserved for Research Projects Carried Out in Partnership between Local or Provincial Service Delivery or Policy Organizations and University-Based Researchers

Child welfare is a knowledge-based domain of practice, policy, and research and should be treated as such. About 10 years ago, a survey of approximately 200 child welfare practitioners, managers, and researchers in Canada was conducted. The respondents were asked, "What do you see as the most important question that research in child welfare should be addressing at present?" It is instructive that most of the respondents agreed that the single greatest need was an answer to the following question: "Are our services to children and their families effective?" If we were to repeat this survey today, the answer would probably not be very different.

Child welfare is a complex, multidisciplinary field that draws on the scientific knowledge and methods of many disciplines, including social work, psychology, sociology, economics, medicine, nursing, and others. To progress, child welfare requires a steady influx of new, valid knowledge. In Ontario, only a few researchers in child welfare are successful in a given year in securing funding for major, multi-year projects from the Social Sciences and Humanities Research Council of Canada (SSHRC). A few others may receive funding from foundations or government. However, these sources are clearly inadequate to support the level of high-quality applied research and evaluation that the expansion of child welfare knowledge and evidence-based interventions demands. We think that child welfare in the province, with a total operational budget of approximately $1.5 billion, merits the annual expenditure of at least 2% of the total budget on applied research and assessment. Such a commitment from MCCSS would yield a yearly pool of $30 million on which the community and research sectors could count and which would transform the field into one of sustained innovation.

An excellent example of provincial support of research is the research program of the Ontario Ministry of Health (MOH). MOH advertises the latter as "designed to support all areas of the ministry with a strong evidence base to enable improvements to the health system." Its research program is multifaceted, including the funding of strategic research aligned with ministry priorities, the translation of knowledge into policy and practice, expert analysis and evidence synthesis, and evidence-related policy and planning. Child welfare would greatly benefit from analogous multifaceted research support. The pertinence of MOH's sponsorship of research has been in evidence during the COVID-19 pandemic in 2020 and 2021. Among other initiatives, the province supported researchers' response to COVID-19 by making available the Ontario Health Data Platform, a set of large databases in the form of an integrated, secure platform.

On its website, the Ontario Ministry of Education (MED) is also publicly committed "to developing and implementing policies, programs, and practices that are evidence-based, research informed, and connected to provincial education goals." MED disseminates the research and evaluation that it sponsors in the form of research briefs that are intended to raise student achievement in literacy and numeracy. MED also publishes research summaries that highlight promising classroom-level teaching practices and convenes an annual Ontario Education Research Symposium, at which papers, presentations, and brief reports attempt to connect research to practice. Again, child welfare is no less complex than education and deserves comparable research support.

These examples from health and education strongly suggest that MCCSS would be wise to expand the kind of cost-effective support that it has afforded the OnLAC Project and help turn child welfare into the knowledge-intensive field it is. A dedicated research fund would enable child welfare to put in place the evolutionary strategy of program development and evaluation that is required (Brown Urban et al., 2014). Mainly formative and qualitative studies would ensure that new programs are able to be implemented and acceptable to stakeholders, while rigorous outcome evaluations would establish their actual effectiveness in practice. Finally, scaling up would transform these programs into long-term components of practice or policy (DuBois, 2020).

8. OnLAC Project Lesson 8: The OnLAC Project Partnership Requires Updating by the University of Ottawa, OACAS, and MCCSS

The long-term support received by the OnLAC Project since the year 2000 from the University of Ottawa, OACAS, and MCCSS (or its predecessors) has enabled us to accomplish much, for which we thank our partners. Like any long-term partnership, however, ours needs updating. Locating the OnLAC Project at a major university, especially in a community-oriented social science research centre in which outcome monitoring and program evaluation have always been prominent, has been a great advantage. It has permitted the OnLAC emphasis on monitoring and evaluation to thrive, and the climate of academic freedom and responsibility has contributed to remarkable stability in the membership of the OnLAC team, despite changes in provincial governments and OACAS leadership. The stability of the project has also benefited from having the same principal investigator since its beginning in 2000, together with long-term, dedicated, and highly knowledgeable and qualified team members. Their rare base of project knowledge and memory has been a crucial resource on which local societies, OACAS, and MCCSS have long drawn and will continue to draw.

The university location of the OnLAC Project has given it the freedom and flexibility to pursue changing priorities as it saw fit, such as a focus on resilience (Flynn et al., 2006). It has also provided local, national, and international opportunities to showcase OnLAC research on child welfare in Ontario. The OnLAC team has produced an extensive body of knowledge in child welfare over the last two decades. This has included annual public reports on Ontario services and outcomes, more than 40 annual confidential reports to local societies concerning their AAR results and performance indicators, several randomized trials of the impact of tutoring on the reading and math skills of young people in care, and dozens of peer-reviewed journal articles, books, book chapters, conference presentations, and technical reports (Miller, Vincent, & Flynn, 2021). Additionally, with the OnLAC team's support, 16 doctoral students in psychology and social work have been able to carry out their thesis research on AAR data, at universities in Ontario (Ottawa, Guelph, and Windsor), the United Kingdom (Oxford), and the United States (Loma Linda).

The partnership between the University of Ottawa and OACAS has been key from the outset. OACAS approved the OnLAC Project from the very beginning as an official board project and has been an indispensable link between local societies and the university. OACAS also facilitated the first OnLAC training sessions, and, until 2017, organized annual data forums in which the sector could learn about and discuss new project initiatives. The forums also gave the OnLAC team a regular platform for disseminating new information and research to the field.

The MCCSS funding each year, provided through OACAS to the OnLAC Project after the initial SSHRC strategic research grant had run its course, has been essential to the ongoing success of the project. Also, the continued commitment of MCCSS and OACAS to the OnLAC Project's service planning, outcome monitoring, and program evaluation functions has communicated that ongoing quality improvement in child welfare practice and policy is a priority in Ontario.

In the future, a three-to-five-year funding commitment by MCCSS would be a major advantage. This would enable the OnLAC team to undertake more "spinoff" initiatives and innovations, possibly with SSHRC or foundation funding, secure in the knowledge that the project would continue, at least in the short to intermediate term. Good examples of spinoff initiatives in the last few years have been the Education Snapshot, described in Chapter 5, and the series of randomized trials of tutoring, described in Chapter 4. As the project evolves and further revises the AAR in the next year or two, the OnLAC team at the University of Ottawa looks to forming a closer, more dynamic, and more effective partnership with local societies, OACAS, and MCCS, for the benefit of young people in care in the province and their families.

This volume aims to contribute to research and practice in child welfare by highlighting the two developmental approaches—Looking After Children: Good Parenting, Good Outcomes, and Child Well-Being—that underpin the OnLAC Project and that we described in Chapter 1. We hope that the book serves as a resource for assessing and improving local and provincial practices and policies and, ultimately, the outcomes and well-being of young people in care. Providing young people with opportunities to acquire as many developmental assets and relationships as possible will contribute markedly to their healthy functioning and resilience. Application of the OnLAC Project lessons described in the present chapter will make this even more likely.

References

Allen, M., and Bissell, M. (2004). Safety and stability for foster children: the policy context. *The Future of Children*, 14(1), 48–73. https://doi.org/10.2307/1602754

Anderson, G. (1997). Introduction: achieving permanency for all children in the child welfare system. *Journal of Multicultural Social Work*, 5(1–2), 1–8. https://doi.org/10.1300/J285v05n01_01

Bai, Y., Ladd, H. F., Muschin, C. G., & Dodge, K. A. (2020). Long-term effects of early childhood programs through eighth grade: Do the effects fade out or grow? *Children and Youth Services Review*, 112, Article 104890. https://doi.org/10.1016/j.childyouth.2020.104890

Brown Urban, J., Hargraves, M., & Trochim, W. M. (2014). Evolutionary evaluation: Implications for evaluators, researchers, practitioners, funders, and the evidence-based program mandate. *Evaluation and Program Planning*, 45, 127–139. https://doi.org/10.1016/j.evalprogplan.2014.03.011

Cameron, C., Höjer, I., Nordenfors, M., & Flynn, R. (2020). Security-first thinking and educational practices for young children in foster care in Sweden and England: A think piece. *Children and Youth Services Review*, 119, Article 105523. https://doi.org/10.1016/j. childyouth.2020.105523

Cleveland, G. (2018). *Affordable for all: Making licensed child care available in Ontario*. [Executive summary]. University of Toronto Scarborough.

Cohen, J. (1977). *Statistical power analysis for the behavioral sciences* (Revised edition). Academic Press.

D'Andrade, A. & Nguyen, H. (2014). The relationship between use of specific services, parental problems, and reunification with children placed in foster care. *Journal of Public Child Welfare*, 8(1), 51–69. https://doi.org/10.1080/15548732.2013.824399

Dubois, D. L. (2020). Supporting volunteerism in youth development programs: Progress and prospects for advancing the knowledge base.

Journal of Youth Development, 15(4), 206–216. https://doi.org/10.5195/jyd.2020.986

Flynn, R. J., Dudding, P. M., & Barber, J. G. (Eds.). (2006). *Promoting resilience in child welfare.* University of Ottawa Press.

Font, S., Berger, L., Cancian, M., & Noyes, J. (2018). Permanency and the educational and economic attainment of former foster children in early adulthood. *American Sociological Review,* 83(4), 716–743. https://doi.org/10.1177/0003122418781791

Font, S., Sattler, K., & Gershoff, E. (2018). Measurement and correlates of foster care placement moves. *Children and Youth Services Review,* 91, 248–258. https://doi.org/10.1016/j.childyouth.2018.06.019

Goldsmith, D., Oppenheim, D., & Wanlass, J. (2004). Separation and reunification: using attachment theory and research to inform decisions affecting the placements of children in foster care. *Juvenile and Family Court Journal,* 55(2), 1–13. https://doi.org/10.1111/j.1755-6988.2004.tb00156.x

Goyette, M. (2022). *Itinérance, judiciarisation et marginalisation des jeunes explacés au Québec* [Homelessness, use of the courts and police, and marginalization of youth formerly placed in out-of-home care in Quebec]. Montréal: École nationale d'administration publique.

Greenberg, B., Miller, M., Flynn, R., Michael, E., & Vincent, C. (2018). *Permanency: Definition, measurement, and outcomes.* Centre for Research on Educational and Community Services, University of Ottawa.

Kovarikova, J. (2017). *Exploring youth outcomes after aging-out of care.* Provincial Advocate for Children & Youth.

Manning, M., Wong, G. T. W., Fleming, C. M., & Garvis, S. (2019). Is teacher qualification associated with the quality of early childhood education and care environment? A meta-analytic review. *Review of Educational Research,* 89(3), 37–415. https://doi.org/10.3102/0034654319837540

Michaud, S. (2001). The National Longitudinal Survey of Children and Youth – Overview and changes after three cycles. *Special Issue on Longitudinal Methodology, Canadian Studies in Population,* 28(2), 391–405. Special Surveys Division, Statistics Canada.

Miller, M. (2021a). *2020 Ontario OnLAC-derived performance indicators 14, 15 & 16.* [Prepared for Ontario Association of Children's Aid Societies.] Centre for Research on Educational and Community Services, University of Ottawa.

Miller, M. (2021b). *Ontario Looking After Children 2020 provincial agency report.* Centre for Research on Educational and Community Services, University of Ottawa.

Miller, M., Vincent, C., & Flynn, R. (2021). *Bibliography of papers, chapters, and conference presentations from the Ontario Looking After Children (OnLAC) Project.* Centre for Research on Educational and Community Services, University of Ottawa.

Pantin, S., Flynn, R. J., & Runnels, V. (2006). Training, experience, and supervision: Keys to enhancing the utility of the Assessment and Action Record in implementing Looking After Children. In R. J. Flynn, P. M. Dudding, and J. G. Barber (Eds.), *Promoting resilience in child welfare* (pp. 281–296). University of Ottawa Press.

Romano, E., Stenason, L., Weegar, K., & Cheung, C. (2020). Improving child welfare's use of data for service planning: Practitioner perspectives on a training curriculum. *Children and Youth Services Review*, 110, Article 1044783. https://doi.org/10.1016/j.childyouth.2020.104783

Rubin, D., O'Reilly, A., Luan, X., & Localio, A. R. (2007). The impact of placement stability on behavioural well-being of children in foster care. *Pediatrics*, 119(2), 336–344. https://doi.org/10.1542/peds.2006-1995

Salazar, A., Jones, K., Amemiya, J., Cherry, A., Brown, E., Catalano, R., & Monahan, K. (2018). Defining and achieving permanency among older youth in foster care. *Children and Youth Services Review*, 87, 9–16. https://doi.org/10.1016/j.childyouth.2018.02.006

Schofield, G., & Beek, M. (2005). Providing a secure base: parenting children in long-term foster family care. *Attachment & Human Development*, 7(1), 3–25. https://doi.org/10.1080/14616730500049019

Statistics Canada. (2019, April 10). Survey on early learning and child care arrangements, 2019. *The Daily*.

Strijker, J., Knorth, E., & Knot-Dickscheit, J. (2008). Placement history of foster children: a study of placement history and outcomes in long-term family foster care. *Child Welfare*, 87(5), 107–124.

Tilbury, C. & Osmond, J. (2006). Permanency planning in foster care: a research review and guidelines for practitioners. *Australian Social Work*, 59(3), 265–280. https://doi.org/10.1080/03124070600833055

Treleaven, S. (2019, November 12). Life after foster care. *Maclean's*. https://www.macleans.ca/society/life-after-foster-care-in-canada/?fbclid=IwAR2f_SNKOP1pRz2LuqHRsDjaN71xmhMVxGKaBoFAAkSqd6xvEWiGoTo3BA8

Walsh, A. (2015). Legal permanency isn't everything: readdressing the need for well-being indicators in child protection courts. *Family Court Review*, 53(2), 326–335. https://doi.org/10.1111/fcre.12151

Appendices

Appendix Table A. Summary of Growth Mixture Model

Class Membership	Class	Proportions	BIC	AIC	VLMR p-value	BLRT p-value	Entropy
1-class	Lc1	-	23708.4	23659.0			
2-class	Lc1	.22	23642.1	23577.9	.00	.00	.71
	Lc2	.78					
3-class	Lc1	.20	23584.0	23505.0	.00	.00	.69
	Lc2	.13					
	Lc3	.67					
4-class	Lc1	.07	23564.3	23470.4	.00	.00	.70
	Lc2	.11					
	Lc3	.14					
	Lc4	.69					

Source: Ontario Looking After Children Project data.

Appendix Table B. Long-term physical health conditions of children in care in Ontario aged 0–5, by Indigenous versus non-Indigenous background (within sex), and sex

Long-Term Physical Health Conditions	Females			Males			Sex		
	Indigenous (n = 126) %	non-Indigenous (n = 310) %	P	Indigenous (n = 157) %	non-Indigenous (n = 356) %	P	Females (n = 436) %	Males (n = 513) %	P
None	60.3	61.9	ns	51.0	49.2	ns	61.5	49.7	.001
Food/digestive allergies	5.6	3.2	ns	7.0	7.6	ns	3.9	7.4	.03
Cerebral palsy	1.6	1.0	ns	1.9	1.4	ns	1.1	1.6	ns
Respiratory allergies/hay fever	0.0	1.3	ns	1.3	1.1	ns	0.9	1.2	ns
Kidney condition/disease	0.0	0.3	ns	1.9	2.2	ns	0.2	2.1	.02
Any other allergies	2.4	1.9	ns	1.1	1.4	ns	2.1	1.6	ns
Blood disorder	0.0	0.6	ns	0.0	0.0	ns	0.5	0.0	ns
Asthma	8.7	4.8	ns	7.6	6.7	ns	6.0	7.0	ns
Bronchitis	0.0	0.3	ns	0.6	0.8	ns	0.2	0.8	ns
Heart condition/disease	1.6	2.6	ns	3.8	2.5	ns	2.3	2.9	ns
Epilepsy	1.6	0.6	ns	0.0	0.3	ns	0.9	0.2	ns
Diabetes	0.8	0.1	ns	0.0	0.0	ns	0.2	0.0	ns
Any other long-term condition	10.3	11.6	ns	10.2	14.0	ns	11.2	12.9	ns

Note. ns = not significant, using continuity correction (for 2 × 2 tables); p-levels are 2-tailed.
Source: Ontario Looking After Children Project data in 2019.

Appendix Table C. Long-term physical health conditions of children in care in Ontario aged 6–9, by Indigenous versus non-Indigenous background (within sex), and sex

Long-Term Physical Health Conditions	Females			Males			Sex		
	Indigenous (n = 83) %	non-Indigenous (n = 181) %	p	Indigenous (n = 104) %	non-Indigenous (n = 249) %	P	Females (n = 264) %	Males (n = 333) %	p
None	49.4	35.9	.05	31.7	25.3	ns	40.2	27.2	.001
Food/digestive allergies	4.8	2.8	ns	5.8	2.4	ns	3.4	3.4	ns
Cerebral palsy	0.0	1.7	ns	1.9	1.6	ns	1.1	1.7	ns
Respiratory allergies/hay fever	1.2	0.6	ns	4.8	2.4	ns	0.8	3.1	ns
Kidney condition/disease	3.6	1.1	ns	1.9	0.8	ns	1.9	1.1	ns
Any other allergies	3.6	1.7	ns	3.8	2.8	ns	2.3	3.1	ns
Blood disorder	0.0	0.6	ns	0.0	0.3	ns	0.4	0.3	ns
Asthma	9.6	3.3	.07	5.8	5.6	ns	5.3	5.7	ns
Bronchitis	1.2	0.0	ns	0.0	0.0	ns	0.4	0.0	ns
Heart condition/disease	1.2	1.1	ns	4.8	2.4	ns	1.1	3.1	ns
Epilepsy	1.2	5.0	ns	1.0	2.8	ns	3.8	2.3	ns
Diabetes	1.2	0.0	ns	1.0	0.0	ns	0.4	0.3	ns
Any other long-term condition	4.8	14.9	.03	16.3	22.1	ns	11.7	20.4	.01

Note. ns = not significant, using continuity correction (for 2 × 2 tables); p-levels are 2-tailed.
Source: Ontario Looking After Children Project data in 2019.

Appendix Table D. Long-term physical health conditions of young people in care in Ontario aged 10–15, by Indigenous versus non-Indigenous background (within sex), and sex

Long-Term Physical Health Conditions	Females				Males				Sex		
	Indigenous (n = 181) %	non-Indigenous (n = 496) %	p		Indigenous (n = 165) %	non-Indigenous (n = 666) %	p		Females (n = 677) %	Males (n = 831) %	p
None	35.4	28.8	ns		26.7	15.9	.01		30.6	18.1	.001
Food/digestive allergies	5.5	3.8	ns		1.2	2.9	ns		4.3	2.5	.08
Cerebral palsy	0.6	2.6	ns		2.4	1.8	ns		2.1	1.9	ns
Respiratory allergies/hay fever	3.1	1.6	ns		3.0	2.3	ns		2.1	2.4	ns
Kidney condition/disease	0.6	1.0	ns		0.6	0.8	ns		0.9	0.7	ns
Any other allergies	5.5	4.2	ns		4.2	2.9	ns		4.6	3.1	ns
Blood disorder	0.0	0.0	ns		0.6	0.8	ns		0.0	0.7	.07
Asthma	2.8	5.0	ns		4.2	5.3	ns		4.4	5.1	ns
Bronchitis	0.6	0.2	ns		0.0	0.2	ns		0.3	0.1	ns
Heart condition/disease	2.2	0.6	ns		1.2	1.2	ns		1.0	1.2	ns
Epilepsy	1.1	2.0	ns		1.8	2.7	ns		1.8	2.5	ns
Diabetes	2.8	0.4	.02		0.6	0.9	ns		1.0	0.8	ns
Any other long-term condition	11.6	8.3	ns		8.5	15.8	.02		9.2	14.3	.01

Note. ns = not significant, using continuity correction (for 2 × 2 tables); *p*-levels are 2-tailed.
Source: Ontario Looking After Children Project data in 2019.

Appendix Table E. Long-term physical health conditions of young people in care in Ontario aged 16+, by Indigenous versus non-Indigenous background (within sex), and sex

Long-Term Physical Health Conditions	Females			Males			Sex		
	Indigenous (n = 73) %	non-Indigenous (n = 326) %	p	Indigenous (n = 67) %	non-Indigenous (n = 382) %	p	Females (n = 399) %	Males (n = 499) %	p
None	28.8	24.8	ns	20.9	20.7	ns	25.6	20.7	ns
Food/digestive allergies	1.4	5.2	ns	1.5	2.9	ns	4.5	2.7	ns
Cerebral palsy	1.4	1.2	ns	1.5	0.5	ns	1.3	0.7	ns
Respiratory allergies/hay fever	1.4	2.8	ns	3.0	2.1	ns	2.5	2.2	ns
Kidney condition/disease	2.7	0.0	.04	0.0	1.3	ns	0.5	1.1	ns
Any other allergies	6.8	3.4	ns	1.5	3.4	ns	4.0	3.1	ns
Blood disorder	0.0	0.6	ns	0.0	0.8	ns	0.5	0.7	ns
Asthma	5.5	6.4	ns	3.0	5.5	ns	6.3	5.1	ns
Bronchitis	2.7	0.3	ns	0.0	0.3	ns	0.8	0.2	ns
Heart condition/disease	0.0	1.8	ns	3.0	2.4	ns	1.5	2.4	ns
Epilepsy	1.4	1.2	ns	1.5	2.4	ns	1.3	2.2	ns
Diabetes	0.0	2.1	ns	0.0	1.8	ns	1.8	1.6	ns
Any other long-term condition	5.5	8.6	ns	10.4	11.8	ns	8.0	11.6	ns

Note. *ns* = not significant, using continuity correction (for 2 × 2 tables); *p*-levels are 2-tailed.
Source: Ontario Looking After Children Project data in 2019.

Appendix F. Fictionalized example of an Education Snapshot

Source: Authors of the Education Snapshot (Elisa Romano, Lauren Stenason, Erik Michael, and Meagan Miller).

Université d'Ottawa | University of Ottawa

OnLAC Assessment and Action Record Education Snapshot

Prepared for:	Agency	Agency File Number	CPIN
	Test Agency	969696	38888888

Written by: Elisa Romano, Lauren Stenason, Meagan Miller and Erik Michael
Original concept by: Elisa Romano, Connie Cheung, Lauren Stenason and Kelly Weegar
Prepared by: Erik Michael

Centre for Research on Educational and Community Services CRECS

crecs.uOttawa.ca

uOttawa

Table of Contents

Introduction

This Assessment and Action Record – 2nd Canadian version (AAR-C2) *Education Snapshot* provides information that can be helpful in better understanding how a youth's context can influence their academic achievement. The information is organized across different levels of influence that include 1) youth's behavioural and emotional functioning; 2) out-of-home placement; and 3) school.

In this way, there is an ecological perspective in understanding how the various systems, and individuals within those systems, can impact a youth's educational success. Systems and individuals closest to the youth have a more direct effect, while systems and individuals further away from the youth (e.g., children's aid society) have an indirect influence on the youth by affecting the systems and individuals most proximal to the youth. These influences are bi-directional, meaning the various systems and individuals not only influence the youth but are also influenced by the youth.

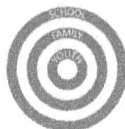

The information in the AAR-C2 *Education Snapshot* is meant to be **integrated into your service planning decisions**, alongside other information that you have about this youth. In addition, issues of equity, diversity, and inclusion must be at the forefront of all service planning decisions. Following an **evidence-informed practice framework** complements your clinical understanding and integrates information from the following four areas:

1. Child, youth, and family considerations (e.g., religion, culture, and their preferences)

2. Case context (e.g., child and family history)

3. Worker, supervisor, and organizational experience (e.g., organizational climate, personal beliefs)

4. Research evidence (e.g., data, evidence-based interventions)

In addition to providing information about the youth's well-being and functioning, the AAR-C2 *Education Snapshot* can also be used as a communication/advocacy tool to be shared with other individuals who play a role in this youth's care.

Scoring

Several of the scores presented in the *Education Snapshot* are expressed in the following way:

- Green suggests functioning that is in line with age-expectations

- suggests difficulties that are more pronounced and need to be monitored

- Red suggests difficulties of sufficient breadth or severity that intervention may be warranted

The *Education Snapshot* is meant to capture aspects of a youth's well-being and functioning from information that is gathered through the AAR-C2. Some ways in which the *Education Snapshot* can be utilized during service planning include:

- Communication/advocacy: information sharing with important stakeholders, especially youth and their caregivers

- Additional source of information to anchor clinical impressions, and to support clinical understanding and judgment

- Presents possible new perspectives and avenues for practice:
  - Longitudinal perspective when multiple years of data for a youth are considered
  - Comparison of a youth's score with agency means

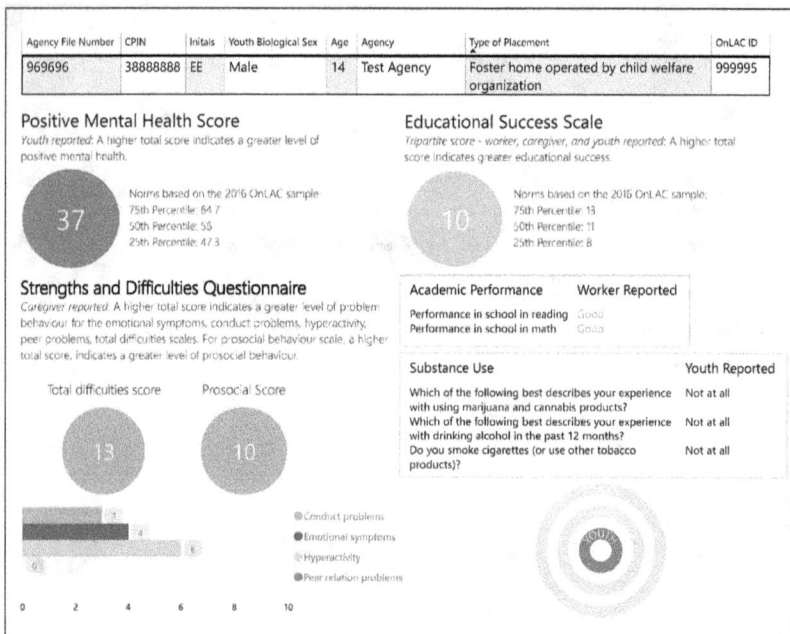

Agency File Number	CPIN	Initals	Youth Biological Sex	Age	Agency	Type of Placement	OnLAC ID
969696	38888888	EE	Male	14	Test Agency	Foster home operated by child welfare organization	999995

Positive Mental Health Score

Youth reported: A higher total score indicates a greater level of positive mental health.

37

Norms based on the 2016 OnLAC sample:
75th Percentile: 64.7
50th Percentile: 55
25th Percentile: 47.3

Educational Success Scale

Tripartite score - worker, caregiver, and youth reported: A higher total score indicates greater educational success.

10

Norms based on the 2016 OnLAC sample:
75th Percentile: 13
50th Percentile: 11
25th Percentile: 8

Strengths and Difficulties Questionnaire

Caregiver reported. A higher total score indicates a greater level of problem behaviour for the emotional symptoms, conduct problems, hyperactivity, peer problems, total difficulties scales. For prosocial behaviour scale, a higher total score, indicates a greater level of prosocial behaviour.

Total difficulties score

13

Prosocial Score

10

- Conduct problems
- Emotional symptoms
- Hyperactivity
- Peer relation problems

Academic Performance	Worker Reported
Performance in school in reading	Good
Performance in school in math	Good

Substance Use	Youth Reported
Which of the following best describes your experience with using marijuana and cannabis products?	Not at all
Which of the following best describes your experience with drinking alcohol in the past 12 months?	Not at all
Do you smoke cigarettes (or use other tobacco products)?	Not at all

Agency File Number	CPIN	Initals	Youth Biological Sex	Age	Agency	Type of Placement	OnLAC ID
969696	38888888	EE	Male	14	Test Agency	Foster home operated by child welfare organization	999995

Relationship with Primary Caregiver

Youth reported: A higher total score indicates a relationship of higher quality with the primary caregiver, as perceived by the young person.

(2)

Norms based on the 2016 OnLAC sample:
75th Percentile: 8
50th Percentile: 7
25th Percentile: 6

Placement Satisfaction

Youth reported: A higher total score indicates a higher level of satisfaction with the current living situation.

(3)

Norms based on the 2016 OnLAC sample:
75th Percentile: 12
50th Percentile: 12
25th Percentile: 9

Confidants

Youth reported: People that the young person feels they can talk to.

Does the young person report having close friends?   Yes

People other than close friends that the youth reports being able to talk to (if blank, then none reported):

Birth father
Birth mother
Birth parent's partner
Child welfare worker
Grandparents
Other
Teacher

Family Adversities

Worker reported: Family adversities experienced by the youth within the last 12 months (if blank, then none reported):

(FAMILY)

Agency File Number	CPIN	Initals	Youth Biological Sex	Age	Agency	Type of Placement	OnLAC ID
969696	38888888	EE	Male	14	Test Agency	Foster home operated by child welfare organization	999995

School Stability
Worker reported:

Changed schools in the last 12 months?   Yes
Total changes in school: Best estimate   2

School Safety
Youth reported:

I feel safe at school   Most or all of the time
I feel safe on my way to and from   Most or all of the time
school
I have experienced bullying at school   Some or one time
or cyberbullying

School Absences
Caregiver reported (if blank, then none reported):

How many days absent from school during the last 12 months?   2
Number of suspensions, if any   1

Main reasons for school absences:

Other
Meeting with social worker or child welfare worker
Illness
Appointments with mental health professional
Appointments with doctor or dentist

Agency File Number	CPIN	Initals	Youth Biological Sex	Age	Agency	Type of Placement	OnLAC ID
969696	38888888	EE	Male	14	Test Agency	Foster home operated by child welfare organization	999995

Developmental Assets

Worker reported: A higher total score indicates that the child welfare worker believes that the young person possesses a greater number of developmental assets. Total scores for external, internal, and total developmental assets are not calculated if more than 10 items in the index were missing a response.

External Assets

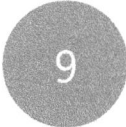

9

Total Developmental Assets

21

0
responses missing

Total Developmental Assets Legend
Green: High assets
Yellow: Medium assets
Red: Low assets

External and Internal Asset Legend
Green: Has asset
Yellow: Uncertain
Red: Does not have asset
Grey: Did not answer

Internal Assets

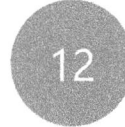

12

After reviewing the information presented in the *Education Snapshot*, you may wish to review the following questions. These questions can serve as a guide for discussing strengths and needs, and for planning for the youth's care. Responses in this worksheet are meant to be used in supervision.

How many green? ☐

How many yellow? ☐

How many red? ☐

Based on these results, what are some areas of strength for this youth? How can these strengths continues to be reinforced?

What are some areas that may require additional supports and what resources are available to address these concerns?

How does this information fit with other information you have about this youth (e.g., observations of and interactions with the youth and other important individuals in the youth's life)?

How does this information inconsistent with other information you have about this youth? What might explain the differences?

What are some issues around equity, diversity, and inclusion that need to be considered?

Is there any additional information needed that might help to plan for next steps?

How do you plan to share the information presented in this *Education Snapshot* with the youth and caregivers?

What are some points that are important to discuss in supervision?

OnLAC Supervision Checklist
AAR Completion Fidelity Checklist

The young person for whom the AAR is being completed:
- ☐ Participated in virtually the entire AAR conversation
- ☐ Participated in only part or none of the AAR conversation

If so, please specify the reason:
- ☐ Refusal
- ☐ Lack of capacity
- ☐ Other (state reason):

Who else took part in the AAR conversation? (Check all that apply)
- ☐ Child welfare worker
- ☐ One foster parent
- ☐ Two foster parents
- ☐ One birth parent
- ☐ Two birth parents
- ☐ Family worker
- ☐ One adult caregiver other than a foster parent
- ☐ Two adult caregivers other than a foster parent
- ☐ FNMI Band or Community representative
- ☐ FNMI Elder or Cultural Teacher
- ☐ Non-caregiving relative
- ☐ Other:

During the administration of the AAR, a good deal of what seemed like frank and useful face-to-face conversation took place between (Check all that apply):
- ☐ Young person and caregiver
- ☐ Young person and child welfare worker
- ☐ Caregiver and child welfare worker

Has the supervisor reviewed the completed AAR?   ☐ Yes ☐ No

AAR Worksheet Question Checklist

- ☐ Based on the AAR *Education Snapshot*, identify the number of green, yellow, and red scores.
- ☐ Based on these results, what are some areas of strength for this youth? How can these strengths continues to be reinforced?
- ☐ What are some areas that may require additional supports and what resources are available to address these concerns?
- ☐ How does this information fit with other information you have about this youth?
- ☐ How does this information inconsistent with other information you have about this youth? What might explain the differences?
- ☐ What are some issues around equity, diversity, and inclusion that need to be considered?
- ☐ Is there any additional information needed that might help to plan for next steps?
- ☐ How do you plan to share the information presented in this *Education Snapshot* with the youth and caregivers?
- ☐ What are some points that are important to discuss in supervision?

In my usual supervision, how often do I discuss the information provided by the AAR with child welfare worker for whom I am responsible:
- ☐ All or most of the time
- ☐ From time to time
- ☐ Rarely or never

Reference Table

Measure	Description	Reported By	User's Manual (AAR-C2-2016)
Total Developmental Assets Profile	A higher total score indicates that the child welfare worker believes that the young person possesses a greater number of developmental assets. Possible range between 0 – 40. See: Scales, P. C. (1999). Reducing risks and building developmental assets: essential actions for promoting adolescent health. *Journal of School Health, 69*, 113-119.	Child Welfare Worker	Page 183
External Developmental Assets Profile	A higher total score indicates that the child welfare worker believes that the young person possesses a greater number of *external* developmental assets. possible range between 0 – 20.	Child Welfare Worker	Page 186
Internal Developmental Assets Profile	A higher total score indicates that the child welfare worker believes that the young person possesses a greater number of *internal* developmental assets. Possible range between 0 – 20.	Child Welfare Worker	Page 188
Positive Mental Health Scale	A higher total score indicates a greater level of positive mental health. Possible score between 0 – 70. See: Keyes, C. L. M. (2006). Mental health in adolescence: Is America's youth flourishing? *American Journal of Orthopsychiatry, 76*, 395-402.	Young Person	Page 65
Strengths & Difficulties Questionnaire (SDQ): Prosocial Behaviour	A higher score indicates a greater level of prosocial behaviour. Possible range between 0 – 10. See: Goodman, R., Ford, T., Simmons, H., Gatward, R., & Meltzer, H. (2000). Using the Strengths and Difficulties Questionnaire (SDQ) to screen for child psychiatric disorders in a community sample. *British Journal of Psychiatry, 177*, 534-539. Goodman, R., Meltzer, H., & Bailey, V. (2003). The Strengths and Difficulties Questionnaire: A pilot study on the validity of the self-report version. *International Review of Psychiatry, 15*, 173-177.	Caregiver	Page 71
SDQ: Total Difficulties	A higher total score indicates a greater level of problem behaviour. Possible range between 0 – 40.	Caregiver	Page 71

Reference Table

Measure	Description	Reported By	User's Manual (AAR-C2-2016)
SDQ: Emotional Symptoms, Hyperactivity, Conduct Problems, Peer Problems	A higher score indicates a greater level of problem behaviour for each subscale. Possible range between 0-10.	Caregiver	Page 71
Placement Satisfaction Scale	A higher total score indicates a higher level of satisfaction with the current living situation. Possible range between 0 – 12. *See:* Flynn, R.J. Robitaille, A., & Ghazal, H. (2006). *Placement satisfaction of young people living in foster or group homes.* In R. Flynn, P. Dudding, & J. Barber, (Eds.), Promoting resilience in child welfare (pp. 191-205). Ottawa, ON: University of Ottawa Press.	Young Person	Page 37
Quality of Relationship with Primary Caregiver Scale	A higher total score indicates a relationship of higher quality with the primary caregiver, as perceived by the young person. Possible range between 0 – 8. *See:* Statistics Canada & Human Resources Development Canada (1999). *National Longitudinal Survey of Children and Youth: Overview of survey instruments for 1998-99, data collection cycle 3.* Ottawa: Authors.	Young Person	Page 40
Educational Success Scale	A higher total score indicates greater educational success. Possible range between 0 – 19. *See:* Tessier, N. G., O'Higgins, A., & Flynn, R. J. (2018). Neglect, educational success, and young people in out-of-home care: Cross-sectional and longitudinal analyses. *Child Abuse & Neglect, 75,* 115–129.	Child Welfare Worker / Caregiver / Young Person	Page 22

Acknowledgements

The OnLAC project has been a joint initiative of the University of Ottawa Centre for Research on Education and Community Services, the Ontario Association of Children's Aid Societies, and local child welfare societies since 2001. In 2006, the Ministry of Children, Community, and Social Services (formerly the Ministry of Children and Youth Services) mandated the use of the OnLAC approach in all Ontario child welfare societies.

This *Education Snapshot* was informed by findings from a Partnership Development Grant from the Social Sciences and Humanities Research Council of Canada (890-2013-0136). The research project was called Improving Ontario Child Welfare's Use of Research to Inform Service Planning and Delivery, and the co-principal investigators were Dr. Elisa Romano (School of Psychology, University of Ottawa) and Dr. Connie Cheung (formerly at the Child Welfare Institute of the Children's Aid Society of Toronto). The project was completed in collaboration with three Ontario child welfare agencies.

We wish to acknowledge the important contributions of many individuals over the years to the project, especially the numerous young people in care, caregivers, practitioners, supervisors, quality-assurance staff, executive personnel, ministry staff, and OnLAC research staff and students who have contributed much to the OnLAC project since the beginning.

Index

Health and Society

Series editor: Position vacant

Health occupies a central place in public debate, and the *Health and Society* series provides a space for dialogue on different fields of expertise (sociology, psychology, political science, biology, nutrition, medicine, nursing, human kinetics, and rehabilitation sciences), generating new insights into health matters from individual as well as global perspectives on population health. The principal domains explored in *Health and Society* are hospitals, communities, medicine, social policies, medico-sanitary institutions, and health systems.

Previous titles in the *Health and Society* collection

Lloyd Hawkeye Robertson, *The Evolved Self: Mapping an Understanding of Who We Are*, 2020.

Sylvie Frigon, ed., *Dance: Confinement and Resilient Bodies / Danse : Enfermenent et corps résilients*, 2019.

Martin Rovers, Judith Malette, and Manal Guirguis-Younger, eds., *Touch in the Helping Professions: Research, Practice and Ethics*, 2018.

Serge Brochu, Natacha Brunelle, and Chantal Plourde, *Drugs and Crime: A Complex Relationship. Third revised and expanded edition*, 2018.

Marie Drolet, Pier Bouchard, and Jacinthe Savard, eds., *Accessibility and Active Offer: Health Care and Social Services in Linguistic Minority Communities*, 2017.

Isabelle Perreault and Marie Claude Thifault, eds., *Récits inachevés : Réflexions sur les défis de la recherche qualitative*, 2016.

Mamadou Barry and Hachimi Sanni Yaya, *Financement de la santé et efficacité de l'aide internationale*, 2015.

For a complete list of the University of Ottawa Press titles, visit:
www.press.uOttawa.ca

www.ingramcontent.com/pod-product-compliance
Lightning Source LLC
Chambersburg PA
CBHW050626280326
41932CB00015B/2541